Unstable Angina

FUNDAMENTAL AND CLINICAL CARDIOLOGY

Series Editor

Samuel Z. Goldhaber, M.D.

Cardiovascular Division
Department of Medicine
Harvard Medical School
and Brigham and Women's Hospital
Boston, Massachusetts

1. *Drug Treatment of Hyperlipidemia,* edited by Basil M. Rifkind

2. *Cardiotonic Drugs: A Clinical Review: Second Edition, Revised and Expanded,* edited by Carl V. Leier

3. *Complications of Coronary Angioplasty,* edited by Alexander J. R. Black, H. Vernon Anderson, and Stephen G. Ellis

4. *Unstable Angina,* edited by John D. Rutherford

Additional Volumes in Preparation

Beta-Blockers in the Management of Cardiac Arrhythmia, edited by Prakash C. Deedwania

Exercise and the Heart in Health and Cardiac Disease, edited by Roy Shephard and Henry S. Miller, Jr.

Cardiopulmonary Physiology in Critical Care, edited by Steven M. Scharf

Adjunctive Therapy for Acute Myocardial Infarction, edited by Eric Bates

Unstable Angina

edited by

John D. Rutherford

Brigham and Women's Hospital
Harvard Medical School
Boston, Massachusetts

Marcel Dekker, Inc. **New York • Basel • Hong Kong**

ISBN 0-8247-8618-1

This book is printed on acid-free paper.

MARCEL DEKKER. INC.
270 Madison Avenue, New York, New York 10016

Current printing (last digit):
10 9 8 7 6 5 4 3 2 1

PRINTED IN THE UNITED STATES OF AMERICA

Series Introduction

John D. Rutherford, M.B., Ch.B., has edited a comprehensive book on unstable angina for this new series of books on Fundamental and Clinical Cardiology. Dr. Rutherford had assembled the talents of world-renowned authorities to discuss the most contemporary aspects of important cardiovascular topics. His book is divided into initial chapters on pathophysiology, middle chapters on practical management aspects of unstable angina, and concluding chapters on areas of continuing controversy. As a practicing cardiologist, I have long sought a book such as this one to aid me in making day-to-day patient management decisions as well as broaden my understanding of underlying pathophysiologic principles. This beautifully produced book will enhance patient care and belongs on the bookshelves of medical libraries and in the offices of cardiologists, internists, family practitioners, cardiac surgeons, and other practitioners who must deal with the challenging issues that arise in patients with unstable angina.

Marcel Dekker, Inc., has done a service by helping to integrate rapidly advancing information for the clinician and clinical researcher. I extend my heartiest congratulations to Dr. Rutherford for the editing of this book and to Marcel Dekker for placing it on the "publication fast track" so that its contents will be timely and topical.

Samuel Z. Goldhaber, M.D.

Foreword

Atherosclerotic coronary artery disease is by far the most common cause of death and a frequent cause of hospitalization and disability in the industrialized world. This form of heart disease encompasses a wide clinical-pathologic spectrum, each end of which has been well defined. At one end of the spectrum are patients with acute myocardial infarction, who now most often are treated with thrombolytic therapy and require mechanical revascularization only occasionally. At the other end are patients with chronic stable angina who usually have atherosclerotic plaques that greatly narrow their epicardial coronary vessels. While these patients often respond to medical measures, when unresponsive they require mechanical revascularization.

Between these two ends of the clinical-pathologic spectrum lie a third group of patients, probably larger than either of the other two: those with unstable angina. This is a common disorder, responsible for some three-quarters of a million hospital admissions in the United States each year. Thus, unstable angina is among the most frequent diagnoses in hospitalized patients in this country at present. It is a serious condition; almost 100,000 patients each year develop acute myocardial infarction within 1 month after the onset of unstable angina. After recovery from the unstable episode, many of the remainder are left with severe chronic stable angina. A group of patients with unstable angina that appears to have a particularly poor prognosis are those who develop this condition shortly after experiencing acute myocardial infarction.

Unstable angina is something of a wastebasket diagnosis. Although it was described early in this century, it has had many names and was referred to as "unstable angina" for the first time only 20 years ago. It probably consists of a number of different conditions, all of which are characterized by severe myocardial ischemia. It is essential that the ambiguity concerning all aspects of unstable angina—pathogenesis, diagnosis, and the many aspects of therapy (established and emerging)—be clarified for physicians, invasive cardiologists, and cardiovascular surgeons. To the extent that this can be achieved, Dr. Rutherford and his talented coauthors have certainly done so. They have also identified those issues surrounding unstable angina which have not yet been clarified. Thus, this fine book provides us simultaneously with both an up-to-date contemporary analysis of this important condition and a blueprint for future clinical investigation.

Eugene Braunwald, M.D.

Hersey Professor of the Theory and Practice of Medicine
Harvard Medical School

Chairman, Department of Medicine
Brigham and Women's Hospital

Boston, Massachusetts

Preface

Unstable angina is a common condition affecting a heterogeneous population of patients. Although there has been a decline in hospitalizations for coronary heart disease nationally, the number of patients discharged from hospital with the diagnosis of unstable angina pectoris has increased. Patients admitted to the hospital with a diagnosis of unstable angina represent a challenge in medical management since many patients will stabilize after a relatively conservative regimen while others will be critically ill and will require intensive medical therapy and, at times, emergency revascularization.

In this book we explore the pathology and pathophysiology of the coronary artery lesions associated with unstable angina pectoris and broadly outline the investigations that might be performed, including cardiac catheterization, ST Holter monitoring, and stress testing, to evaluate and risk-stratify patients. The medical therapy available for treating patients with unstable angina is examined, with emphasis on the choice between nitrates, beta blockers, and calcium antagonists and the known efficacy of antiplatelet and anticoagulant therapy. The pros and cons of thrombolytic therapy are also discussed. Finally, we explore the issues surrounding the choice of either continued medical therapy, percutaneous transluminal coronary angioplasty, or cardiac surgery in the management of patients with unstable angina.

It is our hope that this book will be useful for the practicing internist, cardiologist, and intensive care unit physician who encounter patients with unstable angina, as well as for persons at various stages of training in this field.

John D. Rutherford

Contents

Contributors

John A. Ambrose, M.D. Professor of Medicine and Director of Cardiac Catheterization, Mount Sinai Hospital, New York, New York

Elliott M. Antman, M.D. Director, Samuel A. Levine Cardiac Unit, Cardiovascular Division, Brigham and Women's Hospital, and Associate Professor of Medicine, Harvard Medical School, Boston, Massachusetts

John A. Bittl, M.D. Co-director of Interventional Cardiology, Cardiovascular Division, Brigham and Women's Hospital, and Assistant Professor of Medicine, Harvard Medical School, Boston, Massachusetts

Alan C. Braverman, M.D.* Cardiovascular Division, Brigham and Women's Hospital, and Instructor in Medicine, Harvard Medical School, Boston, Massachusetts

Bernard J. Gersh, M.B., Ch.B., D. Phil. (Oxon.), F.R.C.P., F.A.C.C. Consultant in Cardiovascular Diseases and Professor of Medicine, Mayo Clinic and Mayo Foundation, Rochester, Minnesota

---

**Present affiliation:* Assistant Professor of Medicine, Washington University Medical Center, St. Louis, Missouri.

Craig E. Hjemdahl-Monsen, M.D. Assistant Professor of Medicine, Division of Cardiology, New York Medical College/Westchester County Medical Center, Valhalla, New York

John F. Keaney, Jr., M.D. Cardiovascular Division, Brigham and Women's Hospital and Harvard Medical School, Boston, Massachusetts

Michael J. Landzberg, M.D. Clinical and Research Fellow in Cardiology, Cardiovascular Division, Brigham and Women's Hospital, Boston, Massachusetts

Richard T. Lee, M.D. Director, Cardiac Noninvasive Laboratory, Cardiovascular Division, Brigham and Women's Hospital, Boston, Massachusetts

James E. Muller, M.D. Chief, Cardiology Division, New England Deaconess Hospital, and Associate Professor of Medicine, Harvard Medical School, Boston, Massachusetts

Joseph G. Murphy, M.R.C.P.I., M.R.C.P. Assistant Professor of Medicine, Mayo Clinic and Mayo Foundation, Rochester, Minnesota

Alfred F. Parisi, M.D., F.A.C.C. Professor of Medicine and Chief, Cardiology Division, Program-in-Medicine, Brown University, The Miriam Hospital, and Roger Williams Medical Center, Providence, Rhode Island

John D. Parker, M.D., F.R.C.P.(C.) Department of Cardiology, Brigham and Women's Hospital, and Instructor in Medicine, Harvard Medical School, Boston, Massachusetts

John D. Rutherford, M.B., Ch.B., F.R.A.C.P. Co-director, Clinical Cardiology Service, Brigham and Women's Hospital, and Assistant Professor of Medicine, Harvard Medical School, Boston, Massachusetts

Thomas J. Ryan, Jr., M.D. Cardiovascular Division, Brigham and Women's Hospital, and Clinical and Research Fellow, Harvard Medical School, Boston, Massachusetts

Frederick J. Schoen, M.D., Ph.D. Department of Pathology, Brigham and Women's Hospital, Boston, Massachusetts

Peter H. Stone, M.D. Associate Director, Samuel A. Levine Cardiac Unit, Cardiovascular Division, Brigham and Women's Hospital, and Assistant Professor of Medicine, Harvard Medical School, Boston, Massachusetts

Douglas E. Vaughan, M.D. Co-Director, Center for Research in Thrombolysis, Brigham and Women's Hospital, West Roxbury Veterans Administration Medical Center, and Assistant Professor of Medicine, Harvard Medical School, Boston, Massachusetts

Francine K. Welty, M.D., Ph.D. Instructor in Medicine, Harvard Medical School, and Cardiovascular Division, New England Deaconess Hospital, Boston, Massachusetts

1

Pathology of Unstable Coronary Plaque

Richard T. Lee and Frederick J. Schoen

Brigham and Women's Hospital
Boston, Massachusetts

An understanding of the basic pathology of a disease can guide the development of successful treatments. This principle has been well demonstrated in the acute coronary syndromes, where careful pathologic studies have provided insight into the pathogenesis of acute myocardial ischemia and potential methods of intervention. In this chapter, the basic structure of atherosclerotic lesions will first be reviewed; then, the pathologic considerations of unstable coronary plaque, the lesion responsible for the acute coronary syndromes, will be discussed.

ATHEROSCLEROTIC PLAQUE PROGRESSION

Atherosclerosis is characterized by raised arterial lesions (plaques) consisting of a core of accumulated lipids covered by a cap of tissue derived primarily from the proliferation of cells in the intima (Fig. 1). Lipid deposition and intimal proliferation are not only the hallmarks of atherogenesis but also account for chronic plaque expansion.

Although the components of atherosclerotic lesions can be quite varied, three basic types of lesion are commonly described (1–4). The earliest type is the *fatty streak,* which is present in the aorta of many children by the age of 10. Fatty streaks, which are yellow in color due to intracellular lipid deposits, primarily in macrophages but also in smooth muscle cells beneath the endothelial layer, may be precursors to advanced lesions, but do not themselves cause clinical symptoms. However, the specific relationship between fatty streaks and advanced

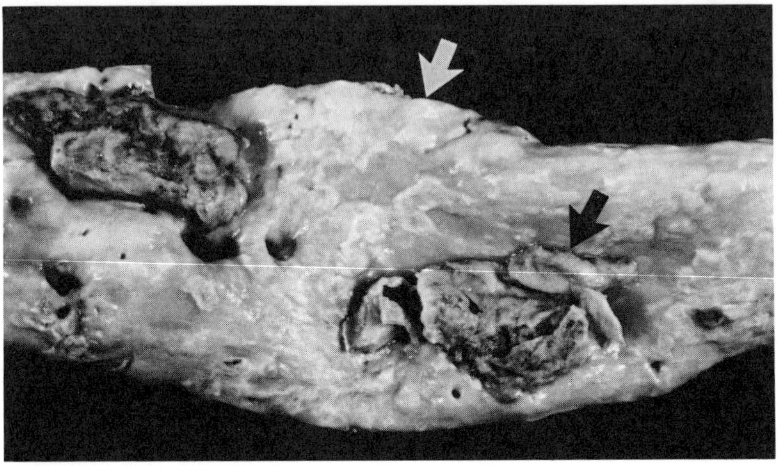

Figure 1 Gross appearance of fibrous uncomplicated atherosclerotic plaque (white arrow) and complicated plaque with superimposed thrombus (dark arrow) from aorta at autopsy. (From Ref. 5 with permission.)

lesions remains uncertain. The second type of atherosclerotic lesion, the *fibrous plaque,* is composed primarily of replications of and connective tissue formation by smooth muscle cells in the intima, although macrophages and other cell types may also be present (Figs. 2 and 3). Fibrous plaques may sometimes be dominated by an extracellular matrix composed of collagen and glycosaminoglycans, with very few cells present. The layer of smooth muscle cells and the extracellular matrix produced by them is called the fibrous cap. A soft lipid pool composed of cellular debris, cholesterol, and other lipids is often present beneath the fibrous cap. The endothelium is usually intact over fibrous plaque. The coronary arterial lesions of stable angina comprise lesions representative of a spectrum of fibrous and complicated plaque (see below).

Complicated lesions are usually identified by degenerative changes such as calcification, necrosis, hemorrhage, or superficial ulceration (Fig. 4). Some complicated lesions have poorly organized thrombotic material below the fibrous cap or a multichanneled arterial lumen; such lesions have probably grown, at least in part, by mural thrombus or plaque hemorrhage. Once a lesion becomes complicated, it is probably more prone to rupture of the fibrous cap, and plaque rupture is generally recognized as the initiating event of most acute coronary syndromes. Thus, we will refer to the plaque with fibrous cap rupture as *unstable plaque,* recognizing that complicated lesions are, or are almost certainly more likely to become, unstable plaques in the future. While the growth of stable lesions proceeds over many years, the plaque probably becomes unstable in

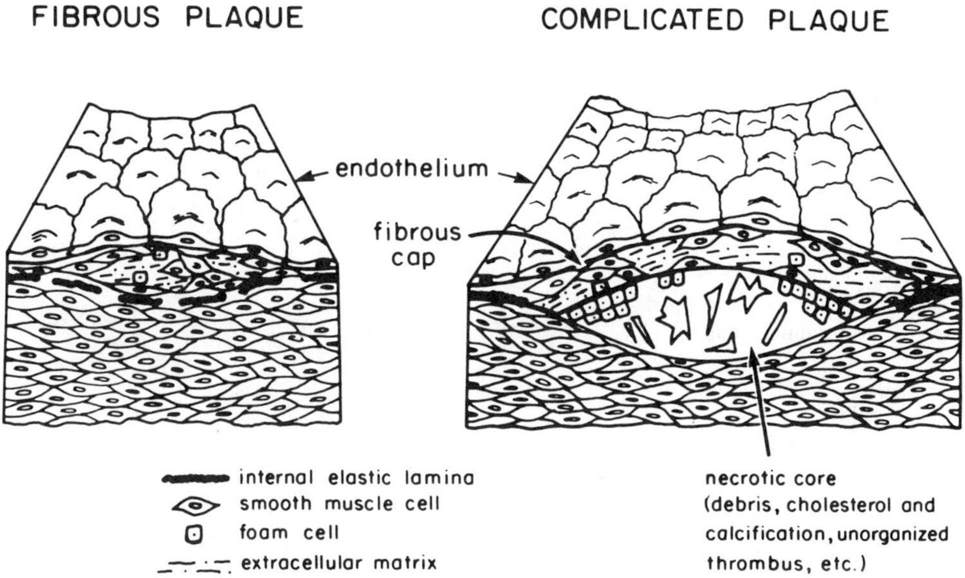

Figure 2 Schematic representation of structure of simple fibrous atherosclerotic plaque (left) and complicated plaque (right). (From Ref. 5 with permission.)

seconds or minutes. It is important to recognize that various interventions such as coronary angioplasty, thrombolysis, and atherectomy, also leave the patient with fissured, unstable plaque (5).

COMPONENTS OF ATHEROSCLEROTIC PLAQUE (Table 1)

Endothelial Cells

Endothelial cells not only serve as a semipermeable barrier in the normal vasculature but also line the surface of most atheromatous lesions. Although in experimental models of atherosclerosis, such as in hyperlipidemic animals, the endothelial surface over plaques is often disturbed, with large areas of denudation and exposure of underlying connective tissue, the endothelium is often preserved into late stages of human lesions. Loss of endothelial cells is associated with adherence of platelets and monocytes (6). Experimental data strongly support the hypothesis that alteration of this endothelial layer is a critical mechanism of atherogenesis (7). Although endothelial injury may be caused mechanically by denudation of previously normal endothelial cells, more subtle forms of endothelial injury ("endothelial dysfunction") may occur without denudation. *Endothelial dysfunction* generally stimulates (a) the production and

Table 1 Atherosclerotic Plaque Components

Cells	
	Endothelial cells
	Smooth muscle cells
	Macrophages
	Lymphocytes
Extracellular matrix	
	Collagen
	Elastin
	Glycosaminoglycans
Other	
	Lipids
	Calcium deposits

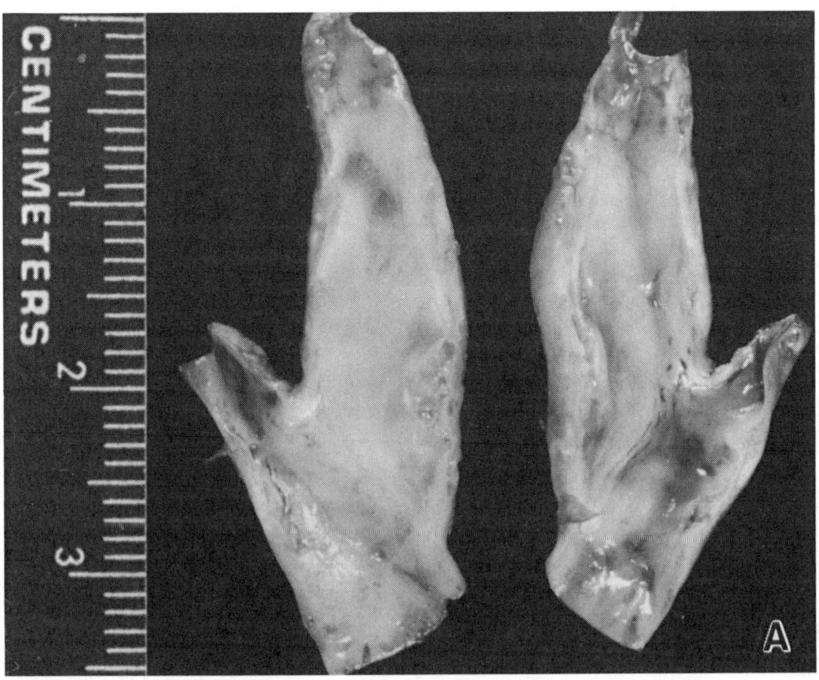

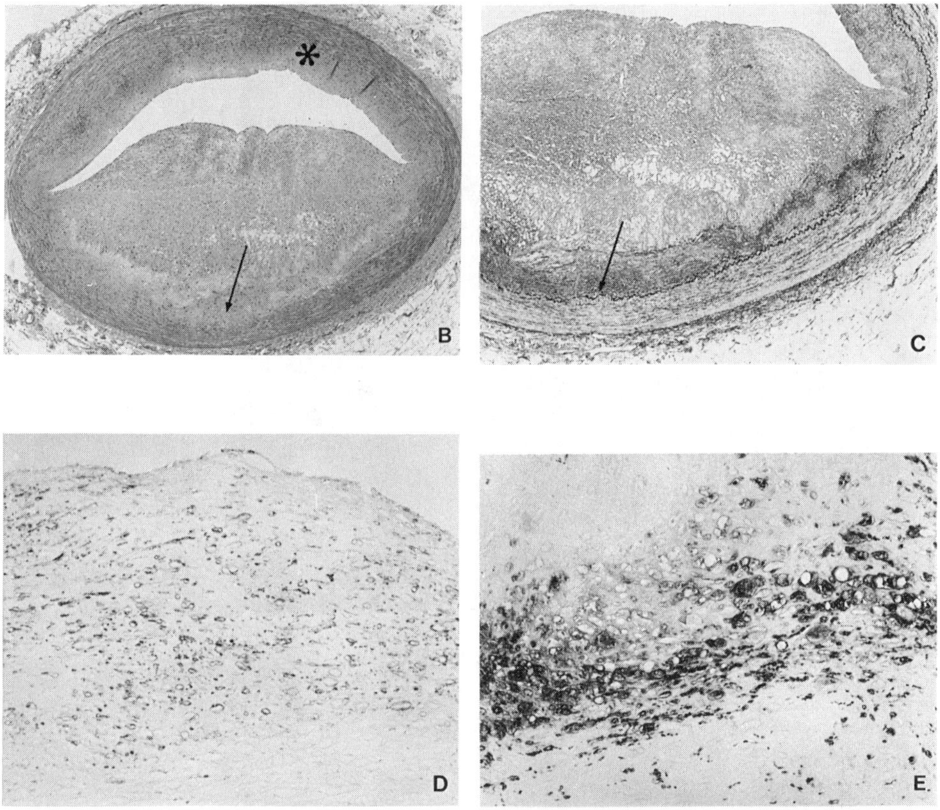

Figure 3 Stable fibrous atherosclerotic plaque and its primary cellular constituents. (A) Gross appearance of carotid plaque removed at endarterectomy. (B–E) Coronary artery obtained at cardiac transplantation. (B) Histologic appearance of moderately obstructive fibrous atherosclerotic plaque. Note the early destruction of the media below the plaque (arrow) and the eccentricity of the lesion with a large plaque-free component (*). Nevertheless, as shown in (C), the internal elastic lamina is relatively intact throughout, with only focal fragmentation (arrows). (D) Smooth muscle cells of lesion shown in (B) stained with antibody directed against muscle cell actin, including smooth muscle cell actin (Mab HHF35). Most of the cells near the lumen are smooth muscle cells. (E) Deep foam cells and other macrophages of lesion shown in (B) stained with antibody directed against a macrophage antigen (Mab MAC56). (B) Hematoxylin and eosin, (C) Elastin stain, (D) and (E) stained with immunoperoxidase technique. (B) Magnification approximately 20×, (C) magnification 40×, (D) and (E) magnification 150×. (A) (From Ref. 5 with permission.)

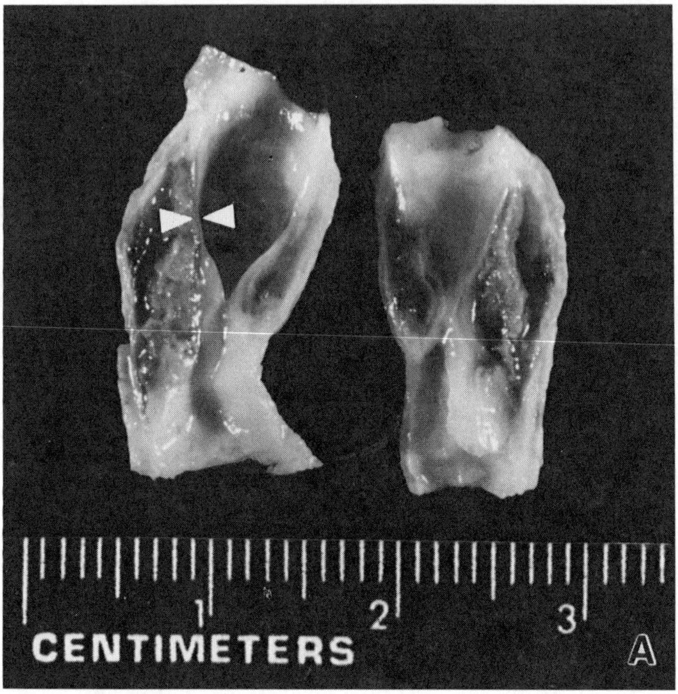
1
2
3
CENTIMETERS
A

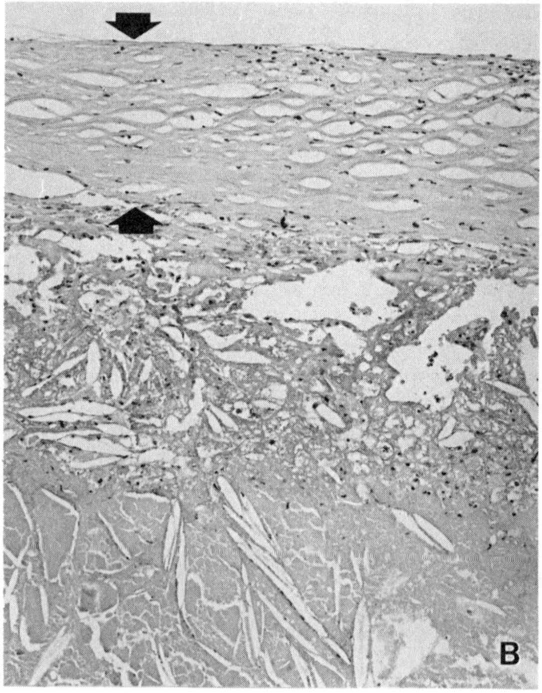
B

secretion of growth factors for smooth muscle cells while decreasing the availability of inhibitory substances, (b) adherence of circulating leukocytes, and (c) thrombogenesis of the vascular lining. Immune mechanisms, hypercholesterolemia, and injury by infectious agents can all promote atherosclerosis. Endothelial cells normally produce substances, such as heparan sulfates, that keep the rate of proliferation of smooth muscle cells to exceedingly low resting levels ($<0.1\%$ per day). Disruption of this natural inhibitory influence can contribute to smooth muscle cell hyperplasia. Moreover, endothelial injury could provide increased opportunities for interactions of the subendothelial vascular wall with platelets or macrophages and result in growth factor release from each of these sources, thereby providing a mitogenic stumulus to smooth muscle cells. Endothelial cells not only regulate the nature of components that reach the subendothelial space, including lipoproteins and other constituents of blood, but also bind and process LDL so that it is recognized and ingested by macrophages and other cells (4).

In addition, it is now recognized that the endothelium functions as an important endocrine organ, secreting a variety of active substances that control blood flow (8,9). It is likely that several of these endothelial hormones, such as endothelium-derived relaxing factor (EDRF), participate in the abnormal vasoreactive state that accompanies unstable angina. Dysfunction of endothelium-mediated vasomotion has been well documented in humans with coronary atherosclerosis (10).

Smooth Muscle Cells

Smooth muscle cells are the dominant cellular component of the media of small-to-medium size arteries, of which the coronary arteries are representative. Normally, smooth muscle cells function as regulators of arterial wall tension, are spindle-shaped resembling fibroblasts, and contain extensive cytoplasmic filaments of actin and myosin. Smooth muscle cell migration to and proliferation in the intima (in response to chemotactic factors and growth stimuli) are key processes in the formation of atherosclerotic plaque (4,11,12). Smooth muscle cells are usually the most numerous cell type in fibrous atherosclerotic plaque, and plaque growth is largely mediated by their proliferation. Smooth muscle cells also can form an extensive connective tissue matrix and can accumulate lipid. Although most foam cells are derived from macrophages, some foam cells are derived from smooth muscle cells. The process of smooth muscle cell

Figure 4 Complicated atherosclerotic plaque removed at carotid endarterectomy. (A) Gross photo. Very thin fibrous cap is seen between arrows. (B) Photomicrograph showing that this lesion is composed of large central zone of necrotic-thrombotic material separated from flowing blood by a very thin fibrous cap (between arrows) which could easily undergo disruption. (B) Hematoxylin and eosin, magnification 60×. (A from Ref. 5 with permission.)

migration and multiplication has been studied extensively by experimental arterial wall injury (3). In response to injury, smooth muscle cells lose the capacity to contract, gain the capacity to divide, and increase their synthesis of extracellular matrix molecules. Structurally, they lose contractile elements and greatly increase rough endoplasmic reticulum, the major organelle involved with protein synthesis. To a large extent, atherogenesis involves smooth muscle cell growth due to disruption of the physiologic balance between smooth muscle cell growth inhibition and growth stimulation, usually endogenously regulated by both promoters (such as platelet-derived growth factor [PDGF]) and inhibitors (such as endothelial cell-derived heparin). In some conditions associated with "accelerated atherosclerosis," such as late restenosis following balloon angioplasty, coronary vein graft intimal hyperplasia and premature arteriosclerosis in patients with cardiac transplants, intense proliferation of and connective tissue synthesis by intimal smooth muscle cells is also found (5).

Monocytes/Macrophages

Monocytes/macrophages (14) are the most numerous and perhaps most important leukocytes in the atheromatous lesion. Adherence of circulating monocytes to the endothelium and the subendothelial migration of these cells are among the earliest events in atherogenesis. Moreover, in large part owing to their ability to accumulate both native and modified LDL and process cholesterol, macrophages are the predominant precursors of foam cells. Although it is difficult to positively identify quiescent macrophages on routinely stained tissues, immunohistochemical staining has demonstrated that cells of macrophage lineage are abundant in atherosclerotic plaque, particularly near the necrotic base of advanced lesions. In addition, macrophages release a number of proteolytic enzymes such as collagenase and elastase that could weaken the fibrous cap.

Lymphocytes

Lymphocytes are present in fatty streaks, fibrous plaque, and complicated plaque. Although T lymphocytes are numerous in atherosclerotic plaque, comprising 20% of cells in fibrous plaque, it is unknown to what extent these cells are immunologically active (14). The possible role of immune mechanisms in atherogenesis is under intense investigation. T lymphocytes produce a number of lymphokines that could participate in atherogenesis.

Platelets

Platelets release their granular constituents following adherence to injured endothelium or subendothelial connective tissue. PDGF, contained in platelet alpha granules and released during this interaction, is a major mitogen for smooth muscle cells. Within minutes following vascular intimal injury, platelet granule constituents can be found deep in the vessel wall. Macrophages and endothelial cells in culture (and likely in vivo) can also secrete growth factors for smooth muscle cells, at least some of which are similar to PDGF (7). Moreover, smooth muscle cells may themselves produce a PDGF-like growth factor, suggesting that these cells may stimulate their own proliferation. Thus, all four principal cells involved in atherogenesis, namely, endothelial cells, smooth muscle cells, monocytes/macrophages, and platelets, can release growth factors (4).

Extracellular Connective Tissue Matrix

The extracellular connective tissue matrix elaborated by intimal smooth muscle cells comprises the predominant mass of many fibrous plaques (15). Collagen types I and III are important components of the fibrous cap; the ratio of collagen to elastin is much higher in atherosclerotic lesions than in normal arterial wall. Collagen is an extremely stiff protein when compared to elastin; this is one reason that fibrous plaques are more resistant to the mechanical deformation than normal vessels. Smooth muscle cells also secrete glycosaminoglycans, whose production is increased in atherosclerotic lesions (16). The most abundant glycosaminoglycan in vascular tissue is chondroitin sulfate B, which may play a role in binding of lipids to the vessel wall. Dystrophic calcification (i.e., deposition of calcium-containing apatitic mineral in injured tissues), a feature of some complicated lesions, occurs in association with cell fragments and within the connective tissue matrix (2). Calcification may be detected noninvasively by fluoroscopy, CT scanning, or, when severe, routine chest radiography. Due to the enhanced ability to detect calcific deposits in arterial lesions, there is renewed interest in coronary artery calcification and its clinical implications.

Lipid Pool

Beneath the fibrous cap, advanced atheromatous lesions generally have a lipid pool (17). The lipid pool is composed of free cholesterol, cholesterol esters, phospholipids, and cellular debris. The majority of the lipid is extracellular, although lipid-laden foam cells may also be found in and around the lipid pool. At body temperature, the lipid pool is most likely in a semifluid state, similar to toothpaste in consistency (18). As discussed below, the structural consequences of a soft lipid pool in an advanced atheromatous lesion may be the disruption of the fibrous cap and the subsequent development of unstable angina.

OTHER BIOPHYSICAL ASPECTS OF ATHEROSCLEROTIC PLAQUE

Although many coronary stenoses are concentric, with atherosclerotic plaque distributed along the entire circumference of the vessel, approximately two thirds are eccentric, with at least part of the lumen wall relatively free of disease

(19,20). There is evidence that this *normal plaque-free arterial wall* at a lesion can enlarge circumferentially, compensating for the potential hemodynamic limitation as the plaque grows. This compensatory mechanism is effective in inhibiting luminal obstruction, at least in early stages of atherosclerosis. One of the mechanisms for this enlargement appears to be thinning of the media, possibly due to atrophy of medial smooth muscle cells (20). The dilatation of the normal arterial wall may be apparent on angiography as a bend in the vessel, as if the normal wall were trying to distance itself from the lesion. In addition, the free arterial wall is more resilient than the stiffer fibrous plaque and probably capable of responding to stimuli that cause vascular spasm. Saner et al. (19) have suggested that changes in luminal caliber during coronary angiography observed by several investigators are due to spasm of this arc of disease-free vessel, and this may be a mechanism for "variable threshold angina."

Arteries have a *vasa vasorum,* a fine bed of capillaries in the adventitia that provide nutrients to the vessel wall. Atherosclerotic coronary arteries are especially rich in vasa vasorum, with heavy concentrations near areas of particularly thickened intima (Fig. 5). Barger et al. (22) have suggested that this fragile capillary bed is involved in the pathogenesis of atherosclerosis, possibly by causing subintimal hemorrhage and increasing plaque internal pressure or by providing enhanced neurotransmitter concentrations to spasm-prone vessels. At the current time, however, a definitive role of the vasa vasorum in the pathogenesis of atherosclerosis or acute coronary ischemia has not been demonstrated.

PATHOBIOLOGY OF THE EARLY LESION

Contemporary concepts of pathogenesis of atherosclerosis are best described by the modified "response-to-injury hypothesis," as formulated by Ross (4,23). The underlying hypothesis suggests that atherogenesis may arise from two interrelated mechanisms: (a) in hypercholesterolemia, monocyte/platelet interaction stimulates smooth muscle cell proliferation through growth factor release; (b) endothelial cells stimulated directly (e.g., hypertension, smoking) may release growth factors that can induce smooth muscle cell migration and proliferation, and perhaps release of cell-stimulating growth factors. In the latter path, the triggering event is likely a subtle, nondenuding endothelial cell injury, manifested by loss of resistance to thrombus formation, expression of surface molecules adhesive to leukocytes, altered matabolism, and impaired selectivity of the permeability barrier. This results in both the adherence of monocytes and their entry into the arterial wall. As discussed, platelets, endothelial cells, and activated macrophages can release chemotactic agents and mitogens for smooth muscle cells, migrate from the media into the injured intima, and secrete large amounts of connective tissue. There is concurrent or subsequent lipid accumulation both intracellularly (in the formation of foam cells) and extracellularly

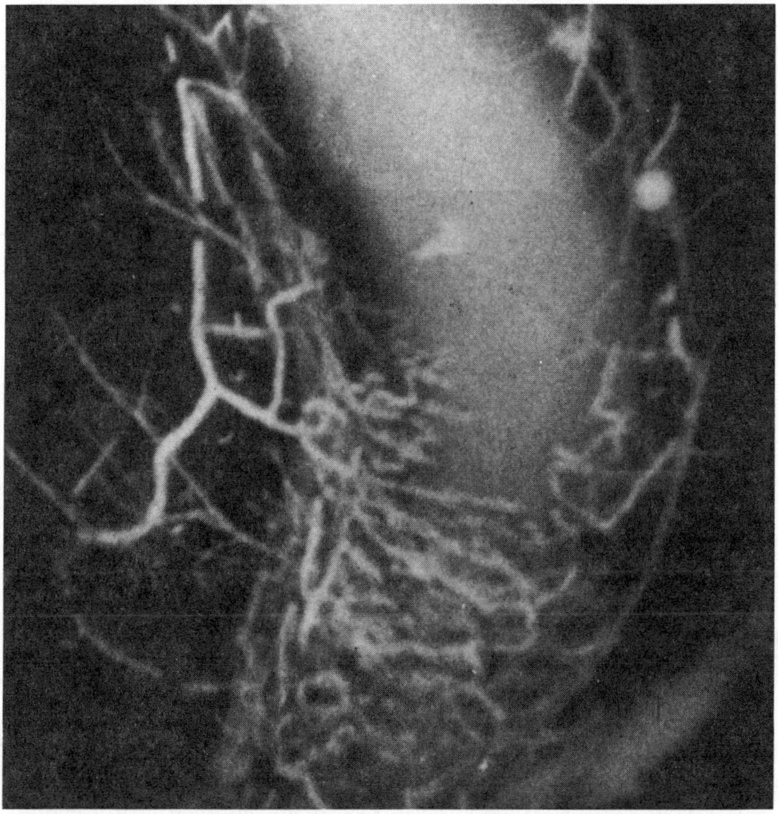

Figure 5 Vasa vasorum of left anterior descending coronary artery in a human with coronary atherosclerosis. Note the dense network of neovasculature in the region of the plaque. (From Barger AC, Beeuwkes R. Am J Cardiol 1990; 66:41G–43G, with permission.)

(trapping of plasma lipoproteins in the connective tissue matrix), cell death with release of intracellular lipids (mostly cholesterol esters), and a chronic inflammatory reaction. Thus, atherosclerosis results from a complex interaction between cells of the blood vessel wall and circulating blood components.

FINDINGS AT AUTOPSY COMPARED TO ANGIOGRAPHY

Several studies have compared angiographic estimation of stenosis severity with necropsy findings (24–26). Although the correlation is generally good, angiography often underestimates the degree of stenosis when compared to autopsy findings. This is particularly true when the coronary arteries are not perfused at physiologic pressure prior to fixation; fixation without pressurization allows the vessel to distort and partially collapse. A second reason that stenoses noted at angiography may appear less severe than in reality is that the stenosis is compared to the caliber of vessel nearby, which may appear angiographically free of disease. However, adjacent segments are often concentrically narrowed by atherosclerosis, so that the percent stenosis of the lesion when compared to the adjacent "normal" vessel underestimates the true severity; this is particularly common when evaluating severe coronary disease. A third reason concerns the ability of the diseased vessel to develop compensatory enlargement in the early stages of plaque formation, so that the severity of disease is underestimated by angiography; this is a common reason for underestimating mild stenoses (26). Moreover, the degree of narrowing described at necropsy is usually the percent reduction in cross-sectional area, not the percent reduction in diameter reported by angiographers.

CHARACTERISTICS OF THE UNSTABLE PLAQUE

The Severity of Stenosis

Pathologic data regarding the severity of coronary stenoses in patients with unstable angina (but without myocardial infarction or sudden death) have been obtained from patients dying during or following coronary bypass surgery. Roberts and Virmani (27) at the National Institutes of Health examined 22 patients with unstable angina and compared them with patients with myocardial infarction or sudden death. Patients with unstable angina had the most severe and extensive atherosclerosis, usually having diffuse three vessel disease. In almost every coronary segment analyzed, at least 25% of the luminal cross-sectional area was reduced by atherosclerosis. In a later study, the NIH investigators found that multiluminal channels were found in 10 out of 10 autopsies following death due to unstable angina; these channels most likely result from organization and recanalization of luminal thrombi (28). The major component of atherosclerotic plaque was a combination of cellular and dense acellular fibrous tissue (>80%). Pultaceous debris accounted for about 8% of plaque in patients with angina pectoris at rest. In contrast, pultaceous debris accounted for 16% of lesion volume in patients with fatal acute myocardial infarction. These studies were, of course, influenced by inadvertent selection bias, because patients with severe coronary disease are probably less likely to survive surgery. However, the data illustrate not only the severity of diffuse coronary disease but also the complexity of plaque composition in many patients with unstable angina.

Pathologic and clinical studies show that (a) plaque disruption usually underlies coronary thrombosis, and (b) plaques that undergo abrupt disruption leading to unstable angina or acute myocardial infarction are often those that previously produced only mild to moderate luminal stenosis. In one study of 166 episodes of

Table 2 Degree of Preexisting Stenosis Under Thrombi Caused by Acute Plaque Change

Stenosis severity (%)	% of cases
30 or less	13
40	13
50	16
60	20
70	15
80 or more	15

Source: Ref. 29.

major coronary thrombi in humans detectable at post-mortem angiography and responsible for death, only 25% occurred over plaques that appeared intact, but 75% occurred over plaques in which the intima was fissured. Most (81%) of the thrombi over intact plaques had preexisting stenosis of >60% in diameter (29). However, the degree of preexisting stenosis at the site of thrombi caused by plaque tears and deeper intimal injury was less and more variable (Table 2). Post-mortem angiographic studies have shown that an eccentric stenosis with a narrow neck and overhanging edges or scalloped borders indicates plaque rupture or hemorrhage, with superimposed partially occluding or recanalized thrombus. Lesions with severe stenosis tend to progress to total occlusion more commonly than do less severe lesions, but severely stenotic lesions often do not produce clinical myocardial infarction, perhaps because of the presence of well-developed collaterals. In angiographic studies, the majority (85%) of infarct-related lesions were not hemodynamically significant at initial study (30). Moreover, following thrombolytic therapy for acute myocardial infarction, the underlying lesion often has <70% diameter stenosis. Patients with angiographically less severe disease may account for as much as two thirds of the patient population who develop unstable angina or acute myocardial infarction. Thus, percent stenosis is not the sole determinant of progression to clinical instability.

Plaque Fissures in Acute Coronary Syndromes

The mechanism of progression of angiographically and pathologically mild stenosis to acute coronary ischemia was elucidated by several classic pathologic studies. In 1926, Benson noted that some coronary thrombi were found over broken atherosclerotic plaques (31). In 1966, Constantinides provided evidence that small fissures were important causes of death in patients with coronary artery disease (32). Studying 22 patients who died at Barnes Hospital in St. Louis, he found by careful serial sectioning that all thrombi were anchored in fissures in the atheromatous wall. Often, these fissures were small (less than 400 μm in length), so that the step serial sections performed by previous investigators were likely to have missed them (Figs. 6 and 7). At that time, it was already well known that trauma to the endothelial surface provoked thrombosis, and Constantinides proposed that the initiating factor in acute coronary ischemia was fissuring of the plaque surface and exposure of thrombogenic subendothelial components (unstable plaque).

In the 1970s, a number of investigators suggested that thrombosis was actually secondary to and not a primary pathophysiologic mechanism of infarction. In patients given radiolabeled fibrinogen as soon as possible following presentation with acute myocardial infarction, radioactivity was detected in the thrombus, supporting the hypothesis that thrombi formed *after* myocardial infarction (33). These studies raised doubts about the plaque rupture–thrombosis hypothesis. However, later studies using similar techniques found that the radiolabel concentrated in the downstream tail of the thrombus, not the head of the thrombus located adjacent to the plaque. Thus, although continued thrombus formation is common during acute myocardial infarction, thrombosis appeared to be present very early, perhaps at the onset of symptoms.

In 1980, DeWood et al. (34) reported that total coronary occlusion by thrombus was present in 87% of patients in the early hours of acute myocardial infarction. Many pathologic, angiographic, and angioscopic studies have now confirmed that intraluminal thrombosis, usually occlusive, is the cause of the majority of acute myocardial infarcts (Fig. 5). Studies of coronary arteries following thrombolysis have also demonstrated underlying plaque fissures with residual intraplaque thrombus (35). In addition, unstable plaques with nonocclusive thrombi appear to be the cause of crescendo angina, while stable angina is typically associated with plaques with smooth surfaces. Thus, unstable angina and transmural infarction may be parts of a continuous spectrum of the consequences of plaque rupture.

The nature of the pathologic lesion in sudden cardiac death is less clear. Unlike acute myocardial infarction, fewer than 10% of patients with sudden cardiac death have coronary thrombi at autopsy in some studies (36). These pathologic data are supported by the clinical observation that many patients who are resuscitated after cardiac arrest will not have evidence of myocardial necrosis. However, when Davies and Thomas (37) carefully examined 100 patients with ischemic cardiac death within 6 hours of symptoms, 74 had coronary thrombi. In addition, among the 26 cases without thrombi, fissured coronary plaques were found in 21. Thus, unstable plaque appears to play an important role in many cases of sudden cardiac death, although the relationship of sudden death and transient coronary thrombotic occlusion is not well defined.

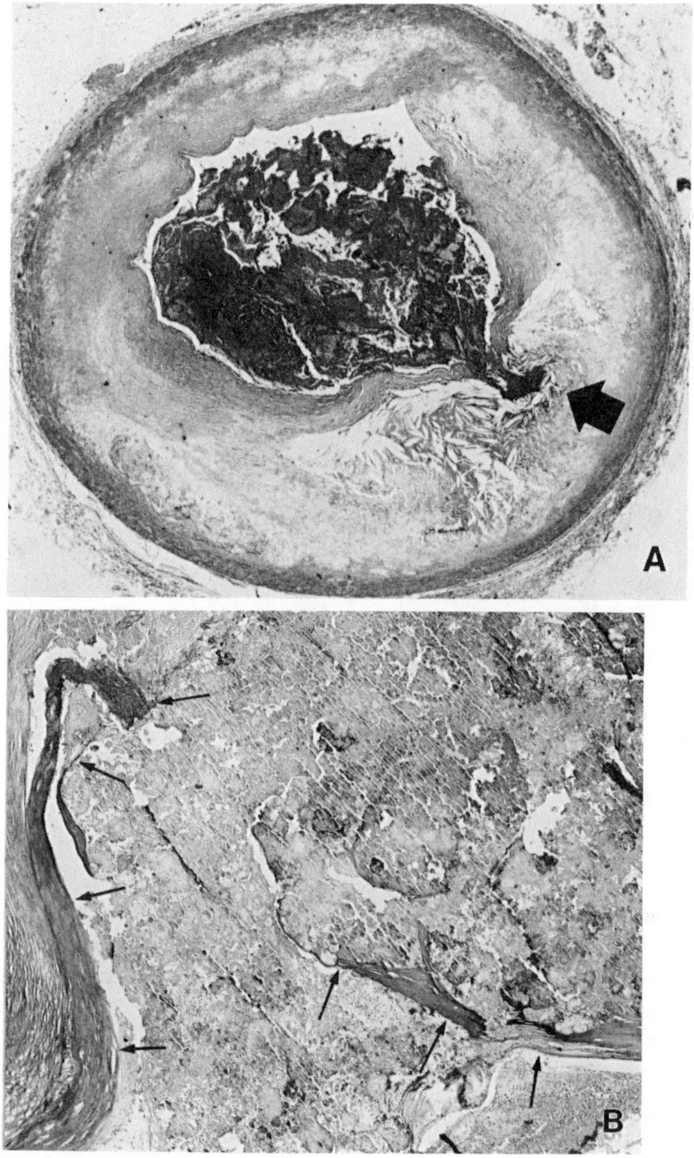

Figure 6 (A) Atherosclerotic plaque rupture. Complicated plaque in human coronary artery, with plaque rupture (arrow) and superimposed complete thrombotic occlusion. Stained with Lendrum stain for fibrin. (B) Disrupted fibrous cap in another coronary arterial plaque with rupture. Fragments of fibrous cap are denoted by arrows. (A) Hematoxylin and eosin, 20×; (B) Elastin stain, 50×.

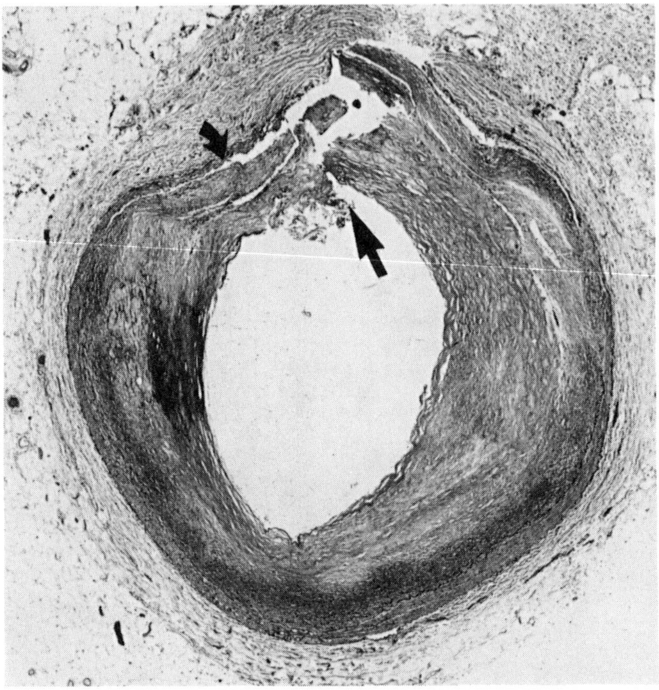

Figure 7 Low power photomicrograph of coronary artery from patient who died several days following coronary angioplasty of this vessel segment. The fracture through the intima and media is at the site designated by a large arrow. A small dissection in the external media at the site is indicated by the small arrow. Elastin stain, approximately 20×.

Histologic evidence of recent plaque fissures is not limited to those patients with acute coronary syndromes. In a group of subjects who died of noncardiac disease, plaque fissures without thrombus were found in 17% of those with atheroma-related diseases such as hypertension or diabetes and 9% of patients without hypertension or diabetes (29). However, although plaque fissures act as a stimulus for the formation of intraluminal thrombi, intraluminal thrombosis in the coronary arteries is probably very rare in noncardiac patients. Although the determinants of outcome following fissuring and whether intraluminal thrombus occurs is uncertain, hemostasis and other poorly understood parameters of the patient probably play a role.

Davies describes three distinct stages in the formation of thrombosis associated with plaque fissuring: (a) small intimal tear allowing continuity between the arterial lumen and the interior of a lipid-rich plaque, leading to a thrombotic mass within the intima; (b) formation of an intraluminal thrombotic component which is nonocclusive, allowing antegrade blood flow over the thrombus; and (c) occlusive luminal thrombosis (27). Mural nonocclusive thrombi are commonly associated with distal embolism of small platelet thrombi within the vascular territory supplied by the coronary artery containing a fissured plaque (38).

The Natural History of Fissured Plaque

If atherosclerotic plaques fissure in everyday life without causing coronary thrombosis, what happens to these plaques? Nonfatal plaque rupture may be an important mechanism of stenosis progression. Plaque rupture is generally followed by hemorrhage into the plaque with some reduction of luminal area. When the stenosis is less than 75%, these intraintimal hemorrhages rarely cause occlusive luminal thrombosis and are possibly asymptomatic. It is possible that this type of plaque rupture tends to heal the injured fibrous cap, causing a further reduction in luminal area. Balloon angioplasty also induces plaque rupture (Fig. 7). This scenario of plaque rupture with rapid smooth muscle cell proliferation is similar to events following the damage caused by percutaneous balloon angioplasty (39). Coronary angioplasty usually results in fracture of the plaque at its weakest point, resulting in longitudinal and circumferential tears in the atheroma and/or vessel wall. In most cases of successful angioplasty, the healing process is probably characterized by reendothelialization and remodeling of the compressed or torn atheroma. However, progressive intimal smooth muscle cell proliferation leads to rapid restenosis in many cases. Thus, postangioplasty restenosis and many cases of unstable angina may share the common pathophysiologic mechanism of the response to intimal injury without occlusive luminal thrombosis. Strategies to change the type or degree of intimal damage or the vascular response to injury such as laser angioplasty, atherectomy, or low molecular weight heparin are currently being evaluated.

The potential outcome of angioplasty is related to the structure of the plaque rupture (5). Plaque fracture and intimal/medial dissection are associated with successful angioplasty, but extensive circumferential or longitudinal dissection can lead to obstructive luminal flaps or compression of less involved segments, respectively. Similarly, unsuccessful thrombolysis may be attributed, in some cases, to complex tears with substantial intraintimal thrombus and an externally compressed lumen, or the presence of a large intimal flap. Moreover, the intimal disruption which occurs during angioplasty is greater and the plaque fissures are usually deeper than those that occur naturally.

An additional type of accelerated atherosclerosis that shares the feature of rapid intimal smooth muscle cell proliferation is coronary vein graft atherosclerosis (7). Atherosclerosis is the major reason that only 60% or less of saphenous vein grafts remain patent after 11 years. The exposure of the vein graft to arterial flow results in endothelial injury with platelet deposition early following surgery despite angiographically normal flow. The reparative process leads to medial smooth muscle cell hyperplasia and connective tissue synthesis; eventually the lipid accumulation and foam cells of typical atherosclerosis develop. Late atherosclerotic lesions in vein grafts are often extremely friable, with thin, poorly formed fibrous caps. Thrombotic occlusion of such vessels is frequently initiated by plaque rupture; emboli can occur spontaneously or can be induced by balloon angioplasty or surgical manipulation of these vessels.

Pathologic Features of the Thrombus

After blood dissects into the intima through the fissure in the plaque surface, a mass of thrombus rich in platelets forms. The most recent part of the thrombus, often the final portion of the thrombus that occludes the vessel, may be identified pathologically as aggregated platelets that can be individually discernible. In patients with unstable angina progressing to fatal myocardial infarction, layered mural thrombi are found in the coronary arteries, suggesting that phases of recurrent thrombosis were responsible for the clinical picture (38). This dynamic nature of thrombosis which is so dependent of the delicate balance between thrombosis and thrombolysis may explain the marked clinical unpredictability seen in many patients with unstable angina.

Microemboli

Necropsy studies have demonstrated another important mechanism of myocardial ischemia in patients with unstable angina. In patients who died of sudden death or infarction, Falk (38) was able to identify fragments of thrombi that had embolized to small intramyocardial arteries, leading to "microinfarcts" in 73% of cases. Although these small infarcts could occur distant from the thrombosed epicardial arteries, they were selectively located in the microcirculation supplied by the thrombosed epicardial vessel. These results are similar to those of Frink et al. (40), who found microemboli in 79% of hearts from patients dying of myocardial infarction. In a larger series of 90 patients, Davies et al. (41) demonstrated that microemboli were more common in patients with unstable angina prior to death than in patients who were stable. Thus, pathologic studies indicate that thrombi are capable of fragmenting and embolizing distally as well as growing intermittently (Fig. 8). These microinfarcts, caused by microemboli, are probably too small to cause a detectable increase in serum cardiac enzymes, and may explain the stuttering clinical course in many patients with unstable angina.

STENOSIS CONFIGURATION AND COMPOSITION DETERMINE PROPENSITY TO RUPTURE

It is likely that both the geometry and the mechanical properties of plaque components influence the tendency of the plaque to fissure. In these concentric stenoses with the entire circumference of the intima involved, it is likely that the

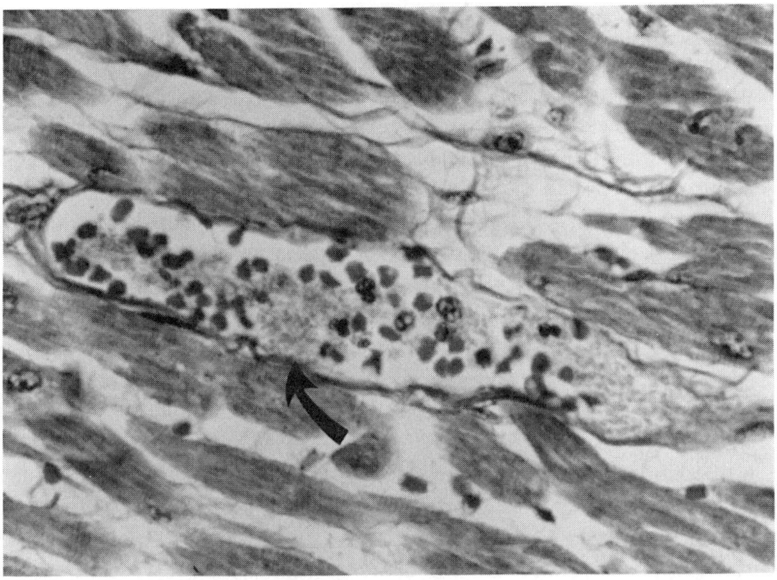

Figure 8 Platelet thromboembolus (arrow) in the myocardium of patient with severe three vessel coronary atherosclerosis, but no apparent acute myocardial infarct, who died suddenly. Hematoxylin and eosin, 375×.

luminal area is relatively constant during the cardiac cycle, due to the increased rigidity of the atheroma compared to the normal vessel. In contrast, eccentric stenoses are probably more susceptible to vascular spasm of the less diseased arc of the vessel, leading to a dynamic reduction in luminal area. It may be difficult to identify eccentric stenoses by angiography, which gives luminal definition but not the location of the internal elastic membrane of the vessel.

Pathologic studies of the relationship of the site of intimal tearing to plaque morphology have provided important clues about the mechanism of plaque rupture. When Richardson et al. (42) studied the ruptured plaques from 85 patients who had died from coronary thrombosis, 67 (79%) were found to be eccentric with a subintimal lipid pool. In these plaques, the intima had torn through the junction of the plaque and the more normal vessel into the lipid pool. Rupture of concentric stenoses was much less common. Thus, the geometry and substructure of the atherosclerotic plaque appears to be a significant factor in determining how the plaque ruptures. However, these studies demonstrate that, in addition to the geometry of the lesion, the mechanical behavior of atherosclerotic plaque components is also important. Although an enormous amount is known about the behavior of normal arteries, surprisingly little is known about the mechanical properties of atherosclerotic tissues.

POST-MORTEM PATHOLOGIC STUDIES

It is clear from the above discussion that pathologic studies have elucidated major features of the natural history of atherosclerotic plaque and its complications. Pathologists examining hearts of patients who have died of coronary artery disease have an ongoing responsibility to carefully dissect specimens and describe lesion morphology to the fullest extent possible in clinically meaningful terms. The exemplary post-mortem angiographic studies of Davies and others have indicated the value of this technique in elucidating plaque morphology. However, quality post-mortem angiograms are not technically feasible in every case. Following fixation of the heart, the coronary arteries should be dissected free and thoroughly decalcified, followed by transverse sectioning at 2–3 mm intervals and gross examination and recording of stenoses. All sections containing occlusions and/or thrombotic deposits or other areas suspicious for acute plaque change should be examined by light microscopy following conventional histologic processing. Critical lesions may be relatively short and multiple areas of interest may be sequential over short distances. In scientific investigations to address research questions, physiologic pressure perfusion and fixation of the coronary arteries, scanning electron microscopy, transmission electron microscopy, immunohistochemistry, and/or morphometric studies may be useful. The pathologic descriptors of atherosclerotic lesions are summarized in Table 3.

Table 3 Atherosclerosis Morphology: Key Features

Geometry
Vessel size
Degree of stenosis
Length of stenosis
Eccentricity of stenosis
Plaque structure
Surface morphology
Presence of endothelium
Fibrous cap thickness/composition
"Soft/hard" core (pultaceous debris)
Calcification
Cellular composition
Relative plaque constituents
Foam cells
Multiple intraluminal vascular channels
Vasa vasorum
Acute plaque change
Intraplaque hemorrhage
Plaque rupture
Mural thrombus

CAN WE PREDICT WHICH PLAQUES WILL RUPTURE?

Characteristics of plaque likely to potentiate rupture are summarized in Table 4. Recognition of specific pathologic features which increase plaque vulnerability to disruption suggests that understanding plaque component morphology and mechanical property correlations may allow prediction of plaques most likely to cause acute myocardial ischemia in the future. Although angiography does not provide sufficient morphologic information to perform a computerized model of the stresses in the diseased vessels, advances in intravascular catheter-tip ultrasound techniques now allow a detailed description of plaque geometry in vivo (43). Thus, with further refinements in intravascular ultrasound, plaques with important stress concentrations and weak areas may be identified in the catheterization laboratory long before they become unstable.

We have recently demonstrated that the mechanical properties of atherosclerotic plaque components can be measured in vitro and are closely related to the underlying microstructure of the plaque (44). However, the task of understanding why plaques rupture will not be a simple one, because the mechanical properties of plaque and its components are complex. Many biological materials are heterogeneous and do not behave like homogeneous elastic solids. Elastic materials deform when a force or pressure is applied and return to the original form when the force is removed. Biological materials are not elastic, but *plastic;* that is, when the force is removed, the material will retain at least some of the deformation. In addition, like most biological materials, plaque components have a high water content, so that the mechanical properties of plaque also reflect interstitial water movement through the extracellular matrix of the plaque. Thus, the response of plaque materials to pressure changes will depend not only on the magnitude of the pressure change but also on the rate at which it is applied. This time-dependent deformation is termed *viscoelasticity*.

Although the mechanical properties of plaques are complicated, a computer technique called finite element analysis now allows complex geometries and mechanical properties to be modeled mathematically. In finite element analysis, small segments of materials ("finite elements") are assigned individual mechanical properties; the computer can then calculate stresses and deformations associated with different pressure changes. Richardson and his colleagues used a simple finite element analysis method to model the stress distribution in the

Table 4 Characteristics of Plaques Likely to Rupture

Soft, with a high proportion of pultaceous debris
Thin fibrous cap
Eccentric lipid pool
Fibrous cap-infiltrating macrophages

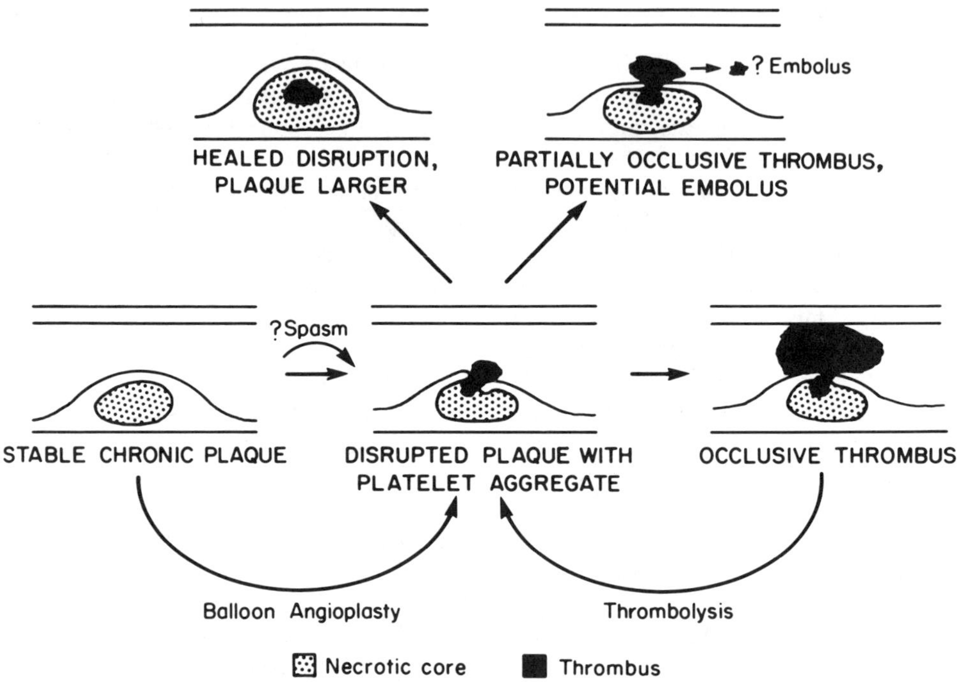

Figure 9 Schematic representation of sequential progression of coronary artery lesion morphology, beginning with stable chronic plaque. This paradigm emphasizes the central role of plaque disruption in both the natural initiation of acute coronary syndromes and the iatrogenic pathology of invasive treatment modalities. Spasm probably contributes to spontaneous plaque disruption. The disrupted plaque is generally present following thrombolysis and balloon angioplasty. Thrombolysis of acutely thrombosed coronary arteries eliminates the bulk of occlusive thrombus, but has little or no effect on the underlying disrupted atherosclerotic lesion. Moreover, balloon angioplasty causes plaque disruption through its basic mechanism: distorted plaque fragments may be a nidus for thrombotic deposits or intimal hyperplasia with restenosis. (From Ref. 5 with permission.)

atherosclerotic plaque and found that the calculated points of maximum stress corresponded to the sites of intimal tearing found in plaques of patients who died of coronary thrombosis. These data suggest that points of high circumferential stress pull the intima apart.

If these points of maximal stress are related to the morphology and histology of the plaque, what determines the answer of plaque rupture? One possibility is that macrophages that are abundant in many atherosclerotic lesions damage the plaque's mechanical integrity (13). Macrophages secrete collagenase, elastase, and other enzymes that digest connective tissue and are commonly found at the site of plaque rupture. Thus, it is possible that macrophages weaken the plaque structure, allowing the stresses in the plaque to tear the intima apart. Proving this hypothesis will be difficult, but with greater understanding of the relationships between the pathology of the plaque and the mechanical properties of plaque components, we should be able to learn much more about why plaques can lie dormant for many years and suddenly grow unstable.

CONCLUSION

Complex interactions between many cell types of the arterial wall and blood components lead to the slow development of atherosclerotic lesions, each of which has its own structural characteristics. It now appears that these characteristics increase the propensity of some plaques to fissure, allowing the exposure of the prothrombotic subintimal plaque components to flowing blood. Stenosis severity is not the sole determinant of structural stability; other factors such as fibrous cap thickness and composition and lipid pool size are probably important. Some plaque fissuring may be subclinical, and fissuring and healing may be one mechanism of stenosis growth. However, once lesions become unstable by fissuring and luminal thrombosis begins, the progression to clinical unstable angina or myocardial infarction is rapid.

REFERENCES

1. Ross R, Glomset JA. The pathogenesis of atherosclerosis (first of two parts). Patho Athero 1976; 295:369–77.
2. Adams DH, Schoen, FJ. In White, RA, ed. Contemporary concepts in atherosclerosis pathology. Atherosclerosis and arteriosclerosis: human pathology and experimental animal methods and models. Boca Raton, FL:CRC Press, 1989:49–86.
3. Munro JM, Cotran RS. The pathogenesis of atherosclerosis: atherogenesis and inflammation. Lab Invest 1988; 58:249–61.
4. Ross R. The pathogenesis of atherosclerosis—an update. N Engl J Med 1986; 314:488–500.
5. Schoen FJ. Interventional and surgical cardiovascular pathology: clinical correlations and basic principles. Philadelphia: W.B. Saunders, 1989.
6. Davies MJ, Woolf N, Rowles, PM, Pepper J. Morphology of the endothelium over atherosclerotic plaques in human coronary arteries. Br Heart J 1988; 60:459–64.
7. Ip JH, Fuster V, Badimon L, Badimon J, Taubman MB, Chesebro JH. Syndromes of accelerated atherosclerosis: Role of vascular injury and smooth muscle cell proliferation. J Am Coll Cardiol 1990; 15:1667–87.
8. Dinerman JL, Mehta, JL. Endothelial, platelet and leukocyte interactions in ischemic heart disease: insights into potential mechanisms and their clinical relevance. J Am Coll Cardiol 1990; 16:207–22.

9. Vane JR, Anggard EE, Botting RM. Regulatory functions of the vascular endothelium. N Engl J Med 1990; 323:27–36.
10. Ludmer, PL, Selwyn AP, Shook TL, Wayne RR, Mudge GH, Alexander RW, Ganz P. Paradoxical vasoconstriction induced by acetylcholine in atherosclerotic coronary arteries. N Engl J Med 1986; 315:1046–51.
11. Ross R, Wight TN, Standness, E, Thiele B. Human atherosclerosis – cell constitution and characteristics of advanced lesions of the superficial femoral artery. Am J Pathol 1984; 114:79–93.
12. Clowes AW, Schwartz SM. Significance of quiescent smooth muscle migration in the injured rat carotid artery. Circulation Res 1985; 56:139–45.
13. Mitchinson MJ, Ball RY. Macrophages and atherogenesis. Lancet 1987:146–48.
14. Jonasson L, Holm J, Skalli O, Bondjers G, Hansson GK. Regional accumulations of T cells, macrophages, and smooth muscle cells in the human atherosclerotic plaque. Arteriosclerosis 1986; 6:131–38.
15. Tan EML, Uitto J. Pathology of the extracellular matrix in atherosclerosis: in vivo and in vitro models. In: White RA, ed. Atherosclerosis and arteriosclerosis: human pathology and experimental animal methods and models. Boca Raton, FL., CRC Press, 1989:87–110
16. Wight TN. Cell Biology of arterial proteglycans. Arteriosclerosis 1989; 9:1–20.
17. Bocan TMA, Schifani TA, Guyton, JR. Ultrastructure of the human aortic fibrolipid lesion. Am J Pathol 1986; 123:413–24.
18. Lundberg B. Chemical composition and physical state of lipid deposits in atherosclerosis. Atherosclerosis 1985; 56:93–110.
19. Saner HE, Gobel FL, Salomonowitz E, Erlien DA, Edwards JE. The disease-free wall in coronary atherosclerosis: its relation to degree of obstruction. Am J Cardiol 1985; 6:1096–99.
20. Glagov S, Weisenberg E, Zarins CK, Stankunavicius R, Kolettis GJ. Compensatory enlargement of human atherosclerotic coronary arteries. N Engl J Med 1987; 316:1371–5.
21. Isner JM, Donaldson RF, Fortin AH, Tischler A, Clarke RH. Attenuation of the media of coronary arteries in advanced atherosclerosis. Am J Cardiol 1986; 58:937–9.
22. Barger AC, Beeuwkes III R, Lainey LL, Silverman KJ. Hypothesis: vasa vasorum and neovascularization of human coronary arteries. N Engl J Med 1984; 310:175–7.
23. Ross R, Glomset JA. The pathogenesis of atherosclerosis (second of two parts). N Engl J Med 1976; 295:420–5.
24. Grondin CM, Dyrda I, Pasternac A, Campeau L, Bourassa MG, Lesperance J. Discrepancies between cineangiographic disease and regent myocardial revascularization. Circulation 1974; 49:703–8.
25. Schwartz JN, Kong Y, Hackel DB, Barthel AG. Comparison of angiographic and postmortem findings in patients with coronary artery disease. Am J Cardiol 1975; 36:174–8.
26. Stiel GM, Stiel LSG, Schofer J, Donath K, Mathey DG. Impact of compensatory enlargement of atherosclerotic coronary arteries on angiographic assessment of coronary artery disease. Circulation 1989; 80:1603–9.
27. Roberts WC, Virmani R. Quantification of coronary arterial narrowing in clinically-isolated unstable angina pectoris. Am J Med 1979; 67:792–9.

28. Kragel AH, Reddy SG, Wittes, JT, Roberts WC. Morphometric analysis of the composition of coronary arterial plaques in isolated unstable angina pectoris with pain at rest. Am J Cardiol 1990; 66:562–7.
29. Davies MJ. A macro and micro view of coronary vascular insult in ischemic heart disease. Circulation 1990; 82:38–46 (Suppl II).
30. Little WC, Constantinescu M, Applegate RJ, Kutcher MA, Burrows MT, Kahl FR, Santamore WP. Can coronary angiography predict the site of a subsequent myocardial infarction in patients with mild-to-moderate coronary artery disease? Circulation 1988; 78:1157–66.
31. Benson RL. The present status of coronary arterial disease. Arch Path 1926; 2:876–916.
32. Constantinides P. Plaque fissures in human coronary thrombosis. J Athero Res 1966; 6:1–17.
33. Erhardt LR, Lundman T, Mellstedt H. Incorporation of 125 I-labelled fibrinogen into coronary arterial thrombi in acute myocardial infarction in man. Lancet 1973; 24;1(800):387–90.
34. DeWood MA, Spores J, Notske R, Mouser LT, Burroughs R, Golden MA, Lang HT. Prevalence of total coronary occlusion during the early hours of transmitral myocardial infarction. N Engl J Med 1980; 303:897–902.
35. Davies MJ. Successful and unsuccessful coronary thrombolysis. Br Heart J 1989; 61:381–4.
36. Davies MJ, Thomas AC: Plaque fissuring—the cause of acute myocardial infarction, sudden ischaemic death, and crescendo angina. Br Heart J 1985; 53:363–73.
37. Davies MJ, Thomas A. Thrombosis and acute coronary-artery lesions in sudden cardiac ischemic death. N Engl J Med 1984; 310:1137–40.
38. Falk E. Unstable angina with fatal outcome: dynamic coronary thrombosis leading to infarction and/or sudden death. Circulation 1985; 71:699–708.
39. Farb A, Virmani R, Atkinson JB, Kolodgie FD. Plaque morphology and pathologic changes in arteries from patients dying after coronary balloon angioplasty. J Am Coll Cardiol 1990; 16:1421–9.
40. Frink RJ, Rooney PA, Trowbridge JO, Rose JP. Coronary thrombosis and platelet/fibrin microemboli in death associated with acute myocardial infarction. Br Heart J 1988; 59:196–200.
41. Davies MJ, Thomas AC, Knapman PA, Hangartner JR. Intramyocardial platelet aggregation in patients with unstable angina suffering sudden ischemic cardiac death. Circulation 1986; 73:418–27.
42. Richardson PD, Davies MJ, Born GVR. Influence of plaque configuration and stress distribution on fissuring of coronary atherosclerotic plaques. Lancet 1989; 941–44.
43. Nishimura RA, Edwards WD, Warnes CA, Reeder GS, Holmes DR, Tajik AJ, Yock PG. Intravascular ultrasound imaging: in vitro validation and pathologic correlation. J Am Coll Cardiol 1990; 16:145–54.
44. Lee RT, Grodzinsky AJ, Frank EH, Kamm RD, Schoen FJ. Structure-dependent dynamic mechanical behavior of fibrous caps from human atherosclerotic plaques. Circulation 1991; 83:1764–70.

2

Triggering and Circadian Variation in the Onset of Unstable Angina

Francine K. Welty and James E. Muller

Harvard Medical School and New England Deaconess Hospital
Boston, Massachusetts

INTRODUCTION

Unstable angina is more likely to occur from 6 a.m. to noon than at other times of the day (1,2) (Fig. 1), as are the related conditions of chronic stable angina, myocardial infarction, and sudden cardiac death (3). Although the onset of unstable angina has not yet been fully investigated, this morning increase suggests that its mechanism is related to the mechanism of onset of the much more extensively studied disorders of myocardial infarction and the transient ischemic episodes that occur in patients with chronic stable angina.

In considering the timing of unstable angina, it is necessary to distinguish between onset of the disorder and the occurrence of individual episodes of transient ischemia once the disorder has begun. In many patients, particularly those with preexistent chronic stable angina, it is impossible to identify an exact moment of onset of unstable angina, but in others, the time and circumstances of the *initial* onset can be determined. Identification of the timing of subsequent episodes is much less difficult, but the pattern may then be altered by the routines of hospitalization and various medications.

With this distinction in mind, it is useful to compare onset of unstable angina with onset of myocardial infarction. First, both conditions are in most cases caused by plaque rupture and subsequent thrombus formation.

Second, although unstable angina is generally associated with a nonocclusive coronary artery thrombus and infarction with an occlusive thrombus, approx-

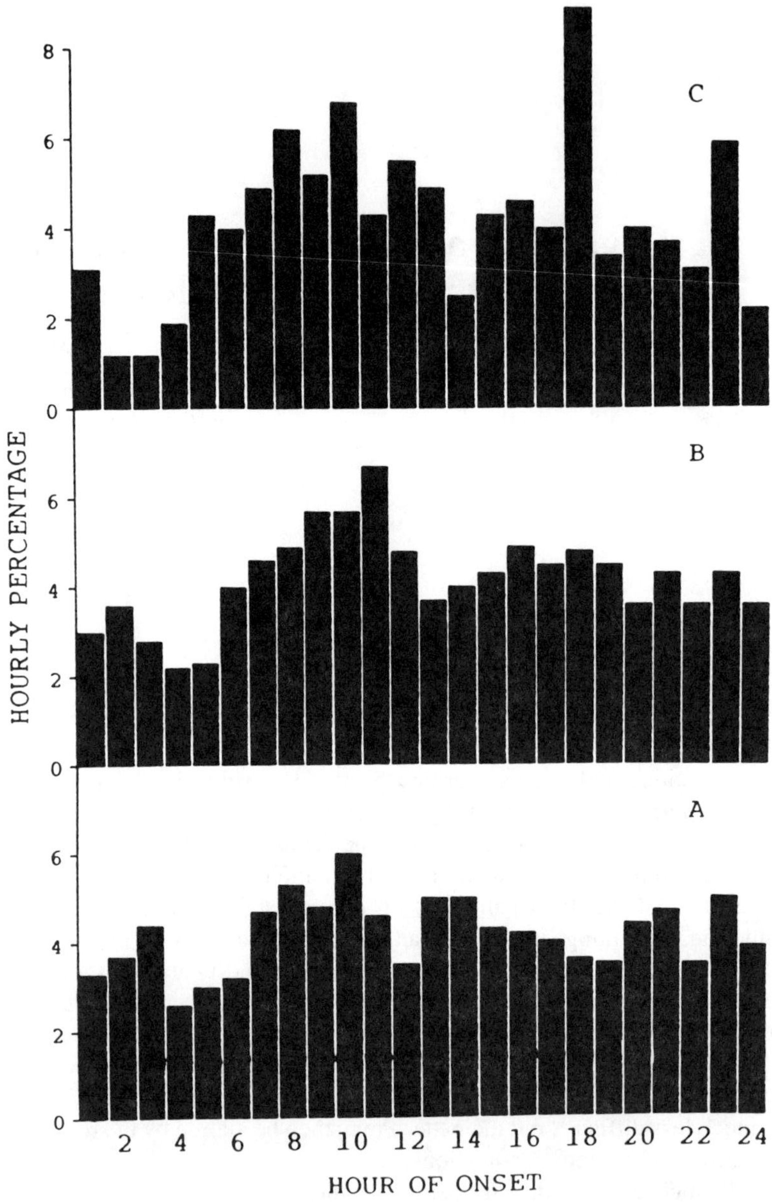

Figure 1 Time of onset of myocardial ischemia due to chronic stable angina, unstable angina, and myocardial infarction. All three conditions show a prominent increase in frequency of onset from 6 a.m. to noon. (Reprinted with permission from Ref. 1.)

imately 20% of cases of unstable angina are caused by the occurrence of an occlusive thrombus in an artery to myocardium well supplied by collateral vessels (4). In these cases the mechanism of onset of unstable angina is likely to be identical to that of myocardial infarction.

Third, as many as one third of cases of myocardial infarction have premonitory symptoms of unstable angina retrospectively identified. Patients prospectively identified with unstable angina progress to infarction in approximately 10% of cases (5).

There are also links between episodes of angina occurring after the onset of unstable angina and those occurring in patients with chronic stable angina. For example, the increases in heart rate and arterial pressure that make the transient myocardial ischemia of stable angina more frequent in the morning may also make unstable angina worse. It is likely, however, that in unstable angina, primary decreases in oxygen supply play a more important role than increases in demand since the thrombus present may grow to produce primary occlusion or produce vasoconstrictor substances.

Given these important interrelationships, it is apparent that much can be learned about onset and subsequent episodes of unstable angina from a review of the rapidly accumulating information about onset of myocardial infarction and the transient ischemia of chronic stable angina.

EPIDEMIOLOGIC EVIDENCE OF THE INCREASED MORNING ONSET OF MYOCARDIAL INFARCTION

Numerous epidemiologic studies now provide undisputed evidence that myocardial infarction is more likely to begin in the morning than at other times of the day. Results from both the MILIS study (6) and from the Intravenous Streptokinase in Acute Myocardial Infarction (ISAM) study (7) demonstrate that myocardial infarction is three times more likely to occur in the morning than in the late evening. The time of first appearance of creatine kinase in plasma was the basis for the determination of the onset of myocardial infarction in both studies. Prior studies using onset of pain as a determination of time of myocardial infarction onset also demonstrated a circadian variation with a peak in the morning; however, these studies were criticized since the morning increase was thought to result from delayed reporting of a myocardial infarction that began while the patient was asleep during the night.

Gilpin et al. reported the pattern of onset of infarction in a study of 4796 patients (8). In the overall population, there was a primary morning peak of onset of infarction and a smaller secondary evening peak. However, subgroup analysis indicated that patients with congestive heart failure or a non-Q myocardial infarction have a primary evening peak. Two relatively equal peaks of onset of infarction were found in smokers, diabetics, women, elderly patients, and those

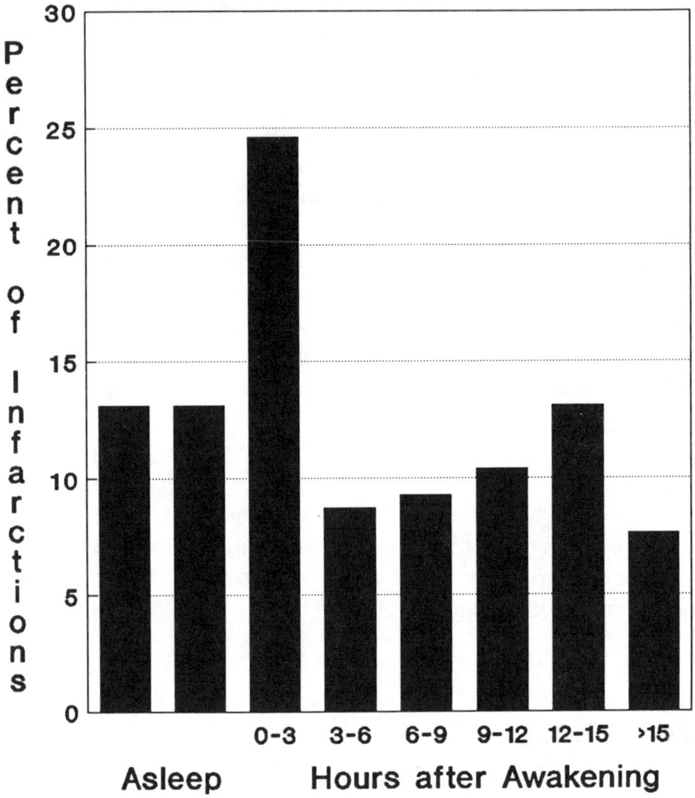

Figure 2 Distribution of the percent of myocardial infarctions occurring while asleep and in successive 3-hour intervals for infarcts with onset after awakening. The frequency of onset is doubled in the first 3 hours after awakening. (From Ref. 10.)

taking beta-blockers. It is interesting to note that in the MILIS and ISAM studies, beta-blockers also attenuated the morning peak of onset of myocardial infarction (6,7).

These early epidemiologic studies have now been extended by more detailed studies in which the wake-time of the patients has been taken into account. In each of the four "wake-time adjusted studies" that have been reported, the authors encountered the remarkably similar finding that the frequency of onset of myocardial infarction is approximately doubled within the first 4 hours after awakening (9–12) (Figs. 2 and 3). Narrowing of the risk period to this interval should facilitate studies of the processes responsible for this increase in the risk of occlusive coronary thrombosis.

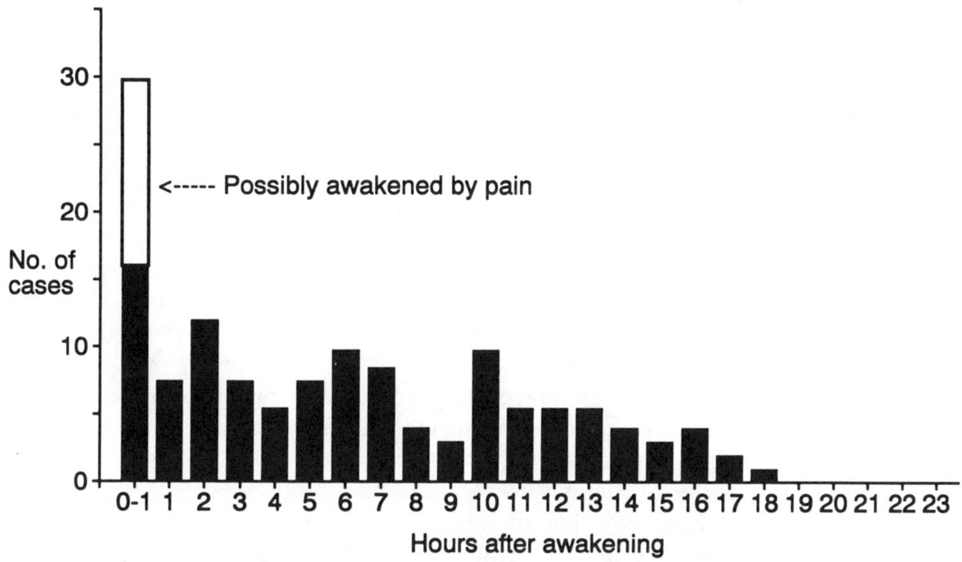

Figure 3 Time of onset of initial symptoms of acute myocardial infarction after awakening. Fifteen of the cases in which symptoms began less than or equal to 1 hour after awakening were possibly awakened by pain. When these cases are excluded, the frequency of onset during the first hour is approximately twice that during subsequent hours. (From Ref. 9.)

Sudden cardiac death, which is often caused by occlusive coronary thrombosis, has also been found to have a circadian pattern with a peak incidence in the morning (13,14). Willich has presented data from a review of the mortality records of the Massachusetts population and the Framingham Heart Study population that indicate that sudden cardiac death occurs with a circadian pattern similar to that of nonfatal infarction with an increase between 6 and 9 a.m. (15). Previous autopsy studies have revealed that one third of the cases of sudden cardiac death are caused by an occlusive coronary thrombus. Stroke, a third condition often resulting from occlusive arterial thrombosis, also has a circadian variation with a similar morning increase (16,17).

TRIGGERING AS THE CAUSE OF THE MORNING INCREASE IN ONSET OF CORONARY THROMBOSIS

From their studies of the clinical features of acute myocardial infarction, Obraztsov and Strazhesko concluded in 1910 that activities frequently triggered infarction onset and presented evidence of onset of infarct after climbing a steep staircase or after a heated card game (18). Their view was challenged during the 1930s as subsequent studies of large numbers of patients failed to reveal obvious precipitating causes of myocardial infarction. Arguments for (19,20) and against (21,22) triggers of infarction were advanced. The controversy subsided in 1960 when Master, with the use of retrospective questionnaires, reported that activities are of little importance in triggering onset of myocardial infarction (23).

The recent documentation of an increase in the onset of infarction in the morning (24) has renewed study of the possibility of triggers of myocardial infarction. Sumiyoshi et al. reported on activities before onset of myocardial infarction of 416 patients admitted to the National Heart Center of Japan from 1977 to 1985 (25). Fifty-three percent of patients without prior angina reported that their infarction began during moderate to heavy exertion, emotional stress, or excitation. Recently, our group has analyzed possible triggers of myocardial infarction as part of the Multicenter Investigation of the Limitation of Infarct Size (MILIS). Forty-eight percent of the patients reported a possible trigger (26), similar to that reported by Sumiyoshi et al. (25). Anecdotal cases relate the onset of infarction with snow shoveling, extreme exertion, and emotional stress (27).

The greatest difficulty in identifying triggers of myocardial infarction and unstable angina arises not from the reports of the activities preceding the infarction but from the collection of the appropriate control data. To obtain control data, Sumiyoshi et al. collected information on the frequency of emotional and physical stress during the month one year prior to the infarction and compared this with the frequency of stress in the month immediately before the infarction. Fifty-eight percent of the patients reported stress during the month prior to the infarction as compared to 34% who reported stress during the control period; however, biased recall and the ability to accurately remember events of 13 months previously are two major problems in interpretation of their results. To collect more meaningful control data, Maclure has proposed that a case-crossover design be utilized in which each patient serves as his or her own control for relatively recent activities (28). This method is being used in an investigation funded by the National Heart, Lung and Blood Institute entitled "Determinants of the Onset of Myocardial Infarction." More than 2000 patients with acute myocardial infarction will be interviewed in an attempt to characterize external triggers of myocardial infarction.

Morning Increase in Physiological Processes That Might Trigger Myocardial Infarction

The underlying cause of most cases of myocardial infarction is a ruptured coronary atherosclerotic plaque. There are a number of systemic physiologic processes that could cause rupture of a vulnerable plaque. The accentuation of these processes following arising could contribute to the morning increase in myocardial infarction onset through a variety of mechanisms.

The morning arterial pressure surge (29) could cause plaque rupture. The increase in coronary arterial tone could worsen the flow reduction produced by a fixed stenosis (30). The elevation of serum cortisol levels above basal levels (even though they are falling compared to the rest of the day) (31) could enhance the sensitivity of the coronary arteries to the vasoconstrictor effects of catecholamines (32), which have a prominent surge after assumption of the upright posture (33). This arterial tone increase, coupled with the morning arterial pressure increase, could lead to increased shear stress (force directed against the endothelium resulting from increased coronary blood flow velocity) (34), predisposing to plaque rupture and increased platelet deposition (35).

Quyyumi et al. have provided support for the contribution of coronary tone to the provocation of ischemia in the morning compared to the afternoon (36). The exercise time to development of 1 mm ST segment depression in patients with stable angina is shorter in the morning than in the afternoon and is associated with an increase in systemic vascular resistance in the morning compared to the afternoon. Hendels et al. (37) used exercise stress testing to study patients with stable angina off their anti-ischemic medications and showed that the time to development of ST segment depression or angina was shortest in the morning compared to other times of the day. Yasue et al. (38) performed exercise stress testing on patients with variant angina and found that they were able to exercise longer in the afternoon and were more likely to develop ST elevation and symptoms in the morning compared to the afternoon. Other studies that have shown no diurnal variation in ischemia generally studied patients while they were taking their antianginal medications.

The increase in blood viscosity (39), the increased platelet aggregability (40) resulting from assumption of the upright posture (33), and a decrease in fibrinolytic activity (41–43) could all produce a state of relative hypercoagulability. Such a thrombotic tendency could increase the likelihood that an otherwise harmless mural thrombus overlying a small plaque fissure would propagate and occlude the coronary lumen.

If the morning arterial pressure surge alone were the dominant factor causing plaque rupture and occlusive thrombus formation, more cases of myocardial infarction during exercise stress testing would be expected, since such tests are frequently performed by individuals with advanced coronary artery disease and associated with major hemodynamic changes. Systolic arterial pressure increases by as much as 100 mmHg during exercise testing, and the double product generally exceeds that observed during the morning arterial pressure surge. However, the incidence of myocardial infarction complicating symptom-limited exercise stress testing is only in the range of 13 per 100,000 (44). This very low incidence could be due to a low likelihood that a plaque vulnerable to rupture is present. Alternatively, the process could be interrupted after plaque rupture by the absence of occlusive thrombus formation due to the increase in fibrinolytic activity with exercise.

The degree to which a 24-hour periodicity of disease onset results from a true, endogenous circadian rhythm versus the daily rest-activity cycle is not fully characterized. Cortisol secretion, for example, is well known to be an endogenous circadian process not dependent on daily activity (31). In contrast, if subjects remain at bed rest (40), the morning increase in platelet aggregability is abolished. Adjustment for time of awakening shows that infarction onset (9) and increases in transient ischemia (1,2) follow awakening, implicating the rest-activity cycle as a major determinant of disease onset. However, the contribution of an endogenous rhythm is not eliminated because adjustment of data for time of awakening also aligns the population for their endogenous circadian rhythms. There may also be an interaction between circadian and rest-activity cycles. For example, assumption of the upright posture leading to sympathetic activation may be more likely to cause significant vasoconstriction when endogenously controlled cortisol levels are high (32).

Although the incidence of onset of myocardial infarction peaks in the morning 2 to 3 hours after awaking, similar physiologic processes probably trigger disease onset throughout the day. The peak morning incidence of infarct onset probably results from the synchronization of the population for triggers in the morning. Synchronization of the population for an additional trigger, such as the evening meal, may be responsible for the secondary evening peak of infarct onset observed in the MILIS data. Exposure of the population to potential triggers is random for the remainder of the day, and no other prominent peaks of incidence are observed.

Circadian (24-hour) cycles are not the only cycles that may provide clues to triggering of disease onset. Giaconi et al. have reported an annual increase in systemic arterial pressure during the winter months (45) during which mortality from ischemic heart disease is also increased (46–48). Thus, the winter increase in arterial pressure and ischemic heart disease onset appears to have a parallel relationship to the morning increase in arterial pressure and disease onset. Other parallel relationships are likely to be identified as this line of research is pursued.

There may also be unusual mechanisms of disease onset occurring in only a minority of the population, such as postural hypotension, which has been suggested as a trigger of stroke onset, causing decreased cerebral perfusion (49). Other possible triggering changes are those associated with acute infectious diseases (50).

Triggers of Onset of Transient Myocardial Ischemia

Myocardial infarction, sudden cardiac death, and stroke are relatively infrequent cardiovascular events compared to the transient ischemic episodes of stable angina. Beamer et al. (1) noted that the transient ischemia of stable angina, like that of unstable angina, is also increased in frequency in the morning with a relative risk of 1.32. The pathophysiology of transient ischemia (as assessed by Holter) is probably more closely related to that of subsequent episodes of unstable angina than to myocardial infarction or sudden cardiac death. The increases in heart rate and blood pressure that make the ischemia of stable angina more frequent in the morning may also make unstable angina episodes worse. With the use of ambulatory Holter monitoring, it has been possible to determine the timing of episodes of transient ischemia with great certainty and eliminate bias resulting from unobserved periods. Since the individual episodes of transient ischemia that follow onset of unstable angina are likely to share mechanisms with the transient ischemic episodes of chronic stable angina, review of the studies of ischemia of chronic angina can serve as a basis for inferences about triggers and pathophysiology of episodes of unstable angina.

Holter monitoring of transient myocardial ischemia of chronic stable angina has demonstrated that the frequency of episodes peaks between 6 a.m. and 12 noon (51–53). By adjusting the timing of episodes for wake-time, Rocco et al. were able to demonstrate that the increase in frequency occurs during the first four hours after awakening (51), a finding similar to that for myocardial infarction (9–12). Rocco used diaries to document the association of possible triggers with transient myocardial ischemia (54). Mental stress was frequently found to be associated with ischemia, as was heavy exercise. Bairey et al. have provided evidence documenting the association of mental stress with myocardial ischemia (55). The effect of mental stress on blood pressure and left ventricular dysfunction as assessed by radionuclide ventriculography was studied in 29 patients with exercise-induced ischemia. Peak systolic arterial pressure was frequently higher during mental stress than during exercise. Seventy-five percent of the patients experienced left ventricular wall motion abnormalities during mental stress.

Mental stress induced LV dysfunction has also been demonstrated using ambulatory radionuclide monitoring (56), a nuclear probe (57), and echocardiography (58). Deanfield et al. used Rubidium-82 uptake during positron emission tomography to show that simply smoking one cigarette causes a decrease in ^{82}Rb uptake at lower levels of myocardial oxygen demand (as measured by heart rate and blood pressure response) than that required to induce ischemia with exercise (59). Therefore, transient ischemic episodes can be triggered by activities that cause coronary vasoconstriction in addition to increases in heart rate and/or systemic arterial pressure (60). The high frequency of triggering of ischemia by mental stress or physical activity is of prime importance, whether it be mediated by an increase in myocardial oxygen demand or a decrease in supply. Further study of triggers of transient myocardial ischemia of stable angina may lead to improved means of prevention of transient ischemia and facilitate efforts to prevent unstable angina, myocardial infarction, and sudden death.

CAUSES AND CONSEQUENCES OF RUPTURE OF AN ATHEROSCLEROTIC PLAQUE

The common denominator linking onset of unstable angina, myocardial infarction, and sudden cardiac death caused by coronary thrombosis is a ruptured atherosclerotic plaque. Since the pioneering work of Constantinides, it is known that a plaque with a fissure underlies the thrombi occluding the vessels (61,62).

Controversy exists over the two major ways in which plaque rupture could occur: rupture of the lumen into the plaque or rupture of the plaque into the lumen. The plaque wall might rupture first due to mechanical stresses from the lumen, and the subsequent exposure of collagen could lead to activation of the coagulation system and platelet aggregation leading to occlusive thrombus formation. Alternatively, the initiating event could be a hemorrhage into the plaque from the vasa vasorum within the plaque (63). Such a hemorrhage could then, possibly by causing an increase in pressure and/or volume inside the plaque, lead to rupture of the plaque wall at a weak area. The resulting exposure of collagen would lead to activation of the coagulation system and platelet aggregation, also leading to occlusive thrombus formation.

Until recently, there was debate as to whether the coronary arteries had significant vasa vasorum, but cinemicrographic studies have now demonstrated extensive neovascularization of intramural coronary atherosclerotic plaques (64). Microsphere studies have shown a fivefold increase in blood flow in the area supplying the plaque compared to the normal media (65). For many years it was thought that coronary luminal pressure was greater than that in the vasa vasorum, thus, causing compression of these small vessels with limited blood flow. However, Heistad and Armstrong have shown that in atherosclerotic monkeys, the vasa vasorum are open and have rapid flow (66). It is possible that the pressure in the vasa may be transmitted from a portion of the vessel proximal to the stenosis and therefore be greater than the pressure in the lumen distal to a significant stenosis. Under such conditions, the morning increase in sympathetic activity and arterial pressure may cause these fragile vessels to rupture leading to a fissure in the plaque. This has been postulated to account in part for the cirdadian variation in myocardial infarction.

The histologic information currently available suggests that rupture from the lumen into the plaque is the more common cause of plaque rupture, but more studies are needed to elucidate the pathologic basis of acute disease onset.

Animal studies have revealed that fissures can be produced in rabbit arteries with advanced atherosclerosis (but not in arteries with early atherosclerosis or in normal vessels) by a sudden surge in blood pressure (induced by an infusion of epinephrine) associated with synergistic endothelial damage and hypercoagulability (created by infusion of Russel viper venom) (67). These fissures resulted in hemorrhage and subsequent thrombus formation thereby sealing the crack. It is not known whether fissures and resulting thrombi in human coronary plaques are caused by surges in blood pressure and/or hypercoagulability alone or whether other factors leading to structural weakening of the atherosclerotic plaque surface or fibrous cap could lead to fracture of the plaque. Changes in the cellular population of the plaque, necrosis, or changes in the collagen structure could all conceivably lead to weakening of the cap of the plaque.

Autopsy studies of accident and suicide victims have revealed the presence of plaque rupture unassociated with clinical symptoms (68). Although it is impossible to be certain that these ruptures occurred before death, it appears likely that plaque rupture can be sealed by thin nonocclusive mural thrombi and can occur without clinical symptoms. This event, although asymptomatic, may lead to an increase in the size and remodeling of the plaque until near occlusive thrombi do form, leading to unstable angina.

MODELS OF PLAQUE RUPTURE

Richardson et al. (69) developed a computer model to examine the distribution of stress in simulated plaques during systole. To obtain direct evidence about plaque fissure, they examined plaques at autopsy in patients who died of coronary thrombosis. Of the 85 patients in whom the type of lesion or site of fissure could be ascertained, 83% had a pool of extracellular lipid in the intima associated with a fissure. Of these, 86% had an eccentric lipid pool and 63% had ruptured at the junction of the plaque cap with the adjoining normal intima. The remaining 37% had a rupture through the center of the cap. There were lipid-filled foam cells at the fissure site in 67% of the cases with lateral tears and 86% of the cases with a fissure through the center of the fibrous cap. Seventeen percent of the 85 plaques had developed a fissure but did not contain a lipid pool. A superficial tear separated a layer of intima from underlying fibrous tissue in 13%. In the remaining few patients, the plaques had torn at the junction of fibrous tissue with calcium within the intima. Therefore, these results indicate that fissuring occurs most often in plaques with eccentric lipid pools and is located at the junction of the lipid pool with the normal intima.

Computer modeling showed that the area of greatest stress is on the plaque cap near the junction with the normal adjacent intima. The majority of fissures occurred at the location of foam cells between collagen strands, suggesting that the intimal layer could be weakened by the presence of foam cells themselves or by enzymatic degradation of connective tissue matrix. It is of note that Constantinides had also noted the infiltration of fissured plaque caps by foam cells (61). Richardson et al. (69) also demonstrated that intimal tears occurred in plaques without an intimal lipid pool, but in these cases, large intraintimal thrombi were not present, presumably due to the absence of a potential space for the thrombus to occupy. These fissures were thought to be less important clinically. Calcified plaques did not appear to fissure as frequently as fibrous plaques.

In morphometric studies of the infarct artery of patients who died after their first myocardial infarction, Gertz and Roberts (70) showed that the atherosclerotic plaques at sites of rupture consisted of approximately 32% pultaceous debris, whereas plaques not associated with rupture contained approximately 5% pultaceous debris. The areas with more extensive pultaceous debris had a correspondingly thinner residuum of fibrous tissue between the pultaceous debris and the arterial lumen. It was postulated that these areas would be more likely to rupture with an increase in shear force than areas with less debris and a thicker fibrous cap.

ABILITY OF AGENTS THAT BLOCK POTENTIAL TRIGGERING PROCESSES TO PREVENT MYOCARDIAL INFARCTION

The efficacy of aspirin therapy and beta-adrenergic blockade in preventing myocardial infarction (71,72) provides indirect support for the theories advanced here. Aspirin is thought to reduce the occurrence of sudden death and myocardial infarction by acting as an antiplatelet agent and preventing coronary thrombosis. Aspirin reduced the overall incidence of myocardial infarction by 44% in the Physician's Health Study (71). However, it was most effective in the morning hours (when platelet activity is increased) during which the aspirin-treated physicians experienced a 59% reduction in myocardial infarction (10). This prevention of infarction by reduction of the platelet activity surge—a potential triggering mechanism—supports the assertion that platelet activity surges are harmful and suggests that increased basal platelet activity may be an unrecognized risk factor for infarction.

Beta blockade eliminated the morning peak of myocardial infarction in both the MILIS and ISAM databases. In the Beta Blocker Heart Attack Trial, 38% of the sudden deaths in the placebo group occurred between 5 a.m. and 11 a.m. compared to only 24% of the deaths in patients treated with propranolol (73). This suggests that the beneficial effect was achieved by blockage of the surge in sympathetic activity in the morning (74). Beta blockade, but not a short-acting calcium blocker, has been shown to decrease the morning surge in silent myocardial ischemia (75). A recent review has summarized the inability of calcium channel-blocking agents to provide a cardioprotective effect (76). The mechanism for prevention of infarction and sudden cardiac death by beta blockade is unknown. It has been suggested that beta-blockers may prevent rupture of atherosclerotic plaques, just as they prevent rupture of the aortic wall in dissecting aortic aneurysm. Other postulated mechanisms include prevention of arrhythmia, cardiac rupture, and effects on sympathetic surges.

THE EFFECT OF LIPIDS ON TRIGGERING MECHANISMS

Brown et al. have shown that a marked decrease in LDL-cholesterol and increase in HDL-cholesterol induced by drug treatment is associated with a decrease in the incidence of clinical events (revascularization for worsening ischemic symptoms, myocardial infarction, and death) despite only a minimal decrease in angiographically measured coronary stenosis (77). Possibly, the decrease in LDL and increase in HDL may have reduced the vulnerability of plaques to rupture by decreasing their lipid content. In addition, the favorable lipid changes may have caused a decrease in platelet aggregability that decreased the tendency for thrombus formation.

An association between lipid levels and the hemostatic system has been appreciated for some time. In 1970, Epstein et al. demonstrated an impaired response of fibrinolytic activity to exercise in patients with type IV hyperlipidemia (78). Carvalho et al. (79) in 1974 demonstrated that the platelets in patients with type II hyperlipidemia undergo aggregation at 1/25 the concentration of epinephrine and 1/3 the concentration of collagen and ADP compared to individuals with normal lipid levels, i.e., they exhibit platelet hyperaggregability.

Shattil et al. (80) in 1975 noted that when the membrane cholesterol content of cholesterol-dipalmitoyl-lecithin liposomes was increased 39%, there was a 35-fold increase in epinephrine-induced platelet aggregation and a 15-fold increase in ADP-induced platelet aggregation. When the membrane cholesterol was decreased 21.4% compared to baseline, there was an 18-fold decrease in epinephrine-induced aggregation. In 1983, Simpson et al. (81) showed that fibrinolytic activity was lower in patients with type IV hyperlipidemia than in subjects with normal lipid levels. Type IV patients also had higher fibrinogen and factor X levels. In 1989, Loscalzo et al. (82) reported that tissue plasminogen activator (t-PA) levels in hypercholesterolemic subjects are twice those of normal subjects. In addition, plasma levels of plasminogen activator inhibitor (PAI) were higher than normal subjects. They suggested that thrombotic tendencies in hypercholesterolemic disorders may be related to abnormal endothelial elaboration of t-PA and PAI. Recently, Richards et al. (83) have shown a difference in the activity of t-PA produced by cultured endothelial cells depending on the type of fatty acids in the medium. The maximum rate of t-PA activity was increased by 22% and 48% with oleate- or linoleate-enriched U937 monocyte cells, respectively, and decreased by 22% with stearate-enriched cells as compared to unmodified monocytes. Thus, *unfavorable lipid content of the blood may* not only increase formation of atherosclerotic plaques, but may also *increase platelet aggregability and decrease the activity of the fibrinolytic system*. These lipid-induced changes in plaque content and hemostatic variables are likely to affect the mechanism of onset of acute cardiovascular disease.

GENERAL THEORY OF TRIGGERING OF CORONARY THROMBOSIS

Our group has proposed a general hypothesis of the manner in which daily activities might trigger coronary thrombosis (3) leading to onset of unstable angina, myocardial infarction, or ischemic sudden cardiac death. The hypothesis (Fig. 4) adds the concept of triggering activities to the general scheme of the role of thrombosis in the acute coronary syndromes advanced by Falk, Davies and Thomas, Fuster, Willerson, and others (84–86).

It is proposed that the initial step in the process leading directly to coronary thrombosis is the development, with advancing age, of what can be termed a vulnerable atherosclerotic plaque. Plaque vulnerability is defined functionally as the susceptibility of a plaque to rupture. Development of such vulnerability is a poorly understood process, but is presumably a dynamic, potentially reversible disorder caused by changes in the constituents of the plaque, its blood supply via vasa vasorum, and/or the functional integrity of the overlying endothelium.

The theory that onset of thrombosis is unrelated to daily activities would presumably attribute disease onset solely to changes in the plaque, and the

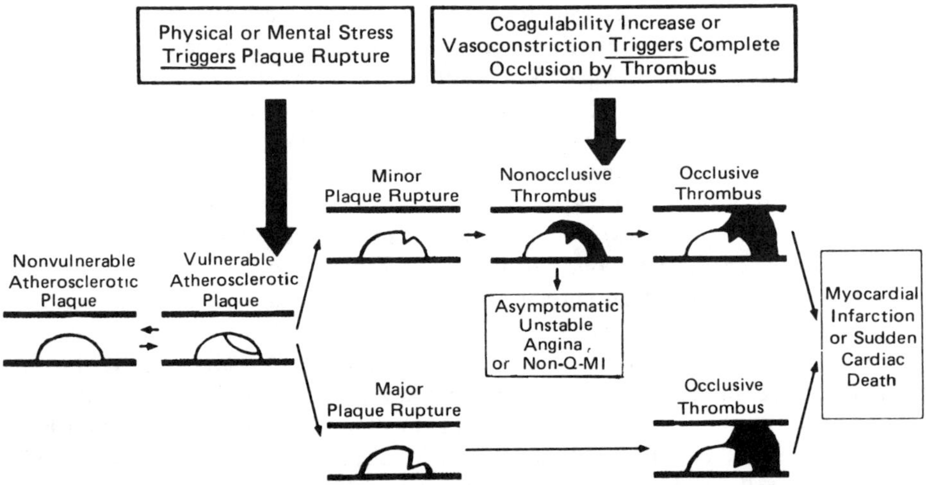

Figure 4 Triggering of coronary thrombosis. A hypothetical model by which daily activities may trigger coronary thrombosis. Three triggering mechanisms, (a) physical or mental stress producing hemodynamic changes leading to plaque rupture, (b) activities causing a coagulability increase, and (c) stimuli leading to vasoconstriction, have been added to the well-known scheme depicting the role of coronary thrombosis in unstable angina, myocardial infarction (MI), and sudden cardiac death. Non-Q = non-Q wave. (Adapted from Ref. 3.)

sequence would, therefore, lead directly from the plaque to occlusive coronary thrombosis without external modifiers. In the present formulation, however, it is proposed that onset might frequently begin when a physical or mental stress or change in lipid content of the blood triggers a hemodynamic change sufficient to rupture a vulnerable plaque. The rupture in the plaque may be major or minor, depending on factors such as the amount and type of collagen exposed (87). A major plaque rupture produces a thrombogenic focus sufficiently intense to cause occlusive coronary thrombosis leading directly to myocardial infarction or sudden cardiac death. A minor rupture leads only to a mural thrombus that fails to produce symptoms or leads to unstable angina or non–Q-wave myocardial infarction. Again, at this point external activities may lead to occlusion of the lumen. For example, a coagulability increase may trigger growth of the thrombus, or vasoconstriction may lead to complete occlusion of an already compromised lumen, leading to infarction or sudden death. Since normal individuals and even patients with coronary artery disease are constantly exposed to potentially triggering activities that do not produce coronary occlusive thrombosis, it seems likely that development of plaque vulnerability together with the conditions for occlusive thrombus formation are the rarest events in this chain of causation.

A clinical observation provides further support that the transition of a plaque to the vulnerable stage with occlusive thrombus formation is a rare event. When myocardial infarction occurs in individuals with double and triple vessel coronary artery disease, the acute event is almost always restricted to the distribution of a single vessel. This suggests that a local feature of the plaque renders it vulnerable to rupture while a systemic increase in coagulability might increase the likelihood that an occlusive thrombus would form.

It is likely that there is an inverse relation between the degree of plaque vulnerability and the intensity of the triggering stimulus required to produce rupture. For instance, an elderly patient with a severe fixed stenosis in a coronary artery and an extremely vulnerable plaque may develop thrombosis with only a minor stress, while a young patient with only a luminal irregularity might require a major stress (such as heavy lifting producing markedly increased arterial pressure) to trigger plaque rupture and coronary thrombosis. Sumiyoshi et al. (25) reported that younger patients were more likely than older patients to report unusual stress before onset, but control data on the relative frequency of unusual stress in older versus younger patients are not available.

Various mixtures of triggering mechanisms may account for thrombosis. For example, the combination of physical exertion (producing a minor plaque rupture) followed by cigarette smoking (producing an increase in coronary artery vasoconstriction and a relatively hypercoagulable state) may be needed to cause disease onset. Thus, the onset of coronary thrombosis, in some cases, may be the result of the unfortunate simultaneous occurrence of several events, each by itself of little consequence but catastrophic when occurring together. The onset of unstable angina with a nonocclusive thrombus can be viewed as a fortunate deviation from the onset of infarction—a deviation in which occlusive thrombus failed to form because of lack of a major stimulus to thrombus or a decreased coagulability of the blood.

SIGNIFICANCE

The primary immediate value of recognition of the circadian variation of onset of unstable angina is the emphasis that can be placed on pharmacologic protection during the morning hours for patients already receiving anti-ischemic and anti-hypertensive therapy. Although no scientific studies have been performed to test the hypothesis, it seems reasonable that long-acting anti-ischemic agents would have an advantage over short-acting agents in providing protection against onset of unstable angina in the morning when the effects of short-acting agents taken the night before may attenuate.

The finding that unstable angina appears to be triggered in the morning raises questions about the desirability of exercise in the morning. At present, the evidence that exercise is beneficial in reducing the risk of coronary artery disease is substantial (88), and although theoretical concerns can be raised, there is no compelling evidence that exercise in the morning is more hazardous than exercise at other times of the day.

Even complete elimination of the morning increase in onset of unstable angina by optimal timing of exercise (if needed) and effective therapy would prevent only a small fraction of the total morbidity and mortality caused by this disorder. Although the incidence of disease onset is greatest in the 6 a.m. to noon period, the majority of episodes of unstable angina (70%) occur at other times of the day, and their prevention requires a broader approach. For this reason, the primary significance of the recognition of circadian variation of disease onset is the support it provides for the broader concept that the onset of unstable angina at any time of the day is frequently triggered by activities of the patient. This concept provides a number of clues to the mechanisms of disease onset—clues that suggest the value of studies ranging from the epidemiologic to the molecular level.

At the basic science level, there is a need for complete characterization of the control mechanisms of potentially adverse and potentially beneficial physiologic changes. When these mechanisms are understood more fully, it may be possible to eliminate unnecessary and potentially detrimental surges in arterial pressure, vasoconstriction, and coagulability that contribute to disease onset and to increase the activity of potentially beneficial processes such as the fibrinolytic system. Further study is also needed of the factors determining plaque vulnerability, and of the possibility that reduction in clinical events achieved by marked lowering of plasma cholesterol (77) might result not only from reduction of the tendency toward coronary artery stenosis, but partially from a reduction in the formation of lipid pools within plaques that might increase the susceptibility of plaques to rupture (69).

A more complete understanding of triggering mechanisms should permit progress in the prevention of unstable angina. The means of prevention would not be elimination of potential triggering activities—an undesirable and unattainable goal—but the design of regimens that can be evaluated in randomized studies for their ability to sever the linkage between a potential triggering activity and development of unstable angina, as well as myocardial infarction and sudden cardiac death.

ACKNOWLEDGMENT

We are grateful for the assistance of Ms. Kathleen Carney in the preparation of the manuscript.

REFERENCES

1. Beamer AD, Lee TH, Cook EF, Brand DA, Rorian GW, Weisberg MC, Goldman L. Diagnostic implications for myocardial ischemia of the circadian variation of the onset of chest pain. Am J Cardiol 1987; 60:998–1001.
2. Behar S, Reicher-Reiss H, Goldbourt U, Koplinsky E and the Principal Investigators of SPRINT, Israel. Circadian variation in pain onset in unstable angina pectoris. Am J Cardiol 1991; 67:91–3.
3. Muller JE, Tofler GH, Stone PH. Circadian variation and triggers of onset of acute cardiovascular disease. Circulation 1989; 79:733–43.
4. DeWood MA, Stifter WF, Simpson CS, et al. Coronary arteriographic findings soon after non-Q wave myocardial infarction. N Engl J Med 1986; 315–415.
5. Scheidt S, Wolk M, Killip T. Unstable angina pectoris. Natural history, hemodynamics, uncertainties of treatment and the ethics of clinical study. Am J Med 1976; 60d(3):409–17.
6. Muller JE, Stone PH, Turi ZG, Rutherford JD, Czeisler CA, Parker C, Poole, WK, Passamani E, Roberts R, Robertson T, Sobel BE, Willerson JT, Braunwald E, and the MILIS Study Group. Circadian variation in the frequency of onset of acute myocardial infarction. N Engl J Med 1985; 313:1315–22.
7. Willich SN, Linderer T, Wegscheider K, Leizorovicz MD, Alamercery I, Schroder R, and the ISAM Study Group. Increased morning incidence of myocardial infarction in the ISAM Study: absence with prior beta-adrenergic blockade. Circulation 1989; 80:853–8.
8. Gilpin EA, Hjalmarson A, Ross JR Jr. Subgroups of patients with atypical circadian patterns of symptom onset in acute myocardial infarction. Am J Cardiol 1990; 66(Suppl):7G–11G.
9. Goldberg R, Brady P, Muller J, Chen Z, deGroot M, Zonneveld P, Dalen J. Time of onset of symptoms of acute myocardial infarction. Am J Cardiol 1990; 66:140–4.

10. Ridker PM, Manson JE, Buring JE, et al. Circadian variation of acute myocardial infarction and the effect of low-dose aspirin in a randomized trial of physicians. Circulation 1990; 82:897–902.
11. Maclure M, Sherwood JB, Andrade S, Goldberg RJ, Tofler GH, Muller JE. Increased risk of myocardial infarction onset within the two hours after awakening (abstract). Circulation 1990; 82(Suppl III):III–281.
12. Willich SN, Loewel H, Lewis M, Arntz R, Loewe A, Schroeder R, and the TRIMM Study Group. Two-fold risk of acute myocardial infarction in three hours following awakening (abstract). Circulation 1990; 82(Suppl III):III–281.
13. Muller JE, Ludmer PL, Willich SN, et al. Circadian variation in the frequency of sudden cardiac death. Circulation 1987; 75:131–8.
14. Willich SN, Levy D, Rocco MB, Tofler GH, Stone PH, Muller JE. Circadian variation in the incidence of sudden cardiac death in the Framingham Heart Study Population. Am J Cardiol 1987; 60:801–6.
15. Willich SN. Epidemiologic studies demonstrating increased morning incidence of sudden cardiac death. Am J Cardiol 1990; 66(Suppl):15G–17G.
16. Tsementizis SA, Gill JS, Hitchcock ER, Gill SK, Beevers DG. Diurnal variation of and activity during the onset of stroke. Neurosurgery 1985; 17:901–4.
17. Marler JR, Price TR, Clark GL, Muller JE, Robertson T, Mohr JP, Hier DB, Wolf PA, Caplan LR, Foulkes MA. Morning increase in onset of ischemic stroke. Stroke 1989; 20:473–6.
18. Obraztsov VP, Strazhesko ND. The symptomatology and diagnosis of coronary thrombosis. Vorobeva VA, Konchalovski MP, eds. Works of the First Congress of Russian Therapists. Comradeship Typography of A. E. Mamontov, 1910; 26–43.
19. Fitzhugh G, Hamilton BE. Coronary occlusion and fatal angina pectoris. Study of the immediate causes and their prevention. JAMA 1933; 100:475–80.
20. Sproul J. A general practitioner's views on the treatment of angina pectoris. N Engl J Med 1936; 215:443–52.
21. Parkinson J, Bedford DE. Cardiac infarction and coronary thrombosis. Lancet 1928; (1):4–11.
22. Phipps C. Contributory causes of coronary thrombosis. JAMA 1936; 106:761–2.
23. Master AM. The role of effort and occupation (including physicians) in coronary occlusion. JAMA 1960; 174:942–8.
24. Muller JE, Stone PH, Turi ZG, Rutherford JD, Czeisler CA, Parker C, Poole WK, Passamani E, Roberts R, Robertson T, Sobel BE, Willerson JT, Braunwald E, and the MILIS Study Group. Circadian variation in the frequency of onset of acute myocardial infarction. N Engl J Med 1985; 313:1315–22.
25. Sumiyoshi T, Haze K, Saito M, Fukami K, Goto Y, Hiramori K. Evaluation of clinical factors involved in onset of myocardial infarction. Japanese Circulation Journal 1986; 50:164–73.
26. Tofler GH, Stone PH, Maclure M, Edelman E, Davis VG, Robertson T, Antman EM, Muller JE, and the MILIS Study Group. Analysis of possible triggers of acute myocardial infarction (MILIS Study). Am J Cardiol 1990; 66:22–7.
27. Muller, JE, Tofler GH, Edelman E. Probable triggers of onset of acute myocardial infarction. Clinical Cardiology 1989; 12:473.

28. Maclure M. The case-crossover design: a method for studying transient effects on the risk of acute events. Am J Epidemiol (submitted 1990).
29. Millar-Craig MW, Bishop CN, Raftery EB. Circadian variation of blood pressure. The Lancet 1978; (1):795–7.
30. Fujita M, Franklin D. Diurnal changes in coronary blood flow in conscious dogs. Circulation 1987; 76:488–91.
31. Weitzman ED, Fukushima D, Nogeire C, Roffwarg H, Gallagher TF, Hellman L. Twenty-four hour pattern of the episodic secretion of cortisol in normal subjects. J Clin Endocr 1971; 33:14–22.
32. Sudhir K, Jennings GL, Esler MD, Korner PI, Blombery PA, Lambert GW, Scoggins B, Whitworth JA. Hydrocortisone-induced hypertension in humans: pressor responsiveness and sympathetic function. Hypertension 1989; 13:416–21.
33. Brezinski DA, Tofler GH, Muller JE, Pohjola-Sintonen S, Willich SN, Schafer AI, Czeisler CA, Williams GH. Morning increase in platelet aggregability: association with assumption of the upright posture. Circulation 1988; 78:35–40.
34. Vita JA, Treasure CB, Ganz P, Cox DA, Fish RD, Selwyn AP. Control of shear stress in the epicardial coronary arteries of humans: impairment by atherosclerosis. JACC 1989; 14:1193–9.
35. Badimon L, Badimon JJ. Mechanisms of arterial thrombosis in nonparallel streamlines: platelet thrombi grow on the apex of stenotic severely injured vessel wall: experimental study in pig model. J Clin Invest 1989; 4:1134–44.
36. Quyyumi AA, Panza JA, Lakatos E, Epstein SE. Circadian variation in ischemic events: causal role of variation in ischemic threshold due to changes in vascular resistance (abstract). Circulation 1988; 78(Suppl II):331.
37. Henkels U, Blumchen G, Ebner F. Zur problematick von Belastungsprüfungen in Abhängigkeit von der Tageszeit bei Patienten mit Koronarinsuffizienz. Herz Kreisal 1977; 9:343–7.
38. Yasue H, Omote S, Takizawa A, Nagao M, Miwa K, Tanaka S. Circadian variation of exercise capacity in patients with Prinzmetal's variant angina: role of exercise-induced coronary arterial spasm. Circulation 1979; 59:938–48.
39. Ehrly AM, Jung G. Circadian rhythm of human blood viscosity. Biorheology 1973; 10:577–83.
40. Tofler GH, Brezinski DA, Schafer AI, Czeisler CA, Rutherford JD, Willich SN, Gleason RE, Williams GH, Muller JE. Concurrent morning increase in platelet aggregability and the risk of myocardial infarction and sudden cardiac death. N Engl J Med 1987; 316:1514–8.
41. Rosing DR, Brakman P, Redwood DR, Goldstein RE, Beiser GD, Astrup T, Epstein SE. Blood fibrinolytic activity in man: diurnal variation and the response to varying intensities of exercise. Circ Res 1970; 27:171–84.
42. Andreotti F, Davies GJ, Hackett DR, Kahn MI, De Bart ACW, Aber VR, Maseri A, Kluft C. Major circadian fluctuations in fibrinolytic factors and possible relevance to time of onset of myocardial infarction, sudden cardiac death and stroke. Am J Cardiol 1988; 62:635–7.
43. Speiser W, Langer W, Pschaick A, Selmayr E, Ibe B, Nowacki PE, Muller-Berghaus G. Increased blood fibrinolytic activity after physical exercise: com-

parative study in individuals with different sporting activities and in patients after myocardial infarction taking part in a rehabilitation sports program. Thrombosis Research 1988; 51:543–55.
44. Rochmis P, Blackburn H. Exercise tests. A survey of procedures, safety and litigation experience in approximately 170,000 tests. JAMA 1971; 217:1061–9.
45. Giaconi S, Ghione S, Palombo C, Genovesi-Ebert A, Marabotti C, Fommei E, Donato L. Seasonal influences on blood pressure in high normal to mild hypertensive range. Hypertension 1989; 14:22–7.
46. Bull GM. Meteorological correlates with myocardial and cerebral infarction and respiratory disease. Br J Prev Soc Med 1973; 27:108–13.
47. Rose G. Cold weather and ischaemic heart disease. Br J Prev Soc Med 1966; 20:97–100.
48. Ornato JP, Siegel L, Craren EJ, Nelson N. Increased incidence of cardiac death attributed to acute myocardial infarction during winter. Coronary Artery Disease 1990; 1:199–203.
49. Dobkin BH. Orthostatic hypotension as a risk factor for symptomatic occlusive cerebrovascular disease. Neurology (in press).
50. Spodick DH, Flessas AP, Johnson MM. Association of acute respiratory symptoms with onset of acute myocardial infarction: prospective investigation of 150 consecutive patients and matched control patients. Am J Cardiol 1984; 53:481–2.
51. Rocco MB, Barry J, Campbell S, Nabel E, Cook EF, Goldman L, Selwyn AP. Circadian variation of transient myocardial ischemia in patients with coronary artery disease. Circulation 1987; 75:395–400.
52. Selwyn AP, Shea M, Deanfield JE, Wilson R, Horlock P. Character of transient ischemia in angina pectoris. Am J Cardiol 1986; 58:21B–25B.
53. Nademanee K, Intarachot V, Josephson MA, Singh BN. Circadian variation in occurrence of transient overt and silent myocardial ischemia in chronic stable angina and comparison with Prinzmetal's angina in men. Am J Cardiol 1987; 60:494–8.
54. Rocco MB. Timing and triggers of transient myocardial ischemia. Am J Cardiol 1990; 66(Suppl):18G-21G.
55. Bairey CN, Krantz DS, Rozanski A. Mental stress as an acute trigger of ischemic left ventricular dysfunction and blood pressure elevation in coronary artery disease. Am J Cardiol 1990; 66(Suppl):28G–31G
56. Breisblatt WW, Weiland FL, McLain JR, Tomlinson GC, Burns MJ, Spaccavento LJ. Usefulness of ambulatory radionuclude monitoring of left ventricular function early after acute myocardial infarction for predicting residual myocardial ischemia. Am J Cardiol 1988; 62:1005–10.
57. LaVeau PJ, Rozanski A, Krantz D, Cornell CE, Cattanach L, Zaret BL, Wackers FJT. Transient left ventricular dysfunction during provocative mental stress in patients with coronary artery disease. Am Heart J 1989; 118:1–8.
58. Gottdiener JS, Krantz DS, McGee A, Oleshansky M, Myerhoff J, Raisen SE, Rozanski A. Echocardiographic assessment of mental stress-induced wall motion abnormalities: comparison with exercise (abstr). J Am Coll Cardiol 1989; 13:158A.
59. Deanfield JE, Shea MJ, Wilson RA, Horlock P, deLandsheere CM, Selwyn AP. Direct effects of smoking on the heart: silent ischemic disturbances of coronary flow. Am J Cardiol 1986; 57:1005–9.

60. Barry J, Selwyn AP, Nabel EG, Rocco MB, Mead K, Campbell S, Rebecca G. Frequency of ST-segment depression produced by mental stress in stable angina pectoris from coronary artery disease. Am J Cardiol 1988; 61:989–93.
61. Constantinides P. Plaque fissure in human coronary thrombosis. J Atheroscler Res 1966; 1:1–17.
62. Constantinides P. Cause of thrombosis in human atherosclerotic arteries. Am J Cardiol 1990; 66(Suppl):37G–40G.
63. Paterson JC. Capillary rupture with intimal hemorrhage as a causative factor in coronary thrombosis. Arch Pathol 1938; 25:474–9.
64. Barger AC, Beeuwkes R III, Lainey LL, Silverman KJ. Hypothesis: vasa vasorum and neovascularization of human coronary arteries. A possible role in the pathophysiology of atherosclerosis. N Engl J Med 1984; 310:175–7.
65. Barger AJ, Beeuwkes R III. Rupture of coronary vasa vasorum as a trigger of acute myocardial infarction. Am J Cardiol 1990; 66:41G–43G.
66. Heistad DD, Armstrong ML. Blood flow through vasa vasorum of coronary arteries in atherosclerotic monkeys. Arteriosclerosis 1989; 6:325–31.
67. Constantinides P. In: Proceedings of Conference on Comparative Atherosclerosis: Los Angeles, January 1964, Chapter 29. New York: Hoeber Publ., 1965.
68. Davies MJ, Thomas AC. Plaque fissuring—the cause of acute myocardial infarction, sudden ischemic death, and crescendo angina. Br Heart J 1985; 53:363–73.
69. Richardson PD, Davies MJ, Born GVR. Influence of plaque configuration and stress distribution on fissuring of coronary atherosclerotic plaques. Lancet 1989; 2:941–4.
70. Gertz SD, Roberts WC. Hemodynamic shear force in rupture of coronary arterial atherosclerotic plaques. Amer J Cardiol 1990; 66:1368–72.
71. The Steering Committee of the Physicians' Health Study Research Group. Final report on the aspirin component of the ongoing Physicians' Health Study. N Engl J Med 1989; 321:129–35.
72. Beta-blocker Heart Attack Trial Research Group. A randomized trial of propanolol in patients with acute myocardial infarction. Mortality results. JAMA 1982; 247:1707–14.
73. Peters RW, Muller JE, Goldstein S, Byington R, Friedman LM for the BHAT Study Group. Propranolol and the morning increase in the frequency of sudden cardiac death (BHAT Study). Am J Cardiol 1989; 63:1518–20.
74. Peters RW, Muller JE, Goldstein S, Byington R, Friedman LM. Propanolol and the circadian variation in the frequency of sudden cardiac death: the BHAT experience (abstract). Circulation 1988; 76(Suppl IV):364.
75. Mulcahy D, Keegan J, Cunningham D, Quyyumi A, Crear P, Park A, Wright C, Fox K. Circadian variation of total ischemic burden and its alteration with anti-anginal agents. Lancet 1988; (2):755–9.
76. Held Ph, Yusuf S, Furberg CD. Calcium channel blockers in acute myocardial infarction and unstable angina: an overview. Br Med J 1989; 299:1187–92.
77. Brown B, Albers JJ, Fisher LD, Schaefer SM, Lin J-T, Kaplan C, Zhao X-Q, Bisson BD, Fitzpatrick VF, Dodge HT. Regression of coronary artery disease as a result of intensive lipid-lowering therapy in men with high levels of apolipoprotein B. N Engl J Med 1990; 323:1289–98.

78. Epstein SE, Rosing DR, Brakman P, Redwood DR, Astrup T. Impaired fibrinolytic response to exercise in patients with type IV hyperlipoproteinemia. Lancet 1970; 2:631–4.
79. Carvalho ACA, Colman RW, Less RS. Platelet function and hyperlipoproteinemia. N Engl J Med 1974; 290:434–8.
80. Shattil SJ, Anaya-Galiando R, Bennett J, Colman RW, Cooper I. Platelet hypersensitivity induced by cholesterol incorporation. J Clin Invest 1975; 55:636–43.
81. Simpson HCR, Mann JI, Meade TW, Chakrabarti R, Stirling Y, Wolf L. Hypertriglyceridemia and hypercoagulability. Lancet 1983; 1:786–92.
82. Mendelsohn ME, Creager MA, Gallagher SJ, Dzau VJ, Loscalzo J. Abnormal tissue plasminogen activator (t-PA) and plasminogen activator inhibitor (PAI) levels in asymptomatic hypercholesterolemic (H) subjects (abstract). Circulation 1989; 80(Suppl II):6.
83. Richards AL, Kuo PC, Weinfeld MS, George D, Loscalzo J. Membrane enrichment with selected fatty acids modulates cell surface binding and activity of tissue plasminogen activator (t-PA) (abstract). Circulation 1990; 82(Suppl III):36.
84. Falk E. Plaque rupture with severe pre-existing stenosis precipitating coronary thrombosis. Br Heart J 1983; 50:127–34.
85. Fuster V, Steele PM, Chesebro JH. Role of platelets and thrombosis in coronary atherosclerotic disease and sudden death. J Am Coll Cardiol 1985; 5(Suppl):175B–184B.
86. Willerson JT, Campbell WB, Winniford MD, Schmitz J, Apprill P, Firth BG, Ashton J, Smitherman T, Bush L, Buja LM. Conversion from chronic to acute coronary artery disease: speculation regarding mechanisms. (Editorial) Am J Cardiol 1984; 54:1349–54.
87. Badimon L, Badimon JJ, Galvez A, Chesebro JH, Fuster V. Influence of arterial damage and wall shear rate on platelet deposition: ex vivo study in a swine model. Arteriosclerosis 1986; 6:312–20.
88. Morris JN, Everitt MG, Pollard R, Chave SPW. Vigorous exercise in leisure time: protection against coronary heart disease. Lancet 1980; 2:1207–10.

3

Angiographic Morphology of Unstable Plaque

John A. Ambrose

Mount Sinai Hospital
New York, New York

Craig E. Hjemdahl-Monsen

New York Medical College/Westchester County Medical Center
Valhalla, New York

INTRODUCTION

The clinical syndrome of unstable angina is recognized by the new onset of low workload or rest angina or by a dramatic change in the frequency or severity of preexistent angina. While the clinical presentations are rather characteristic, the angiographic findings in terms of disease severity and extent are similar to stable angina. However, subtle, qualitative differences in the angiographic appearance of lesions can be demonstrated in patients with unstable angina.

Pathologic data have shown evidence of plaque disruption or fissuring with variable amounts of superimposed thrombus in the majority of patients with the acute coronary syndromes of unstable angina, myocardial infarction, and sudden death. This "unstable" plaque appears to play a crucial role in the pathophysiology of these syndromes. Activated platelets at the site of disruption that release vasoconstrictor substances and fibrin formation may intermittently decrease perfusion or permanently occlude the coronary lumen. In this chapter, we review qualitative angiographic studies that have demonstrated a specific morphology in all of these syndromes. This morphology is likely the angiographic representation of the disrupted atherosclerotic plaque with superimposed thrombus formation.

EXTENT OF ANGIOGRAPHIC DISEASE IN UNSTABLE ANGINA

Early studies evaluating the extent and severity of coronary artery disease in patients with unstable angina failed to demonstrate a significant difference from patients with stable angina (1,2). These studies found similarities in both the number of diseased vessels and in the severity of stenosis as measured by percent diameter reduction. There have been a number of observations regarding the distribution of disease in unstable angina. Among patients with unstable angina in one study (3), a high prevalence (25%) of left main stenosis was found. Other studies have indicated a wide range of patients (12–52%) in whom single vessel coronary artery disease was found (4,5). In most studies, a majority of patients had multivessel disease. Nonobstructive or normal coronary arteries have been found consistently in 10–15% of patients. Differences that have been found may be related to the population undergoing study. These differences are likely related to the group of patients being studied and not necessarily related to the underlying pathophysiology of unstable angina. For example, younger patients with unstable angina could be expected to have a higher prevalence of single vessel disease than elderly patients. Additionally, as unstable angina does not represent a homogeneous syndrome but includes patients with similar yet varied clinical presentations (6), it is not surprising that differences in coronary anatomy may be present between studies.

QUALITATIVE ANGIOGRAPHY

Numerous pathologic studies (7–11) helped to develop the concept of plaque disruption and thrombus formation as being central to the pathophysiologic basis of the acute coronary syndromes. Analysis of lesion morphology on coronary angiography has also been useful in proving this concept pre-mortem. Before discussing the angiographic studies that systematically looked at the qualitative or morphologic aspects of coronary artery disease in patients with unstable angina, we should elaborate on what is meant by qualitative angiography.

While percent diameter stenosis, percent area reduction, minimal luminal diameter or area, and number of diseased vessels have been used to quantify coronary artery disease severity, there are a multitude of other characteristics of atherosclerotic plaque that can be determined from the coronary angiogram. The length of the atherosclerotic plaque, its eccentricity, the smoothness of its borders, and the presence of lucencies proximal to, within, or distal to the plaque represent some of the aspects of coronary stenoses that were not commonly considered in early angiographic studies of unstable angina. The aspects of qualitative angiography that are most important are derived from analysis of the lesion edges silhouetted by the contrast agent. Some of these chracteristics can be measured in much the same way as percent stenosis. There are other parameters that are more difficult to directly measure and are therefore subject to observer variation and interpretation. It is the less than quantitative nature of many of these parameters that lead us to talk about qualitative angiography. These qualitative aspects of the coronary plaque make up what is considered as the coronary morphology. As coronary morphology requires analysis of the entire contour of the lesion, total occlusions cannot be characterized.

The angiographic requirements necessary for qualitative assessment of coronary morphology parallel those of quantitative angiography. State-of-the-art imaging chains capable of high resolution are necessary to distinguish the subtle edge details often required for proper analysis of morphology. Because edge details are frequently seen in only one projection, multiple projections are usually required to ensure proper assessment of morphologic properties. In order to see the lesions edges clearly, lesions must be imaged in a plane orthogonal to the long axis of the lesion to avoid foreshortening of the lesion. Also, views that avoid vessel overlap are necessary. The coronary must also be adequately filled with contrast to avoid potential artefacts that may occur due to streaming of dye and other factors. Finally, coronary angiograms often must be projected at four- to fivefold magnification to enable appropriate visualization of the coronary morphologic features. From a practical standpoint, this involves projecting the angiograms on a separate screen to enable adequate magnification.

ANGIOGRAPHIC STUDIES

Unstable Angina

A description of the lesion borders represents a major component of morphologic or qualitative analysis. The first methodical analysis of coronary morphology was performed on a group of 110 consecutive patients undergoing coronary angiography (12). The patients were determined to have either stable or unstable angina by history. The coronary angiograms were reviewed by observers blinded to the history of the patient. Significant lesions ($\geq$50% and $<$100% diameter stenosis) were then classified according to their qualitative appearance. The classification scheme (Fig. 1) used to specify the morphology was as follows:

1. Concentric stenosis: a symmetric narrowing of a coronary artery. The borders of the lesion are smooth or only slightly irregular.
2. Eccentric stenosis: an asymmetric narrowing of a coronary artery. Two subgroups are noted:
   a. Type I: an asymmetric stenosis with smooth borders and a broad neck.
   b. Type II: an asymmetric stenosis usually in the form of a convex intraluminal obstruction with a narrow base or neck due to one or more overhanging edges or borders that are irregular or scalloped.

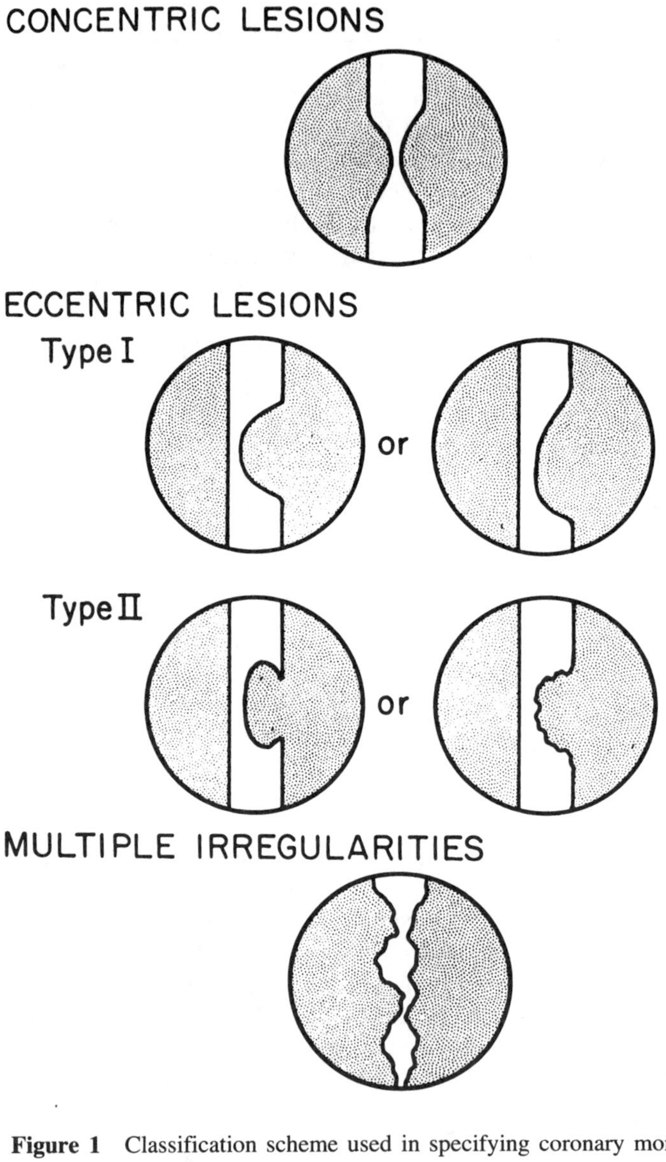

Figure 1 Classification scheme used in specifying coronary morphology. (From Ref. 12.)

3. Multiple irregularities: three or more closely spaced, serial, and severe (≥70% diameter stenosis) lesions in a coronary artery. This includes arteries with severe diffuse irregularities or arteries in which the segment of a coronary artery between two severe obstructions also exhibit significant diffuse luminal irregularities.

Of all lesions ≥50% and <100% narrowed, there were 54% Type II eccentric lesions in those patients with unstable angina and only 7% of these lesions in patients with stable symptoms. If only the artery responsible for the ischemic symptoms was considered, that is, the "angina-producing artery," 71% of arteries were found to show the Type II eccentric morphology in patients with unstable symptoms compared to 16% in patients with stable symptoms. The significant difference in patients with stable versus unstable angina represented a specific morphology that could be identified with the clinical syndrome and was found in the majority of patients.

To appreciate the significance of this specific coronary morphology, one must refer to the post-mortem angiographic study of Levin and Fallon (13). These investigators studied patients dying of myocardial infarction or post–bypass surgery. They correlated the post-mortem angiograms of patients to the pathologic findings. They determined that stenoses with irregular borders on angiogram often demonstrated plaque rupture or partially occlusive thrombi upon histologic examination. The lesions with irregular borders appear similar to the Type II lesions of patients with unstable angina. It was therefore not unreasonable for Ambrose et al. (12) to propose that the Type II eccentric lesions might be the angiographic representation of a disrupted atheroslcerotic plaque with superimposed thrombus. These angiographic-pathologic correlations have also been confirmed by Onodera et al. (14), who found irregular narrowing and filling defects on the coronary angiograms of patients following thrombolysis. Rupture and hemorrhage of the atherosclerotic plaque were found on post-mortem examination.

Observations by other investigators have corroborated the findings of a specific coronary morphology in patients with unstable angina (15,16). The classification schemes and designation of the coronary morphology were somewhat different, however, the "T" lesions described by Haft et al. (15) and the complex lesions described by Williams et al. (16) represent a similar qualitative appearance of the atherosclerotic plaque that is a specific finding in patients with unstable angina.

The Type II eccentric lesions may have an overhanging edge which results in a common shape, sometimes giving the appearance of a "cresting wave" (Fig. 2). Another common feature to Type II eccentric lesions is that of sharp angulation of the lesions (Fig. 3). This is in contrast to the smooth borders of obstructive lesions that are found in stable patients or in the non–ischemia-producing arteries of patients with unstable angina.

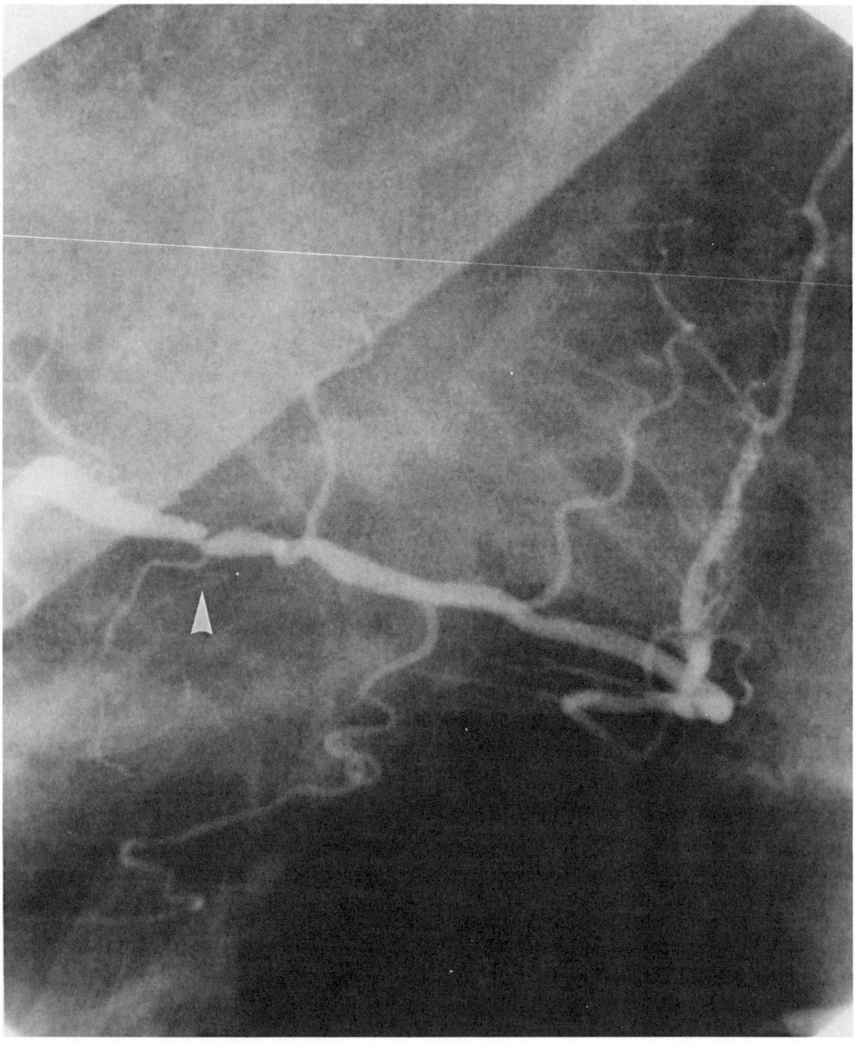

Figure 2 Complex right coronary artery stenosis (arrow) with an overhanging edge that gives the appearance of a "cresting wave."

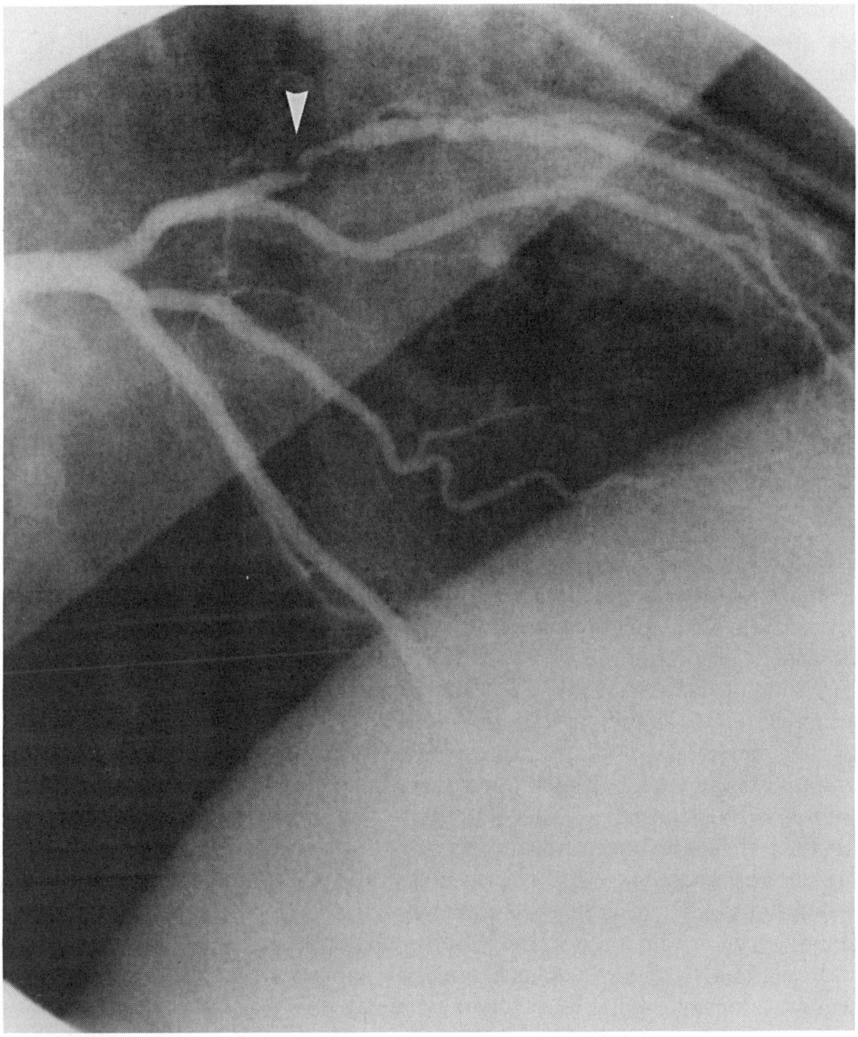

Figure 3 Complex circumflex artery stenosis (arrow) that is eccentric with rather sharp angulations to the margins of the lesion.

Since the initial description of coronary morphology by Ambrose et al. (12), there have been several refinements to the classification scheme. Pathologic studies have found that most obstructive coronary stenoses are eccentrically located. The morphology of the lesion responsible for unstable angina is also most often eccentric. However, in some cases a concentric narrowing on angiography manifests other findings consistent with a disrupted plaque such as scalloped or irregular borders. These lesions are not common, but are considered to represent the same pathophysiologic process as the typical Type II eccentric lesion. We therefore now prefer to classify these concentric or eccentric irregular plaques as complex lesions and distinguish these from simple lesions (smooth concentric or eccentric lesions).

Intracoronary Thrombi

The importance of intracoronary thrombi as a component of the angiographic morphology of unstable plaque has been shown by several studies (17–21). Angiographically, intracoronary thrombi are intraluminal lucencies or filling defects proximal, within, or distal to a coronary stenosis (Fig. 4). The reported prevalence of intracoronary thrombi in patients with unstable coronary syndromes varies from 1 to 85%. The wide variation noted may be due to differences in the selection of patients and prior treatment of patients with antithrombotics and/or thrombolytic agents. If patients are studied within 24 hours of an episode of rest pain, the highest rate of intracoronary thrombi is noted. The definitions used for intraluminal thrombus also vary from study to study, explaining part of the wide variation in this finding. There is no standardized definition for an intracoronary thrombus when the "culprit" or angina-producing lesion is <100% occluded. This is the rule rather than the exception in patients with unstable angina, occurring in about 80–90% of cases. For our purposes, we consider an intracoronary thrombus as a radiolucent filling defect either proximal to or distal to a stenosis that is surrounded by contrast on at least three sides. Filling defects within a lesion are considered in terms of its coronary morphology. Using this definition, we have noted intraluminal filling defects to be more common after myocardial infarction than in patients with unstable angina. Their incidence in unstable angina is <20%. These defects can be seen with lesions that otherwise appear either simple or complex. While complex plaques undoubtedly contain intraluminal thrombus, the angiographic distinction between complex plaques and intraluminal filling defects as proposed should allow for standardization in describing angiographic findings in these syndromes.

Myocardial Infarction

Pathologic studies (9,10) in patients dying suddenly after a recent bout of unstable angina or myocardial infarction have found disruption of an

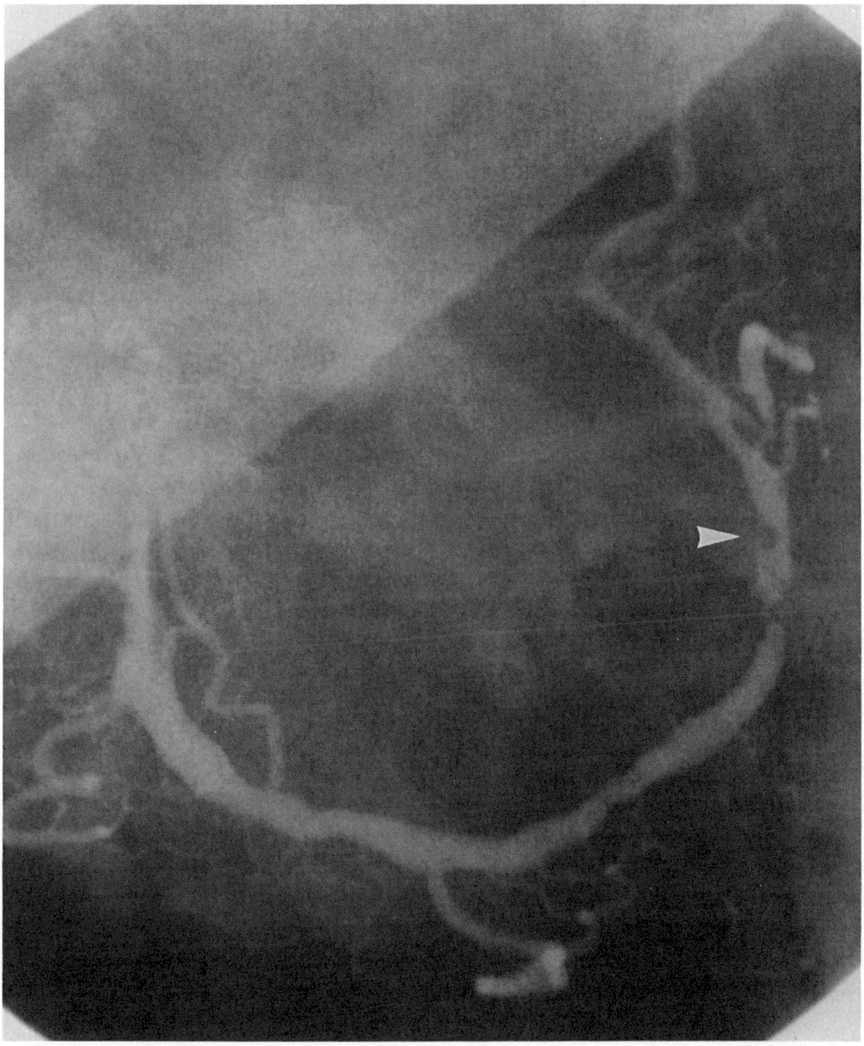

Figure 4 Distal right coronary artery stenosis with intraluminal filling defect (arrow) distal to the stenosis.

atherosclerotic plaque with superimposition of thrombus. Therefore, it was anticipated that the angiographic morphology found in patients with unstable angina might also be seen in patients with myocardial infarction and patent infarct-related arteries. This would serve to link the pathophysiology of unstable angina and myocardial infarction as well as add further credence to the notion that complex lesions represent the angiographic equivalent of a disrupted atherosclerotic plaque.

Angiographic features of myocardial infarction in the early hours following the onset of symptoms have demonstrated a high rate of total occlusion. The studies of DeWood et al. (22) showed 84% of patients with coronary occlusion if studied within 6 hours of symptoms. Further morphologic analysis of these lesions in the early hours post-myocardial infarction is therefore limited. If patients are given thrombolytic therapy or are studied several days following acute myocardial infarction, patency of the infarct vessel is often achieved. This represents dissolution of the occlusive thrombus. The obstruction that remains following exogenous or endogenous thrombolysis would be expected to disclose a similar complex morphology. Angiographic analysis was done for a group of 41 such patients with acute or recent (<3 months) infarction in whom the infarct-related artery was nontotally occluded allowing for a determination of coronary morphology. In this group of patients, in which some received intracoronary thrombolytic therapy with streptokinase, the Type II eccentric lesion was seen in 66% of infarct-related arteries but in only 11% of noninfarct vessels with obstructive lesions. Similar complex lesions were found in a study reported by Davies et al. (23) in patients with acute myocardial infarction who received streptokinase treatment. Additionally, these investigators found the degree of lesion complexity to be inversely related to the time following the infarction. Serial angiography following myocardial infarction in a subgroup of patients studied by these authors demonstrated a remodeling of the coronary plaque which resulted in a less complex lesion on the later angiogram. This suggests a dynamic nature to the morphology of the coronary lesion following thrombolysis. This change or remodeling may be due to further endogenous lysis of thrombus at the site of the complex plaque.

Non–Q Wave Infarction

Non–Q wave infarction represents a clinical syndrome whose pathophysiology lies somewhere between unstable angina and Q-wave myocardial infarction. While non-Q infarction is defined by the absence of Q waves on electrocardiogram following myocardial infarction, it does not necessarily imply nontransmural necrosis. The extent of myocardial necrosis in non-Q myocardial infarction, however, is usually less than in Q wave infarction. There are a number of factors that may modulate the size of an infarct and lead to a smaller infarct in non-Q infarction. These include the presence of recruitable collaterals, a transient period of occlusion followed by spontaneous lysis that limits the extent of necrosis, or a prolonged supply/demand imbalance in a patient with obstructive coronary disease that results in subendocardial necrosis.

While the number of diseased vessels is similar in patients with unstable angina, Q wave, and non–Q wave infarction (24), the frequency of total occlusion on angiography within hours or days of non-Q infarction is between that of unstable angina and Q wave infarction (24–26). The angiographic morphology of patients with patent infarct-related arteries studied after non-Q infarction shows a 65% prevalence of Type II eccentric (complex) lesions. This finding also supports the pathophysiologic mechanism that underlies all these acute coronary syndromes—that is, disruption of an atherosclerotic plaque with superimposed thrombus.

Sudden Death

There are few clinical data evaluating angiography in survivors of sudden cardiac death. However, pathologic data have shown disruption of an atherosclerotic plaque with superimposed thrombus in many of these patients (9,10). Electrical instability associated with a lethal arrhythmia is the suspected mode of death in most patients with sudden death. The substrate for the electrical instability may be related to prior infarction and left ventricular dysfunction in some patients. In others, death may be the first manifestation of coronary artery disease. In any event, coronary artery disease has been found in most survivors of sudden death (27). Patients with left ventricular dysfunction as the substrate for a lethal arrhythmia would be expected to have a persistent electrical instability following successful resuscitation. In patients in whom disruption of an atherosclerotic plaque plays a causal role, the electrical instability would not necessarily remain fixed.

Two studies (28,29) have compared the angiographic morphology of survivors of sudden death to the persistent electrical instability as assessed by programmed electrical stimulation. Stevenson et al. (28) found a complex lesion similar to the Type II eccentric lesion in 64% of sudden death survivors in whom ventricular tachycardia could not be induced by programmed stimulation, compared to finding complex morphology in only 25% of patients who were inducible. Lo et al. (29) found similar lesions in 50% of survivors without inducible arrhythmias compared to only a 19% prevalence in patients with inducible ventricular tachycardia. Thus, the angiographic morphology seen in the unstable coronary syndromes is also present in some patients with sudden death. Therefore, the unstable plaque may be related to the mechanism of electrical instability in these patients. Conceivably, sudden complete coronary occlusion or distal embolization of thrombotic debris with associated induction of fractionated electrical potentials may be a direct result of acute rupture of an atherosclerotic plaque.

UNSTABLE PLAQUE AND THE PROGRESSION OF CORONARY ARTERY DISEASE

One of the more interesting observations regarding the pathogenesis of acute coronary syndromes relates to how a plaque progresses; i.e., how coronary anatomy changes in patients with clinically silent or stable symptoms to become unstable anatomy. Much of the data addressing this issue comes from studies of selected patients in whom an angiogram was available both before and after the onset of the acute coronary syndrome. While angiography underestimates the degree of coronary narrowing when compared to pathologic examination, these angiographic studies indicate that many acute lesions in unstable angina and acute myocardial infarction originate from vessels that previously appeared to have insignificant lesions.

Angiographic Progression to Unstable Angina

Moise et al. (30) compared a group of such patients with unstable angina with a group of control patients with stable symptoms who had serial angiograms. Seventy-six percent of patients with a diagnosis of unstable angina had angiographically determined progression on the second angiogram compared to only 33% in the control stable angina patients. In 38% of unstable patients the progression to lesions that were obstructive occurred on previously "healthy" or nonobstructive segments. Similarly, Ambrose et al. (31) noted progression in the angiographic severity of 75% of patients with unstable angina in whom an angiogram prior to the onset of the unstable symptoms was available for review. In 72% of these patients, the lesion responsible for the unstable syndrome had less than a 50% diameter stenosis on the initial angiogram.

Angiographic Progression to Myocardial Infarction

Progression of plaque in patients with acute myocardial infarction shows a similar tendency to develop from a nonobstructive (<50%) lesion. In studies involving serial angiograms, Little et al. (32) found nonobstructive lesions in 66% of patients prior to myocardial infarction. Ambrose et al. (33) noted a similar progression from nonobstructive to obstructive disease in 48% of patients with myocardial infarction. Results of angiographic studies following successful thrombolysis also indicate that in about 15% of patients there appears to be a nonobstructive lesion. Brown et al. (34), by carefully examining the postthrombolysis angiograms of 32 patients following successful thrombolysis, could identify an underlying stenosis of <60% severity in 66% of patients. Hackett et al. (35) found 47% of patients with residual stenoses <60% in patients undergoing successful thrombolysis with their first myocardial infarction. Recently, Van Lierde et al. (36) quantitatively analyzed percent diameter narrowing 10–14 days following transmural myocardial infarction in patients with patent infarct-related arteries. Whether the patient received thrombolytic therapy or the infarct-related artery opened secondary to endogenous thrombolysis, the median diameter stenosis was 58%.

There are some studies, however, that refute the notion that myocardial infarction commonly occurs from plaques that are not severe (37–39). These studies found infarction to occur more commonly in lesions that previously had significant (>70%) obstruction. The development of a new total occlusion may in fact be more common in lesions that are more severe to start. However, progression from a severe stenosis to total occlusion may not necessarily be associated with clinical Q wave infarction but may be clinically silent or associated with unstable angina or a non–Q wave myocardial infarction. Ambrose et al. (33) compared a group of patients with myocardial infarction to a group of patients with new total occlusions without infarction who had a prior angiograms for review. The percent stenosis on the initial angiogram was 48% for the infarct group compared to 74% for the group with new total occlusions but without clinical infarction. Analysis of the infarct group also revealed differences between those patients with Q wave and non–Q wave infarction. The stenosis on initial angiography in patients with Q wave infarction averaged 34%, while patients with non–Q wave infarcts had an 80% stenosis seen on the initial angiogram. It may be that while there is a tendency of severe lesions to progress to total occlusion over time, the clinical significance of this progression may be less due to the likely development of collateral circulation to limit or prevent the infarct.

These retrospective observations of disease progression in selected patients with serial angiography have been confirmed in a prospective, randomized study of antiplatelet therapy at the Mayo Clinic (40). There were 283 patients comprising a low risk medically treated group that had two angiograms nearly 5 years apart. Repeat angiography showed 85% of lesions responsible for intervening myocardial infarctions originated from lesions less than 75% on the initial angiogram. Lesions initially >75% were more likely to progress to total occlusion, but were less likely to be associated with a clinical myocardial infarction.

ANGIOGRAPHIC MORPHOLOGY AND PROGNOSIS

The syndrome of unstable angina often portends further cardiac events in the short period following its onset. Unfortunately, there are few data regarding the prognostic importance of identifying a Type II eccentric or complex lesion in patients with or without unstable coronary syndromes. Since these lesions are seen in a high percentage of ischemia-producing arteries in patients with unstable angina, it is conceivable that they might be predictive of patients with a high likelihood of developing further clinical events. However, this has not yet been clearly demonstrated. A few studies have focused on how the angiographic morphology affects prognosis or response to treatment.

Angiograms of 118 patients in the CASS registry in patients that developed anterior myocardial infarction during the 3-year follow-up period were compared to a group of 141 control patients without infarction. Multivariate analysis of multiple angiographic features revealed percent stenosis and lesion roughness of the anterior descending artery to be highly predictive of the risk of developing anterior myocardial infarction (41). However, patients were not restudied after infarction. Therefore, the precise site of infarction could not be determined. In another study evaluating the response to medical therapy in a group of 69 patients with unstable angina, Sansa et al. (42) found that patients who failed to respond to medical therapy for unstable angina had a significantly higher prevalence of intracoronary thrombus and multiple and eccentric stenoses in the angina-producing arteries than those patients responsive to medical therapy. Patients who did respond to medical therapy had more frequently occluded angina-producing arteries. Freeman et al. (43) randomized a group of patients with unstable angina to either early or late elective angiography and evaluated the effect of complex morphology and intracoronary thrombus on the in-hospital cardiac event rate. Patients with coronary thrombus, complex lesion morphology, or multiple-vessel disease had more cardiac events including death, myocardial infarction, and need for urgent revascularization than the patients without those features.

"QUANTITATIVE" MEASURES OF ANGIOGRAPHIC MORPHOLOGY

The subjectivity of angiographic morphology probably represents the major limitation of this qualitative method of angiographic analysis. While reproducibility determinations by blinded observers can be demonstrated in some laboratories, classification of coronary lesions based on their morphology can be difficult particularly if angiographic images are technically inadequate. Also, despite the high specificity for the Type II eccentric or complex lesion in identifying unstable plaque, angiographic analysis may fail to accurately categorize a lesion as a ruptured plaque with superimposed thrombus. In a study by Sherman et al. (44) using angioscopy during coronary bypass surgery, intracoronary thrombus or complex plaque was seen in all patients with unstable angina and recent rest pain, while only 20% of these patients were correctly identified to have complex plaque or intraluminal thrombus by angiography.

Efforts to quantify lesion irregularity were first proposed by Wilson et al. (45). The degree of luminal irregularity by measurement of serial arterial diameters within a lesion was made in 25 patients with recent myocardial infarction or unstable angina and in 15 patients with chronic stable angina. While there were only small differences between groups with respect to percent stenosis measurements, there was a significant difference in the luminal irregularity in patients with recent infarction or unstable angina compared to patients with chronic stable angina. This "ulceration index" represented a quantitative means of assessing coronary morphology that was not subject to observer bias.

Perhaps the most ambitious attempt at quantifying coronary morphology has been developed by Kalbfleisch et al. (46). These investigators made use of a system of automated edge detection to delineate the borders of a coronary lesion by digitization of selected coronary angiographic images. From the borders of the lesion derived from the automated edge detection scheme, curvature and fractal analysis was performed. Five parameters were derived from this analysis that were felt to be associated with lesion complexity. When these parameters were applied to a group of patients with unstable angina and a control group with stable angina, four of the five parameters were found to be significantly different in the group with unstable angina. The results of this study have to be qualified, however, as there were differences in the two groups with respect to the severity of disease. In addition, while according to Kalbleisch et al. (46) the classification scheme of Ambrose et al. (12), failed to show a difference between the two groups, the reported sensitivity and specificity of this technique were similar to what we and others have reported using a purely qualitative approach. Nevertheless, a method to quantify lesion complexity free from inter- and intraobserver variability that is inherent in visual inspection of coronary lesions was developed.

Although quantitative methodologies remove some of the subjective nature to the determination of coronary morphology, no single quantitative parameter yet developed encompasses all of the factors that are considered in the visual determination of coronary morphology. For example, the automated quantitative technique just described considers each edge of a lesion independently. It therefore would be rather insensitive to eccentricity as a component of coronary morphology. Similarly, vessel borders must be continuous. Therefore, filling defects or other features, such as lucency, that result in discontinuities of the vessel borders cannot be directly measured. Finally, no quantitative technique can judge whether the lesion was analyzed using adequate angiographic projections.

OTHER ANGIOGRAPHIC FEATURES OF UNSTABLE PLAQUE

Another angiographic observation relating to the unstable plaque is represented by the way in which complex plaques undergo angioplasty. If the Type II eccentric plaque is the angiographic representation of a ruptured atherosclerotic plaque with superimposed thrombus, one might anticipate that this type of lesion would be softer than other lesions consisting mainly of fibrous tissue. Hjemdahl-

Monsen et al. (47) studied a group of 29 lesions in 27 patients in whom angioplasty was performed. The diameter of the balloon was measured during balloon inflation at various incremental pressures. The amount of dilation as reflected by the identation of the balloon was compared for Type II eccentric lesions and non–Type II eccentric lesions. There was a significant difference in the amount of dilation achieved at low inflation pressures in lesions with Type II eccentric lesions. This suggests that these lesions are more distensible. This may be due to the different nature of these lesions compared to non–Type II eccentric lesions. One possible explanation for this finding is that the lesions are softer owing to the presence of thrombus within the plaque. Another observation of this study was the presence of "elastic recoil" following angioplasty. Elastic recoil was defined as the ratio of the diameter of the angioplasty balloon, at the site of the lesion, at maximal inflation to the immediate postangioplasty lesion diameter. This represented the extent of apparent loss of lumen diameter immediately following dilation. While 3-mm balloons were used for all lesions, the extent of elastic recoil was found to be related to the diameter of the balloon at maximal inflation pressure, especially in patients with complex plaques. This may have been due to reversible stretching of the arc of "normal wall" that may be found in these plaques.

CONCLUSIONS

A specific angiographic morphology is found in patients with an unstable plaque. This finding can be demonstrated by qualitative assessment of the coronary angiogram. Correlation with pathologic studies would suggest that the eccentric irregular lesions seen in patients with the unstable plaque, whether from unstable angina, myocardial infarction, or sudden death, represent disruption of a preexisting atherosclerotic plaque with superimposed thrombus. Angiographic morphology may be important in understanding coronary artery disease progression. Lesion appearance may also be important in predicting future clinical events. While qualitative techniques of analysis are subject to inter- and intraobserver variation as all strictly visual methods are, attempts at quantifying the irregularities seen in these lesions may prove useful in the future.

REFERENCES

1. Alison HW, Russell RO Jr, Mantle JA, Kouchoukos NT, Moraski RE, Rackleu CE. Coronary anatomy and arteriography in patients with unstable angina pectoris. Am J Cardiol 1978; 41:204–9.
2. Fuster V, Frye RL, Connolly DC, Danielson MA, Elveback LR, Kurkland LT. Arteriographic patterns early in the onset of the coronary syndromes. Br Heart J 1975; 37:1250–5.

3. Plotnick GD, Greene HL, Carliner NH, Becker LC Fisher ML. Clinical indicators of left main coronary artery disease in unstable angina. Ann Intern Med 1979; 91:149–53.
4. Victor MF, Likoff MJ, Mintz GS, Likoff W. Unstable angina pectoris of new onset: a prospective clinical and arteriographic study of 75 patients. Am J Cardiol 1981; 47:228–32.
5. Conti CR, Brawley RK, Griffith LSC, Pitt B, Humphries JO, Gott VL, Ross RS. Unstable angina pectoris: morbidity and mortality on 57 consecutive patients evaluated angiographically. Am J Cardiol 1973; 32:745–50.
6. Braunwald E. Unstable angina. A classification. Circulation 1989; 80:410–4.
7. Blumgart HL, Schlesinger MJ, Davis D. Studies on relation of the clinical manifestations of angina pectoris, coronary thrombosis and myocardial infarction to the pathological findings. Am Heart J 1940; 19:1–91.
8. Constantinides P. Plaque fissures in human coronary thrombosis. J Atheroscler Res 1966; 6:1–17.
9. Davies MJ, Thomas AC. Thrombosis and acute coronary artery lesions in sudden cardiac ischaemic death. N Engl J Med 1984; 310:1137–40.
10. Falk E. Unstable angina with fatal outcome: dynamic coronary thrombosis leading to infarction and/or sudden death. Circulation 1985; 71:699–708.
11. Davies MJ, Thomas AC. Plaque fissuring—the cause of acute myocardial infarction, sudden ischaemic death, and crescendo angina. Br Heart J 1985; 53:363–73.
12. Ambrose JA, Winters SL, Stern A, Eng A, Teichholz LE, Gorlin R, Fuster V. Angiographic morphology and the pathogenesis of unstable angina pectoris. J Am Coll Cardiol 1985; 5:609–16.
13. Levin DC, Fallon JT. Significance of the angiographic morphology of localized coronary stenoses. Histopathologic correlations. Circulation 1982; 66:316–20.
14. Onodera T, Fujiwara H, Tanaka M, Wu DJ, Matsuda M, Takemura G, Ishida M, Dawamura A, Dawai C. Cineangiographic and pathological features of the infarct related vessel in successful and unsuccessful thrombolysis. Br Heart J 1989; 61:385–9.
15. Haft JI, Goldstein JE, Niemiera ML. Coronary arteriographic lesion of unstable angina. Chest 1987; 92:609–12.
16. Williams AE, Freeman MR, Chisholm RJ, Patt NL, Armstrong PW. Angiographic morphology in unstable angina pectoris. Am J Cardiol 1988; 62:1024–7.
17. Bresnahan DR, Davis DR, Holmes DR Jr, Smith HC. Angiographic occurrence and clinical correlates of intraluminal coronary artery thrombus: role of unstable angina. J Am Coll Cardiol 1985; 6:285–89.
18. Vetrovec GW, Cowley MJ, Overton H, Richardson DW. Intracoronary thrombus in syndromes of unstable myocardial ischemia. Am Heart J 1981; 102:1202–08.
19. Capone G, Wolf NM, Meyer B, Meister SG. Frequency of intracoronary filling defects by angiography in angina pectoris at rest. Am J Cardiol 1985; 56:403–6.
20. Mandelkorn JB, Wolf NM, Sing S, Shechter JA, Kersh RI, Rodgers DM, Workman MB, Bentivoglio LG, LaPorte SM, Meister SG. Intracoronary thrombus in nontransmural myocardial infarction and in unstable angina pectoris. Am J Cardiol 1983; 52:1–6.

21. Vetrovec GW, Leinbach RC, Gold HK, Cowley MJ. Intracoronary thrombolysis in syndromes of unstable ischemia: Angiographic and clinical results. Am Heart J 1982; 104:946–52.
22. DeWood MA, Spores J, Notske R, Mouser LT, Burroughs R, Golden MS, Lang HT. Prevalence of total coronary occlusion during the early hours of transmural myocardial infarction. N Engl J Med 1980; 303:897–902.
23. Davies SW, Marchant B, Lyons JP, Timmis AD, Rothman MT, Layton CA, Balcon R. Coronary lesion morphology in acute myocardial infarction: demonstration of early remodeling after streptokinase treatment. J Am Coll Cardiol 1990; 16:1079–86.
24. Huey BL, Gheorghiade M, Crampton RS, Beller GA, Kaiser DL, Watson DD, Nygaard TW, Craddock GB, Sayre SL, Gibson RS. Acute non-Q wave myocardial infarction associated with early ST segment elevation: evidence for spontaneous coronary reperfusion and implications for thrombolytic trials. J Am Coll Cardiol 1987; 9:18–25.
25. Ambrose JA, Hjemdahl-Monsen CE, Borrico S, Gorlin R, Fuster V. Angiographic demonstration of a common link between unstable angina pectoris and non-Q wave acute myocardial infarction. Am J Cardiol 1988; 61:244–7.
26. DeWood MA, Stifter WF, Simpson CS, Spores J, Eugster GS, Judge TP, Hinnen ML. Coronary arteriographic findings soon after non-Q wave myocardial infarction. N Engl J Med 1986; 315:417–23.
27. Weaver WD, Lorch GS, Alvarez HA, Cobb LA. Angiographic findings and prognostic indicators in patients resuscitated from sudden cardiac death. Circulation 1976; 54:895–900.
28. Stevenson WG, Wiener I, Yeatman L, Wohlgelernter B, Weiss JN. Complicated atherosclerotic lesions: a potential cause of ischemic ventricular arrhythmias in cardia arrest survivors who do not have inducible ventricular tachycardia? Am Heart J 1988; 116:1–6.
29. Lo Y-SA, Cutler JE, Blake K, Wright AM, Kron J, Swerdlow CD. Angiographic coronary morphology in survivors of cardiac arrest. Am Heart J 1988; 115:781–5.
30. Moise A, Theroux P, Taeymans Y, Descoings B, Lesperance J, Waters DD, Pelletier GB, Bourassa MG. Unstable angina and progression of coronary atherosclerosis. N Engl J Med 1983; 309:685–9.
31. Ambrose JA, Winters SL, Arora RR, Eng A, Riccio A, Gorlin R, Fuster V. Angiographic evolution of coronary artery morphology in unstable angina. J Am Coll Cardiol 1986; 7:472–8.
32. Little WC, Constantinescu M, Applegate RJ, Kutcher MA, Burrows MT, Kahl FR, Santamore WP. Can coronary angiography predict the site of a subsequent myocardial infarction in patients with mild-to-moderate coronary artery disease? Circulation 1988; 78:1157–66.
33. Ambrose JA, Tannenbaum MA, Alexopoulos D, Hjemdahl-Monsen CE, Leavy J, Weiss M, Borrico S, Gorlin R, Fuster V. Angiographic progression of coronary artery disease and the development of myocardial infarction. J Am Coll Cardiol 1988; 12:56–62.
34. Brown BG, Gallery CA, Badger RS, Kennedy JW, Mathey D, Bolson EL, Dodge HT. Incomplete lysis of thrombus in the moderate underlying atherosclerotic lesion

during intracoronary infusion of streptokinase for acute myocardial infarction: quantitative angiographic observations. Circulation 1986; 73:653–61.
35. Hackett D, Davies G, Maseri A. Pre-existing coronary stenoses in patients with first myocardial infarction are not necessarily severe. Eur Heart J 1988; 9:1317–23.
36. Van Lierde J, De Geest H, Verstraete M, Van de Werf F. Angiographic assessment of the infarct-related residual coronary stenosis after spontaneous or therapeutic thrombolysis. J Am Coll Cardiol 1990; 16:1545–9.
37. Moise A, Lesperance J, Theroux P, Taeymans Y, Goulet C, Bourassa MG. Clinical and angiographic predictors of new total coronary occlusion in coronary artery disease: analysis of 313 nonoperated patients. Am J Cardiol 1984; 54:1176–81.
38. Ellis S, Alderman E, Cain K, Fisher L, Sanders W, Bourassa M, and the CASS Investigators. Prediction of risk of anterior myocardial infarction by lesion severity and measurement method of stenoses in the left anterior descending coronary distribution: a CASS registry study. J Am Coll Cardiol 1988; 11:908–16.
39. Neill WA, Wharton TP, Fluri-Lundeen J, Cohen IS. Acute coronary insufficiency—coronary occlusion after intermittent ischemic attacks. N Engl J Med 1980; 302:1157–62.
40. Webster MWI, Cheseboro JH, Smith HC, Frye RL, Holmes DR, Reeder GS, Bresnahan DR, Nishimura RA, Clements IP, Bardsley WT, Grill DE, Bailey KR, Fuster V. Myocardial infarction and coronary artery occlusion: a prospective 5-year angiographic study. J Am Coll Cardiol 1990; 15:218A.
41. Ellis S, Alderman EL, Cain K, Wright A, Bourassa M, Fisher L, and the participants of the Coronary Artery Surgery Study (CASS). Morphology of left anterior descending coronary territory lesions as a predictor of anterior myocardial infarction: a CASS registry study. J Am Coll Cardiol 1989; 13:1481–91.
42. Sansa M, Cernigliaro C, Bolognese L, Bongo SA, Rossi L, Rossi P. Angiographic morphology and response to therapy in unstable angina. Clin Cardiol 1988; 11:121–6.
43. Freeman MR, Williams AE, Chisholm RJ, Armstrong PW. Intracoronary thrombus and complex morphology in unstable angina. Relation to timing of angiography and in-hospital cardiac events. Circulation 1989; 80:17–23.
44. Sherman CT, Litvack F, Grundfest W, Lee M, Hickey A, Chaux A, Kass R, Blanche C, Matloff J, Morgenstern L, Ganz W, Swan HJC, Forrester J. Coronary angioscopy in patients with unstable angina pectoris. N Engl J Med 1986; 315:913–9.
45. Wilson RF, Holida MD, White CW. Quantitative angiographic morphology of coronary stenosis leading to myocardial infarction or unstable angina. Circulation 1986; 73:286–93.
46. Kalbfleisch SJ, McGillem MJ, Simon SB, DeBoe SF, Pinto IMF, Mancini GBJ. Automated quantitation of indexes of coronary lesion complexity: comparison between patients with stable and unstable angina. Circulation 1990; 82:439–47.
47. Hjemdahl-Monsen CE, Ambrose JA, Borrico S, Cohen M, Sherman W, Alexopoulos D, Gorlin R, Fuster V. Angiographic patterns of balloon inflation during percutaneous transluminal coronary angioplasty: role of pressure-diameter curves in studying distensibility and elasticity of the stenotic lesion and the mechanism of dilation. J Am Coll Cardiol 1990; 16:569–75.

4

Pathophysiology of Unstable Angina: Other Considerations

Douglas E. Vaughan

Brigham and Women's Hospital
West Roxbury Veterans Administration Medical Center
and Harvard Medical School
Boston, Massachusetts

INTRODUCTION

Under normal circumstances, coronary blood flow can increase severalfold to meet increased cardiac metabolic demands. In individuals with stable angina pectoris, the coronary supply is able to meet metabolic demands at rest but is limited in its capacity to increase coronary blood flow under more stressful circumstances. In contrast, in the syndrome of unstable angina pectoris, there appears to be a primary decrease in the capacity of coronary circulation to deliver blood, even in the absence of increased metabolic demands. Accordingly, unstable angina is viewed as a "supply-side" problem.

The supply of blood to a particular myocardial region can be jeopardized by an abnormality in the conduit (coronary arteries), the carrier (blood), or both. The experimental and clinical evidence relating abnormalities in these two factors to the development of unstable angina will be reviewed in this chapter.

UNSTABLE ANGINA AS A SUPPLY PROBLEM

Myocardial oxygen requirements are quite sensitive to changes in metabolic demand, which in turn vary in relation to the heart rate, contractility, and loading conditions. If unstable angina is initiated by alterations in blood supply, then none of these three determinants of myocardial oxygen consumption should increase prior to the onset of pain.

As recently as 15 years ago, it was thought that increases in myocardial oxygen demand, albeit transient, were responsible for the development of pain at rest in patients with unstable angina. Two clinical studies were fundamentally important in altering this perception of the pathogenesis of unstable angina. The first of these, by Figueros et al. (1), was performed by analyzing continuous hemodynamic and electrocardiographic changes in patients hospitalized after experiencing chest pain at rest. In many patients, reproducible episodes of pain were always preceded by ischemic electrocardiographic changes and evidence of left ventricular dysfunction, including increases in pulmonary artery pressure and a fall in the stroke volume index. At the onset of the electrocardiographic and hemodynamic changes, the double product (used as an indicator of myocardial oxygen demand) was unchanged in the majority of patients studied. These data were cautiously interpreted as indicative of a spontaneous reduction in myocardial perfusion as a primary mechanism of rest angina.

These findings were confirmed and extended in a study the following year by Chierchia et al. (2). In this study, which was adventurous by current standards, six patients hospitalized for recurrent episodes of angina at rest were selected for investigation. Coronary sinus oxygen saturation was continuously monitored together with left ventricular ($n = 4$) or aortic pressure ($n = 2$). A total of 135 episodes of chest pain with associated ST-changes were monitored. A fall in coronary sinus oxygen consumption consistently preceded the ECG and hemodynamic changes that occurred with pain. The fall in coronary sinus oxygen saturation was never preceded by any detectable increase in the hemodynamic determinants of myocardial oxygen consumption (Fig. 1). These findings, together with those of Figueros, convincingly demonstrate that an alteration in oxygen delivery (i.e., supply) may be the proximate cause of angina at rest.

Several factors, alone or in combination, may act to diminish the flow of blood to the myocardium and contribute to the development of unstable angina. Included among these factors are plaque morphology, coronary vascular tone, and hemostatic variables.

PLAQUE MORPHOLOGY AND PROGRESSION OF ATHEROSCLEROSIS

Structural impediments to flow are frequently detected in patients with unstable angina pectoris. As discussed earlier in this volume, rupture of an atherosclerotic plaque is thought to play a major role in the development of acute cardiovascular syndromes, including both unstable angina and myocardial infarction. Pathologic examination of coronary arteries from individuals that have died shortly after developing unstable angina frequently display disrupted atherosclerotic plaques (3). Ruptured plaques are not frequently seen in patients with stable angina

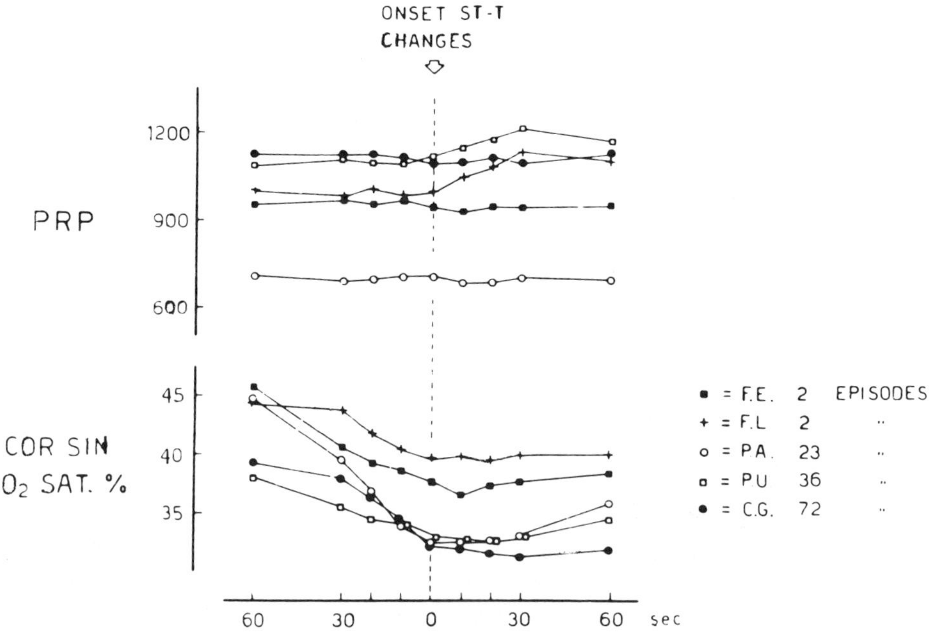

Figure 1 Behavior of coronary sinus O_2 saturation (CSO_2S) and pressure-rate product (PRP $\times$ 1^{-2}) in five patients who showed ECG changes on anterior leads. Each point represents the mean of the values measured in all the recorded episodes. Time 0 refers to the onset of ST-T changes. A drop in CSO_2S precedes the onset of ST-segment changes in the absence of any detectable changes in myocardial oxygen consumption. (Courtesy of S. Chierchia, et al. [Ref. 2]. Reprinted by permission of the American Heart Association.)

pectoris, even though the severity of coronary artery stenosis can be, and is often, more severe in these individuals than in patients with unstable angina.

There is widespread recognition of the role of plaque rupture in unstable angina (4). The sequence of events leading to plaque rupture has been described in the studies of Davies and Thomas (5) and reviewed in the preceding section of this text. Atherosclerotic plaques typically encompass only part of the circumference of a coronary artery. On the luminal surface of the plaque a fibrous cap is frequently seen, and underneath this lies a mass of fatty deposits. The plaques that appear most prone to rupture are relatively soft and those in which the lipid is eccentrically located. Rupture itself is preceded by a thinning of the fibrous cap and usually occurs at the junction between the fibrous cap and the normal vessel wall. The forces that directly initiate plaque rupture are not well defined, but may be related to increased shear stress. The recently reported circadian early morn-

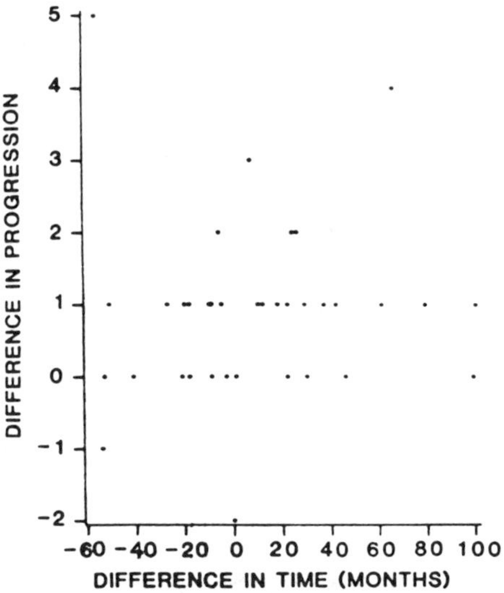

Figure 2 Relation between progression of coronary atherosclerosis and interval between studies. For each pair of patients, the difference in the number of coronary segments in which the disease progressed is plotted against the difference in the time elapsed between the two studies. A positive value on the *y* axis indicates that progression was more extensive in the patient with unstable angina, and a negative value indicates that it was more marked in the paired patient with stable angina. On the *x* axis a positive value indicates a longer interval for the patient with unstable angina, and a negative value a shorter interval. No correlation exists between differences in disease progression and differences in the interval between studies. (Courtesy of A. Moise, et al. [Ref. 7]. Reprinted by permission of the *New England Journal of Medicine*.)

ing increase in occurrence of ischemic cardiac events has led to the suggestion that catecholamine surges may also play a role (6).

This acute alteration in plaque morphology has been recognized in angiographic studies as well. Interestingly, it is difficult to segregate patients into stable or unstable categories on the basis of the number of diseased vessels or severity of stenoses. However, angiographic studies performed in patients with preexisting stable angina demonstrated that disease progression is present in three out of four patients that destabilize (Fig. 2) (7,8). This often corresponds to the presence of an eccentric angiographic coronary artery lesion. As described by Ambrose and colleagues, a coronary obstruction with a narrow neck and an overhanging edge is five times more common in patients with unstable angina than in patients with stable angina (9).

THROMBUS FORMATION

A second structural factor that serves to impede coronary flow is intraluminal thrombus formation. Currently, thrombi are perceived as playing a primary role in the pathogenesis of unstable angina (10,11). Severe injury of an arterial vessel, as seen following plaque rupture, leads to the exposure of the arterial media to blood. In the media, fibrillar collagen is present and exposure to collagen can initiate platelet activation and adhesion. Activated platelets provide a surface that enhances thrombin formation, which in turn stimulates further platelet activation and aggregation. Independently, the exposure of tissue factor and other substances in the damaged vessel wall can lead to activation of both the intrinsic and extrinsic clotting cascades.

Several angiographic studies have provided evidence that intracoronary thrombus is related to the syndrome of unstable angina, especially when angiography is performed soon after the occurrence of rest pain (12,13) (Fig. 3).

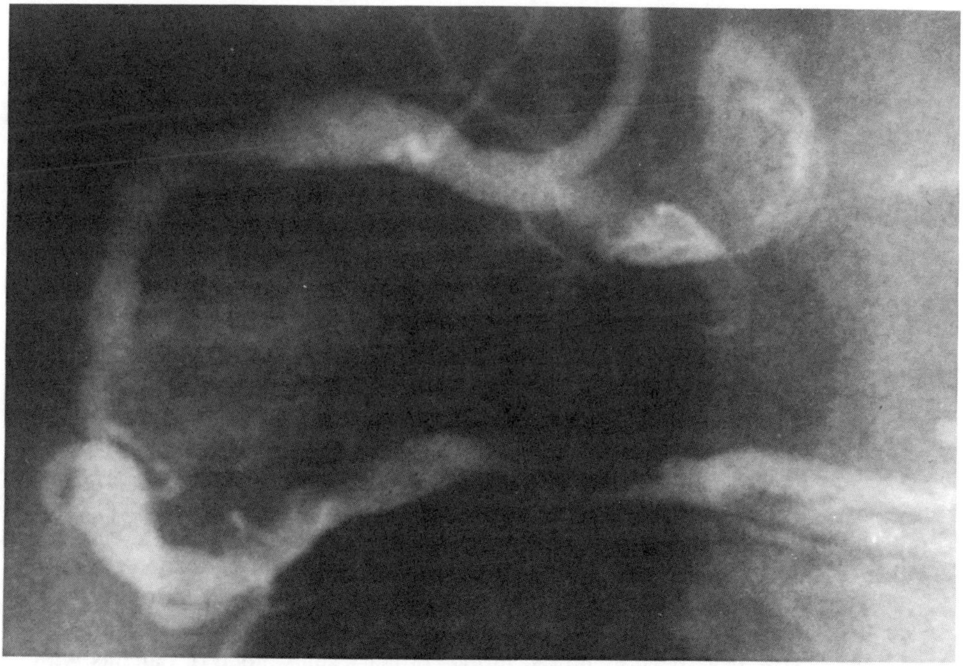

Figure 3 Coronary arteriogram obtained within 6 hours of pain in a patient with unstable angina. Note evidence of thrombus in the right coronary artery. (Angiogram provided courtesy of John Bittl, M.D.)

The recent development of angioscopic devices has permitted investigators to directly visualize the coronary arteries of individuals with unstable angina. Almost uniformly, angioscopy reveals the presence of thrombi, even in unstable angina patients that do not appear to have thrombi by coronary angiography (14). Several other pieces of evidence indicate that thrombus, or a prothrombotic process, is present in patients with unstable angina. Theroux and colleagues (15) described elevated levels of fibrinopeptide A in patients with unstable angina. Fibrinopeptide A (FPA) is produced by the action of thrombin on fibrinogen and circulates in plasma with a very short half life (3–5 minutes). Accordingly, elevated levels of FPA are generally interpreted as indicative of active thrombosis. Elevations in other markers of coagulation activity have been observed in patients with unstable angina, including fibrin-related antigen, D-dimer, and fibrin monomer (16). Evidence of platelet activation (as quantified by thromboxane B_2 levels) has also been reported (17) (Fig. 4).

ABNORMAL CORONARY VASCULAR TONE

Coronary blood flow is regulated by several different factors, including neural, hormonal, autoregulatory, and metabolic factors. It is beyond the scope of this chapter to review the complexities of regulation of myocardial perfusion, but specific areas deserve attention for potentially participating in the pathogenesis of unstable angina.

Vasoconstriction, albeit inappropriate, can rapidly and effectively jeopardize the flow of blood to the heart. Indeed, this may play a role in the pathogenesis of unstable angina, and can be initiated by at least three different mechanisms: (a) increased production of vasoconstricting substances, (b) failure of local production of counter-regulatory vasodilators, and (c) paradoxical vasoconstriction to substances that normally vasodilate. It seems highly probable that the same local factors that promote thrombus formation can also participate in the production of vasoconstrictive substances in selected areas. Probably the best characterized candidate is thromboxane A_2 (TxA_2). This substance is synthesized and released by aggregating platelets. As discussed previously, platelets adhere to and are activated by the ruptured atherosclerotic plaque. As if platelet accumulation and thrombus formation were not enough, aggregating platelets add "insult to injury" by secreting a powerful vasoconstrictor, TxA_2. A focal overproduction of TxA_2 in the coronary vasculature may well contribute to the development of unstable angina. Indeed, increased levels of the major metabolite of thromboxane A_2, termed TxB_2, have been identified in the coronary sinus blood of patients with unstable angina (18), while simultaneous systemic levels of TxB_2 were normal (Fig. 5).

It is now abundantly clear that the vascular endothelium plays more than a passive role in the maintenance of coronary blood flow. The endothelium is a primary location for the production of a variety of vasoactive substances, both

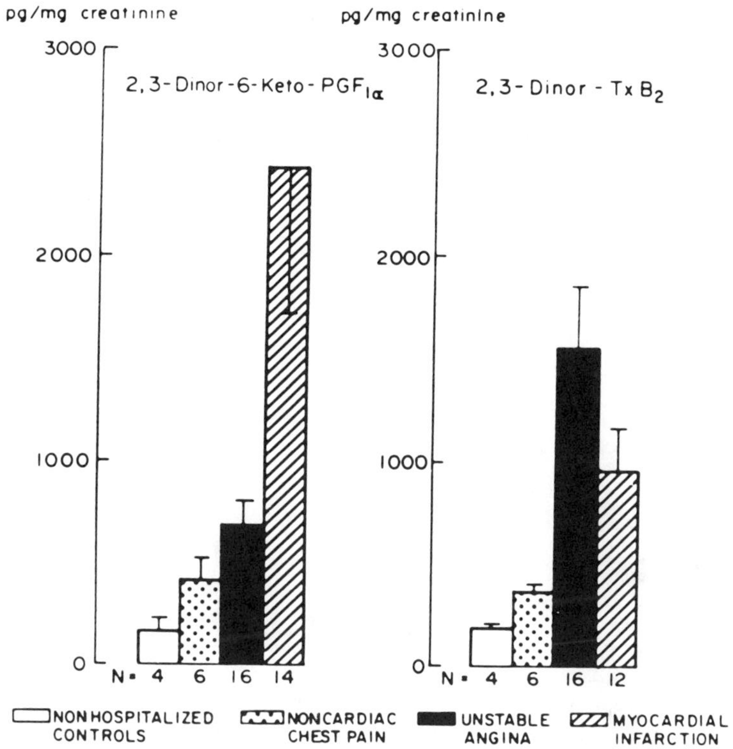

Figure 4 Peak urinary metabolite excretion in controls and in patients with unstable angina or myocardial infarction. Peak 2,3-dinor-6-keto-prostaglandin $F_1\alpha$ excretion was highest in patients with myocardial infarction ($p < 0.025$ vs. patients with unstable angina and $p < 0.01$ vs. controls), whereas 2,3-dinor-thromboxane B_2 excretion was highest in patients with unstable angina ($p < 0.05$ vs. patients with myocardial infarction and $p < 0.01$ vs. controls). PG, prostaglandin; and Tx, thromboxane. Mean ± SEM. (Courtesy of D. J. Fitzgerald et al. [Ref. 17] Reprinted by permission of the *New England Journal of Medicine*.)

dilatory and constrictive in function. Several endothelial-derived factors appear to play important roles in modulating vascular tone.

Prostacyclin

The first vasodilatory substance derived from endothelium to be recognized was prostacyclin (PGI_2) (19). This prostaglandin is the major cyclooxygenase product of arachidonate metabolism in vascular endothelium and is a potent vasodilating and platelet inhibitory compound. Factors known to stimulate the production and release of prostacyclin include bradykinin, thrombin, arachidonic acid, and

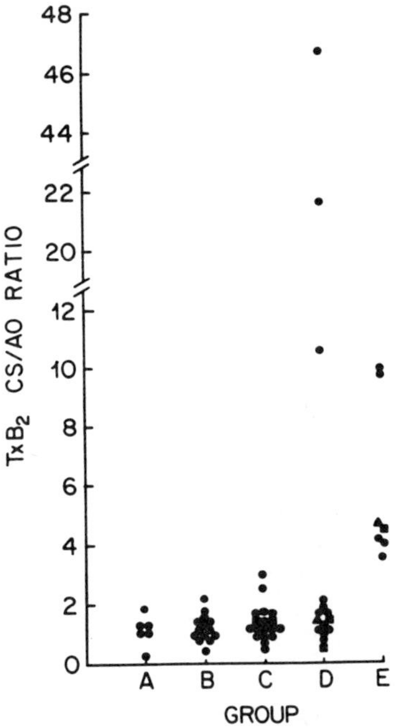

Figure 5 Ratios of thromboxane B_2 (TxB_2) in coronary sinus and in ascending aorta (CS/AO) in five groups of patients. Each point represents data from one patient. Squares identify patients who received a cyclooxygenase inhibitor within 5 days of study, and triangles patients with coronary arterial spasm. In Groups A (valvular and congenital ischemic heart disease), B (chest pain syndrome without ischemic heart disease), and C (ischemic heart disease without chest pain for at least 96 hours), all patients had TxB_2 CS/AO ratios of 3.1 or lower. Group D (ischemic heart disease with chest pain 24 to 96 hours before study) had a bimodal distribution: 12 patients had low TxB_2 ratios, whereas three had very high ratios. Group E (ischemic heart disease and chest pain within 24 hours before study) had TxB_2 CS/AO ratios (range, 3.5 to 9.9) that were higher than those of Groups A, B, and C ($p < 0.05$). (Courtesy of P. D. Hirsh et al. [Ref. 18]. Reprinted by permission of the *New England Journal of Medicine*.)

adenine nucleotides. Prostacyclin has a $t_{1/2}$ of 2–3 minutes in the circulation and is rapidly broken down to 6-keto-$PGF_{1\alpha}$. The synthesis and secretion of prostacyclin, which is dependent upon cyclooxygenase activity, can be reduced by aspirin, which acetylates and deactivates the enzyme. The ability of endothelial cells to synthesize cyclooxygenase de novo serves as the fundamental biochemical explanation for the relatively selective and therapeutically divergent effects of aspirin on platelet and endothelial prostaglandin synthesis. The platelet arachidonic pathway preferentially elaborates thromboxane A_2, which, in contrast to prostacyclin, is a potent vasoconstrictive and platelet proaggregatory compound. Since platelets lack the biosynthetic machinery to synthesize new proteins, the acetylation and inhibition of platelet cyclooxygenase by aspirin cannot be overriden. Thus, aspirin appears to push the thromboxane/prostacyclin balance in the direction of prostacyclin production, although the optimal dose and frequency of aspirin administration has not yet been clarified.

Prostacyclin acts directly on smooth muscle cells in the vascular wall to induce vasodilation. Prostacyclin first binds receptors on the surface of smooth muscle cells and initiates a sequence of events leading to increased intracellular levels of cAMP. This is followed by a decrease in cytosolic calcium concentrations, thereby promoting muscular relaxation and vasodilation. It is tempting to speculate that a local deficiency of prostacyclin production may contribute to the development of unstable angina. This concept, though currently unproven, derives from the notion that diseased or damaged endothelial cells, adjacent to an atherosclerotic coronary plaque, would be unable to produce adequate amounts of prostacyclin, thus tipping the local microenvironmental balance toward vasoconstriction and platelet aggregation. It has recently been demonstrated that the half-life of prostacyclin is regulated in plasma by an interaction with high density lipoprotein (20). It appears that apolipoprotein A-I (apo A-I), which is a major apolipoprotein of HDL, stabilizes prostacyclin in plasma and prolongs both the chemical and biological half-life of prostacyclin. Decreased stability of prostacyclin may theoretically play a role in the pathogenesis of thrombus formation, since a shortened half-life of this prostanoid may lead to inadequate prostacyclin activity at sites of vascular damage. When patients with unstable angina were compared with normal controls and patients with stable angina pectoris, Aoyema and colleagues (20) found that prostacyclin was least stable in patients with unstable angina and corresponded with low levels of HDL-associated ApoA-I.

Endothelial-Derived Relaxing Factor

Endothelial cells produce a second vasodilatory substance, termed endothelial-derived relaxation factor (EDRF). The existence of EDRF was first proposed by Furchgott and Zawadzki, who showed that acetylcholine-induced vascular relaxation was dependent upon the presence of endothelium (21). It now appears certain that EDRF is either nitric oxide or a nitrosothiol (22). EDRF is produced in endothelial cells in response to multiple different stimuli, both chemical and physical, including acetylcholine, bradykinin, histamine, blood flow, ADP, by aggregating platelets. EDRF is very labile and has a half-life measured in seconds following release into the blood and into adjacent structures. EDRF has several effects, all of which are apparently mediated through increased levels of cyclic GMP in target cells, including platelet inhibition and smooth muscle relaxation. In the absence of functional endothelium (as in a diseased

Table 1 Speculative Endothelial Mechanisms in Preventing Unstable Angina

	Effects
Endothelial Synthetic Products	
Prostacyclin	Vasodilator Inhibits platelet aggregation
EDRF	Same as prostacyclin
Tissue plasminogen activator	Converts plasminogen to plasmin: enhances fibrinolysis
Endothelial Surface Structures	
Heparan sulfate	Activates ATIII → inhibits thrombin
Fibrinolytic receptors	Co-localize t-PA and plasminogen → enhances fibrinolysis
Thrombomodulin	Binds thrombin and enhances the production of activated protein C

atherosclerotic coronary), substances that normally induce EDRF release and vasodilation (like acetylcholine or platelet secretory products) can instead act directly upon smooth muscle and promote paradoxic vasoconstriction (23). Thus, the relative lack of EDRF production in a vascular locale bereft of healthy endothelium can influence the tendency towards arterial vasoconstriction and, thus, may play a role in the transient decreases in blood supply that occur in unstable angina.

Endothelin

Endothelial cells have been shown to elaborate vasoconstrictor substances as well. The first such factor, identified by Yanagisawa and colleagues (24), was termed endothelin. It is now apparent that at least three separate endothelin isopeptides are present in humans (25). Endothelial cells are apparently only responsible for the synthesis of endothelin-1, which is a small coiled peptide 21 amino acids in length.

The most striking property of endothelin-1 is its long-lasting vasoconstricting action. In fact, it appears to be the most potent pressor substance known. Endothelin is thought to act by binding to a specific membrane receptor, which leads to the activation of phospholipase C and increased cystolic calcium levels. At the present time, preliminary evidence is available demonstrating that increased endothelin-1 levels are present in patients with unstable angina (26), and elevated levels have been demonstrated in patients with acute myocardial infarction (27), which is viewed as having a pathogenesis similar to that of unstable angina. EDRF serves as a counterregulatory vasodilator opposing the vasoconstrictor effects of endothelin.

Even in the absence of increased levels of endothelin (or other vasoconstrictors for that matter), a deficient production and release of EDRF could conceivably shift the tonic balance in a vessel toward vasoconstriction. Given the recent intense interest in endothelin, it seems likely that synthetic antagonists of it will soon be developed for use in a variety of cardiovascular disorders, including unstable angina. If endothelin antagonists prove to have a beneficial therapeutic effect in treating patients with this syndrome, it would constitute compelling evidence that this vasoconstrictor plays a role in the pathogenesis of unstable angina.

IMPAIRED FIBRINOLYSIS

The topic of endothelial dysfunction prompts a discussion of other more speculative mechanisms that may participate in the pathogenesis of unstable angina. For example, humans have the capacity to rapidly dissolve thrombi that form in the vasculature (27). Fibrinolysis occurs when plasmin cleaves fibrin and converts it into soluble degradation products. Plasmin is formed by the action of tissue plasminogen activator (t-PA) on plasminogen, which itself is inactive. t-PA, like prostacyclin and EDRF, is synthesized and secreted by endothelial cells. The fibrinolytic system is poised to react to thrombus formation on a microenvironmental level. When thrombi are found, local hypoxia and acidosis likely follow, and both of these conditions stimulate healthy endothelium to secrete t-PA. Paradoxically, thrombin, which activates platelets and is responsible for the conversion of fibrinogen to fibrin, also stimulates endothelial cells to generate t-PA. It is tempting to speculate that a paucity of functional endothelium in the vicinity of a ruptured plaque may play a permissive role in thrombus development and the pathogenesis of unstable angina, by virtue of their inability to respond to local stimuli and provide focally enriched concentrations of t-PA. Endothelial cells also express receptors in their surface that bind t-PA (28) and plasminogen (29). This co-localization of tissue fibrinolytic components enhances their activity, and again, in the absence of healthy, intact endothelium with functional receptors for fibrinolytic proteins, a focal fibrinolytic deficiency may develop and contribute to thrombus formation.

Thrombin also stimulates the release of plasminogen activator inhibitor-1 (PAI-1) from endothelial cells. PAI-1 is a rapid inhibitor of t-PA in plasma and elevated levels of PAI-1 have been identified in youthful survivors of acute myocardial infarction (30). Increased levels of PAI-1 could potentially tip a precarious balance between coagulation and fibrinolysis towards thrombosis and thereby play a role in the development of unstable angina. This is highly speculative at the present time, given the lack of prospective data relating elevated levels of PAI-1 to the development of unstable angina or acute myocardial infarction.

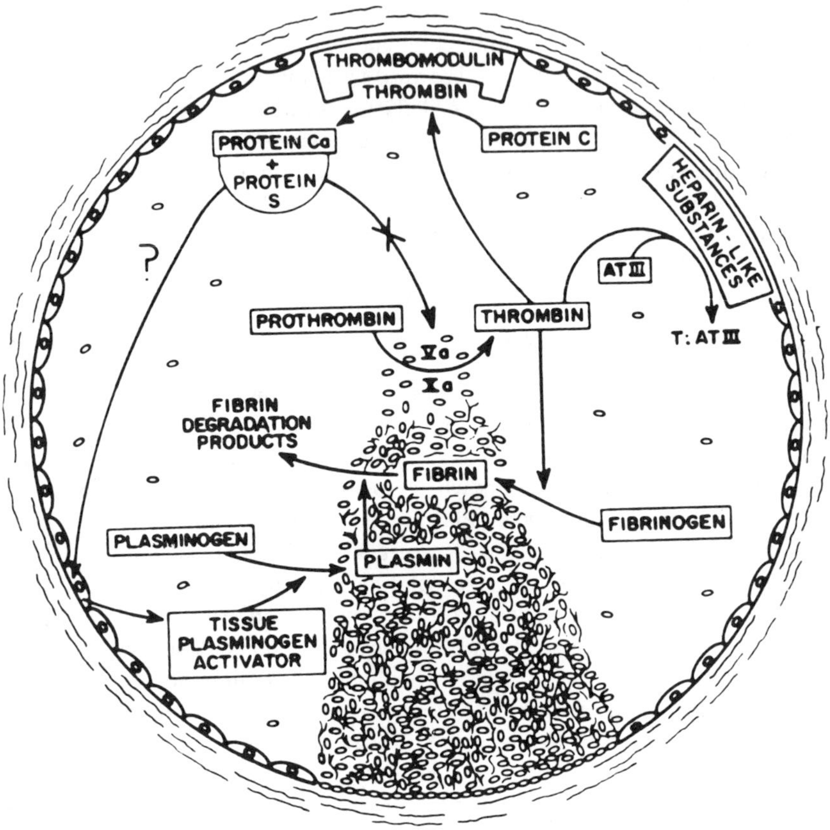

Figure 6 Formation of the hemostatic plug at the site of vascular injury. Three major physiologic anticoagulant mechanisms—antithrombin II (AT III), protein C, and the fibrinolytic system—are activated to limit clot formation to the site of damage and to prevent generalized thrombosis. T = thrombin. (Courtesy of A. I. Schafer [Ref. 33]. Reprinted by permission of the *Annals of Internal Medicine*.)

Endothelium also plays an important role in endogenous anticoagulant mechanisms (Fig. 6). The surface of healthy endothelium is coated with glycosaminoglycans, including heparan sulfate. The endogenous inhibitor of thrombin, antithrombin III, binds to and is activated by heparan sulfate. Again, in the absence of healthy endothelium, there may be a relative lack of heparan sulfate, which in turn may yield inadequate levels of activated antithrombin III and a focal predisposition towards thrombosis. Endothelial cells participate in endogenous anticoagulation through additional mechanisms. Endothelial cells express a receptor for thrombin, termed thrombomodulin (31). After bound by thrombomodulin, the substrate specificity of thrombin is converted so that it no longer has coagulant activity and it preferentially converts protein C to activated protein C (protein Ca). Protein Ca has potent anticoagulant effects due to its rapid inactivation of coagulation factors V and VIII. In fact, the binding of thrombin to thrombomodulin enhances the rate of generation of protein Ca nearly 30,000-fold (32).

CONCLUSIONS

A primary decrease in coronary blood flow appears to be an important initiating factor for the development of unstable angina. Clearly, structural impediments, including plaque rupture and thrombus formation, play a pivotal role in diminishing the flow of blood through involved coronaries. Multiple factors probably contribute to this process and may occur at a microenvironmental level. In an atherosclerotic coronary artery, the substrate exists for dynamic equilibrium shifts away from vasodilation toward vasoconstriction and away from anticoagulation towards thrombosis. Future advancements in our ability to treat unstable angina will depend on a more precise elucidation of the multiple factors that contribute to the impairment of blood flow in an atherosclerotic coronary microenvironment and our ability to manipulate them.

ACKNOWLEDGMENT

The author is the recipient of a Clinician-Scientist Award from the American Heart Association, Dallas, Texas, and a Merit Review Award from the U.S. Veterans Administration.

REFERENCES

1. Figueros J, Singh BN, Ganz W, Charuzi Y, Swan HJC. Mechanism of rest and nocturnal angina: observations during continuous hemodynamic and electrocardiographic monitoring. Circulation 1979; 59:955–68.
2. Chierchia S, Brunelli C, Simonetti I, Lazzari M, Maseri A. Sequence of events in angina at rest: primary reduction in coronary flow. Circulation 1980; 61:759–68.
3. Falk E. Plaque rupture with severe pre-existing stenosis precipitating coronary thrombosis: characteristics of coronary atherosclerotic plaques underlying fatal occlusion thrombi. Brit Heart Journal 1983; 50:127–34.
4. Fuster V, Badimon L, Cohen M, Ambrose JA, Badimon JJ, Chesbro J. Insight into the pathogenesis of acute ischemic syndromes. Circulation 1988; 77:1213–20.
5. Davies MJ, Thomas AC. Plaque fissuring: the cause of acute myocardial infarction, ischemic death, and crescendo angina. Brit Heart Journal 1985; 53:363–73.
6. Tofler GH, Brezinski D, Schafer AI, Cxeisler CA, Rutherford JD, Willich SN, Gleason RE, Williams GH, Muller JE. Concurrent morning increases in platelet

aggregability and the risk of myocardial infarction and sudden cardiac death. N Engl J Med 1987; 316:1514–8.

7. Moise A, Theroux P, Taeymans Y, Descoings B, Lesperance J, Waters DD, Pelletier GB, Bograssa MG. Unstable angina and progression of coronary atherosclerosis. N Engl J Med 1983; 309:685–9.
8. Ambrose JA, Winters SL, Arora RR, Ricio A, Gorlin R, Fuster V. Angiographic evolution of coronary artery morphology in unstable angina. J Am Coll Cardiol 1986; 7:472–8.
9. Ambrose JA, Winters SL, Stern A, Eng A, Teichholz LE, Gorlin R, Fuster V. Angiographic morphology and the pathogenesis of unstable angina. J Am Coll Cardiol 1985; 5:609–16.
10. Falk E. Unstable angina with fatal outcome: dynamic coronary thrombosis leading to infarction and/or sudden death. Circulation 1985; 71:699–708.
11. Levin DC, Fallon JT. Significance of the angiographic morphology of localized coronary stenoses. Histopathological correlations. Circulation 1982; 66:316–20.
12. Capone G, Wolf NM, Meyer B, Meister SG. Frequency of intracoronary filling defects by angiography in angina pectoris at rest. Am J. Cardiol 1985; 56:403–6.
13. Freeman MR, Williams AE, Chisholm RJ, Armstrong PW. Intracoronary thrombus and complex morphology in unstable angina. Circ 1989; 80:17–23.
14. Sherman CT, Litvak F, Grundjest W, Lee M, et al. Coronary angioscopy in patients with unstable angina pectoris. N Engl J Med 1986; 315:913–9.
15. Theroux P, Latour JG, Leger C, DeLara J. Fibrinopeptide A and platelet factor levels in unstable angina pectoris. Circulation 1987; 75:156–62.
16. Kruskal JB, Commerford PJ, Franks JJ, Kirsch RE. Fibrin and fibrinogen-related antigens in patients with stable and unstable coronary artery disease. N Engl J Med 1987; 317:1361–5.
17. Fitzgerald DJ, Roy L, Catella F, Fitzgerald GA. Platelet activation in unstable coronary disease. N Engl J Med 1986; 315:983–9.
18. Hirsh PD, Hillis LD, Campbell WB, Firth BG, Willerson JT. Release of prostaglandins and thromboxane into the coronary circulation in patients with ischemic heart disease. N Engl J Med 1981; 304:685–91.
19. Moncada S, Gryglewski R, Bunting S, Vane JR. An enzyme isolated from arteries transforms prostaglandin endoperoxides to an unstable substance that inhibits platelet aggregation. Nature (Lond) 1976; 263:663–5.
20. Aoyema T, Yoshiki Y, Morishita H, Kawai C. Prostaglandin I_2 half-life regulated by high density lipoprotein is decreased in acute myocardial infarction and unstable angina pectoris. Circulation 1990; 81:1784–91.
21. Furchgott RF, Zawadzki JV. The obligatory role of endothelial cells in the relaxation of arterial smooth muscle by acetylcholine. Nature (Lond) 1980; 288:373–6.
22. Ignarro LJ. Biological actions and properties of endothelium-derived nitric oxide formed and released from artery and vein. Circ Res 1989; 65:1–21.
23. Ludmer PL, Selwyn AP, Shook TL, Wayne RR, Mudge GH, Alexander RW, Ganz P. Paradoxical vasoconstriction induced by acetylcholine in atherosclerotic coronary arteries. N Engl J Med 1986; 315:1046–51.
24. Yanagisawa M, Kurihara H, Kimura S, Tomobe Y, Kobayashi M, Mitsui Y,

Yazoki Y, Goto K, Masaki T. A novel potent vasoconstrictor peptide produced by vascular endothelial cells. Nature 1988; 332:411–5.

25. Inoue A, Yanagisawa M, Kimura S, Kasayu Y, Miyauchi T, Goto K, Masaki T. The human endothelin family: three structurally and pharmacologically distinct isopeptides predicted by three separate genes. Proc Natl Acad Sci USA 1989; 86:2863–7.
26. Arendt RM, Wilbert-Lampen U, Hencke L. Increased plasma endothelin in patients with hyperlipiproteinemia and stable or unstable angina. Circ 1990; 82:III-248 (Abstract).
27. Bachmann F. Fibrinolysis. In: Verstraete M, Vermylen J, Lijnen R, Arnout J, eds. Thrombosis and haemostasis 1987. Leuven University Press, 1987:227–65.
28. Hajjar KA, Hamel NM, Harpel PC, Nachman RL. Binding of tissue plasminogen activator to cultured endothelial cells. J Clin Invest 1987; 80:1712–9.
29. Hajjar KA, Harpel PC, Jaffe EA, Nachman RL. Binding of plasminogen to cultured human endothelial cells. J Biol Chem 1986; 261:11656–62.
30. Hamsten A, Wiman B, DeFaire U, Blomback M. Increased plasma levels of a rapid inhibitor of tissue plasminogen activator in young survivors of myocardial infarction. N Engl J Med 1985; 313:1557–63.
31. Esmon CT, Owen WG. Identification of an endothelial cell cofactor for thrombin-catalyzed activation of protein C. Proc Natl Acad Sci USA 1981; 78:2249–52.
32. Clouse LH, Comp PC. The regulation of hemostasis: the protein C system. N Engl J Med 1986; 314:1298–1304.
33. Schafer AI. The hypercoaguable states. Ann Int Med 1985; 102:814–28.

5

Clinical Presentation of Unstable Angina

John D. Rutherford

Brigham and Women's Hospital and Harvard Medical School
Boston, Massachusetts

Unstable angina is a common condition. A major hospital discharge survey suggested that, while there was a decline in hospitalizations for coronary heart disease and reduced discharges from hospital with the diagnosis of chronic ischemic heart disease, between 1984 and 1986 the number of discharges with the diagnosis of unstable angina pectoris doubled. For both unstable and stable angina pectoris in the elderly population, more women than men were affected (1). "Unstable angina," which is the unpredictable occurrence of myocardial ischemia in a crescendo or accelerated pattern, effects a heterogeneous population of patients (2). It has been proposed by Braunwald that we should classify patients based on the severity of the clinical circumstances that provoke the unstable angina and whether the symptomatic ischemic episodes are accompanied by transient electrocardiographic changes (Table 1). This classification notes whether rest pain is present, whether episodes of pain have occurred within the preceding 48 hours, and whether the angina is provoked by conditions such as anemia, fever, infection, or tachyarrhythmias. In addition, patients with unstable angina may have a history of a prior myocardial infarction or known single- or multivessel coronary artery disease on the one hand; alternatively, this may be their initial presentation with coronary artery disease. They may be taking no medical therapy or may be suffering severe, transient episodes of myocardial ischemia despite a combination of medications including nitrates, calcium channel antagonists, beta-blocking agents, aspirin, and intravenous heparin or nitroglycerin. Furthermore, unstable angina can also occur within

Table 1 Classification of Unstable Angina

SEVERITY
Class I: New onset, severe or accelerated angina. Patients with angina of less than 2 months duration, severe or occurring three or more times per day, or angina that is distinctly more frequent, and precipitated by distinctly less exertion. No rest pain in the last months.
Class II: Angina at rest. Subacute. Patients with one or more episodes of angina at rest during the preceding month but not within the preceding 48 hr.
Class III: Angina at rest. Acute. Patients with one or more episodes at rest within the preceding 48 hr.
CLINICAL CIRCUMSTANCES
Class A: Secondary unstable angina. A clearly identified condition extrinsic to the coronary vascular bed that has intensified myocardial ischemia, e.g., anemia, infection, fever, hypotension, tachyarrhythmia, thyrotoxicosis, hypoxemia secondary to respiratory failure.
Class B: Primary unstable angina.
Class C: Postinfarction unstable angina (within 2 weeks of documented myocardial infarction).
INTENSITY OF TREATMENT
1. Absence of treatment or minimal treatment.
2. Occurring in presence of standard therapy for chronic staple angina (conventional doses of oral beta-blockers, nitrates, and calcium antagonists).
3. Occurring despite maximally tolerated doses of all three categories of oral therapy, including intravenous nitroglycerin.

Source: Adapted from Ref. 2. Reproduced by permission.

days or weeks of a documented myocardial infarction, and in this circumstance the management will differ from that proposed for a patient with their first symptoms of coronary artery disease. In contrast to chronic stable angina pectoris, where an increase in demand for myocardial oxygen commonly precedes the onset of angina, patients with unstable angina may have a primary decrease in myocardial oxygen supply caused by increases in coronary vasomotor tone (vasoconstriction) (3,4), rapid progression of coronary artery stenosis, or "activation" or "destabilization" of an atherosclerotic plaque. Clinical studies have suggested that certain patients with unstable angina have evidence of increased aggregation of platelets (5), and the presence of an active thrombotic process is suggested by increased serum concentrations of fibrin-related antigen and D-dimer (the major breakdown of fragment of fibrin) (6), all changes that are not seen in patients with chronic stable angina. Pathologic (7,8) and angiographic studies (9–18) have suggested the presence of coronary artery thrombus in patients with unstable angina. Thrombus has also been observed using coronary angioscopy in patients undergoing revascularization surgery for unstable angina pectoris (17). The morphology of the coronary artery lesion associated with the clinical syndrome of "unstable angina" tends to be eccentric and irregular rather than symmetric and smooth-bordered and may be associated with filling defects which are assumed to be caused by coronary thrombi (10–12,18). Since recent episodes of rest angina can be associated with nonocclusive intracoronary thrombi (16,18), it is logical that certain patients will be treated aggressively with heparin, antiplatelet therapy, and, perhaps in the future, thrombolytic therapy. In patients presenting early after the onset of rest angina or especially in those who have rest angina despite a full conventional medical regimen, there is a high incidence of coronary thrombi (16), which itself is a strong predictor of subsequent adverse cardiac events including death, myocardial infarction, and the need for urgent revascularization.

In patients with no prior history of coronary artery disease who present with unpredictable crescendo, accelerated or rest angina, a conservative approach initially is reasonable. Such patients are usually hospitalized, and therapy is initiated with aspirin, nitrates, and/or beta-blockers, and/or calcium antagonists, while secondary causes of unstable angina such as anemia or infection are excluded.

Many patients will rapidly stabilize on a full medical regimen, and risk stratification will be subsequently performed by noninvasive assessment of ventricular function and some form of stress testing (exercise electrocardiography, thallium scintigraphy, dipyridamole imaging) will be undertaken. In those patients with normal ventricular function who have an excellent exercise capacity or evidence of ischemia only at a high workload, a conservative approach may be adopted. In those who have evidence of moderate or severe left ventricular dysfunction or a poor exercise capacity and evidence of extensive ischemia at a low workload, then angiography with a view to revascularization will be considered. The details of both invasive and noninvasive work-up will be considered in Chapters 6, 7, and 8.

REFERENCES

1. Feinleib M, Havlik RJ, Gillum RF, Pokras R, McCarthy E, Moien M. Coronary heart disease and related procedures. National Hospital Discharge Survey Data. Circulation 1989; 79(6 Pt2)1:13–18.
2. Braunwald E. Unstable angina: a classification. Circulation 1989; 80:410–14.
3. Maseri A. Pathogenic mechanisms of unstable angina as a guideline to individual patient management and prognosis. Am J Med 1986; 80(Suppl 4C):48–55.
4. Chierchia S, Brunelli C, Simonetti I, Lazzari M, Maseri A. Sequence of events in angina at rest: primary reduction in coronary blood flow. Circulation 1980; 61:759–68.
5. Grande P, Grauholt A, Madsen JK. Unstable angina pectoris. Platelet behaviour and prognosis in progressive angina and intermediate coronary syndrome. Circulation 1990;(Supp I):16–19.

6. Kruskal J, Commerford P, Franks J, Kirsch R. Fibrin and fibrinogen-related antigens in patients with stable and unstable coronary artery disease. N Engl J Med 1987; 317:1361–5.
7. Davies MJ, Thomas AC, Knapman PA, Hangartner JR. Intramyocardial platelet aggregation in patients with unstable angina suffering sudden ischemic cardiac death. Circulation 1986; 73:418–27.
8. Falk E. Unstable angina with fatal outcome: dynamic coronary thrombosis leading to infarction and/or sudden death. Autopsy evidence of recurrent mural thrombosis with peripheral embolization culminating in total vascular occlusion. Circulation 1985; 71:699–708.
9. Ambrose JA, Hjemdahl MC, Borrico S, Sherman W, Cohen M, Gorlin R, et al. Quantitative and qualitative effects of intracoronary streptokinase in unstable angina and non-Q wave infarction. J Am Coll Cardiol 1987; 9:1156–65.
10. Holmes D, Hartzler G, Smith H, Fuster V. Coronary artery thrombosis in patients with unstable angina. Br Heart J 1981; 45:411–16.
11. Vetrovec GW, Leinbach RC, Gold HK, Cowley MJ. Intracoronary thrombolysis in syndromes of unstable ischemia: angiographic and clinical results. Am Heart J 1982; 104:946–52.
12. Capone G, Wolf N, Meyer B, Meister S. Frequency of intracoronary filling defects by angiography in angina pectoris at rest. Am J Cardiol 1985; 56:403–6.
13. de Zwaan C, Bar F, Janssen J, de Swart H, Vermeer F, Wellens H. Effects of thrombolytic therapy in unstable angina: clinical and angiographic results. J Am Coll Cardiol 1988; 12:301–9.
14. Mandelkorn JB, Wolf NM, Singh S, Shechter JA, Kersh RI, Rodgers DM, Workman MB, Bentivoglio LG, LaPorte SM, Meister SG. Intracoronary thrombus in nontransmural myocardial infarction and in unstable angina pectoris. Am J Cardiol 1983; 52:1–6.
15. Bresnahan D, Davis D, Holmes D, Smith H. Angiographic occurrence and clinical correlates of intraluminal coronary artery thrombus: role of unstable angina. J Am Coll Cardiol 1985; 6:285–9.
16. Freeman M, Williams A, Chisholm R, Armstrong P. Intracoronary thrombus and complex morphology in unstable angina: relation to timing of angiography and in-hospital cardiac events. Circulation 1989; 80:17–23.
17. Sherman CT, Litvack F, Grundfest W, Lee M, Hickey A, Chaux A, Kass R, Blanche C, Mattloff J, Morgenstern L. Coronary angioscopy in patients with unstable angina pectoris. N Engl J Med 1986; 315:913–19.
18. Gotoh K, Minamino T, Katoh O, Hamano Y, Fukui S, Hori M, Kusuoka H, Mishima M, Inoue M, Kamada T. The role of intracoronary thrombus in unstable angina: angiographic assessment and thrombolytic therapy during ongoing anginal attacks. Circulation 1988; 77:526–34.

6

Cardiac Investigations: Cardiac Catheterization and Intra-aortic Balloon Counterpulsation

John D. Parker

Brigham and Women's Hospital and Harvard Medical School
Boston, Massachusetts

INTRODUCTION

Over the past decade, management approaches to the patient with unstable angina have changed significantly. Despite important improvements in medical therapy, myocardial revascularization procedures are now employed much more frequently in the care of these patients. This fact, coupled with the recognition that selective coronary angiography and left ventriculography can be carried out safely in the majority of patients with unstable coronary syndromes, has led to a marked increase in the number of patients with unstable angina undergoing cardiac catheterization.

In this chapter a number of issues concerning the approach to cardiac catheterization of the patient with unstable angina will be addressed. The typical angiographic findings in patients with unstable angina will be reviewed along with their prognostic implications. Timing and indications for cardiac catheterization will be discussed with particular attention given to the management of the patient who is extremely unstable. Finally, the risks and utility of intra-aortic balloon counterpulsation in the setting of unstable angina will be summarized.

ANGIOGRAPHIC FINDINGS IN UNSTABLE ANGINA

There have been numerous reports concerning the severity of coronary artery disease in patients presenting with unstable angina (1–5). In interpreting the results of these investigations it is important to recall that unstable angina represents a wide spectrum of clinical disorders. Investigations that have included *all* patients presenting with unstable angina have generally demonstrated a distribution and severity of coronary artery disease which is similar to that seen in patients with stable angina and in those who have previously suffered a myocardial infarction (1–3). These studies reveal a roughly equal distribution of single-, double-, and triple-vessel coronary artery disease. As in stable angina, the left anterior descending artery is the most commonly affected vessel. Patients with unstable angina do appear to have a higher incidence of left main coronary artery stenoses. A review of several investigations suggests that the incidence of significant left main coronary artery disease is approximately 15%, which is higher than that reported for stable angina patients (1–5).

It is now known that in any given population with unstable angina, the expected angiographic findings and extent of coronary artery disease are highly variable, being dependent on the patient's history and mode of presentation (Table 1). Patients who experience unstable angina superimposed on a history of chronic stable angina (a syndrome which has been termed crescendo angina) have been shown to have a high incidence of multivessel and left main coronary artery disease. This pattern of unstable angina is seen in about 50% of individuals presenting with unstable angina, and this population has a high incidence of severe multivessel coronary disease. Double- or triple-vessel coronary artery disease will be found in approximately 60%, left main stenoses will be seen in more than 20%, while single-vessel disease is seen in about 10% (4). By contrast, when coronary angiography is carried out in the subset of patients where unstable angina is the first clinical manifestation of coronary artery disease (new-onset angina), a different distribution of coronary artery disease is found (4,5). In this setting, fully 50% of patients will have single-vessel coronary artery disease, and in the majority of these cases the left anterior descending coronary is the involved vessel. Therefore, this clinical distinction has important management implications in terms of assessing patients as potential candidates

Table 1 Extent of Coronary Artery Disease Assessed by Arteriography

Coronary artery disease	Group 1: angina of recent onset, N = 84, N(%)	Group 2: crescendo angina, N = 134, N(%)
Left main	6(7)	28(21)
Triple-vessel	16(19)	56(42)
Double-vessel	19(23)	25(19)
Single-vessel	35(42)	15(11)
No or minimal disease	8(9)	10(7)

Source: Ref. 4 with permission.

for revascularization procedures. The patient with new-onset angina is much more likely to have disease amenable to percutaneous transluminal angioplasty, whereas the patient with crescendo angina is more likely to require coronary artery bypass surgery.

In approximately 5–10% of patients with the clinical diagnosis of unstable angina, angiography will reveal normal coronary anatomy (1–5). In some of these patients the diagnosis of angina pectoris is incorrect, while in the remainder coronary spasm or abnormalities of the intramyocardial vascular bed represent the cause of ischemic episodes.

Morphology of Coronary Stenoses and Unstable Angina

In 1980 De Wood et al. provided definitive evidence that total coronary occlusion by thrombus was present in the vast majority of patients in the early hours after acute myocardial infarction (6). This pivotal investigation provided confirmation of the important role of coronary thrombosis in the pathogenesis of acute myocardial infarction, a finding which has now been confirmed by several pathologic angiographic, and angioscopic studies. Shortly thereafter, attention was focused on the clinical syndrome of unstable angina, and it was soon recognized that coronary thrombosis also played an important role in the pathogenesis of this disorder.

Previous pathologic investigations had suggested that coronary thrombosis was commonly associated with underlying complicated atherosclerotic plaque (7,8). In 1982, Levin and Fallon first compared the post-mortem angiographic morphology of coronary stenoses with histologic findings in a group of patients who had died from complications of a myocardial infarction or coronary artery bypass surgery (9). These authors found that coronary stenoses could be divided into two different types based on their angiographic morphology. Type I stenoses manifested smooth borders, were generally concentric with an hourglass configuration, and were not associated with intraluminal lucencies. Histologic sections of these lesions revealed uncomplicated stenoses with fatty or fibrous plaques, intact intimal surfaces, and no superimposed thrombus (Fig. 1). Angiographically, type II lesions demonstrated irregular borders and/or intraluminal lucencies. Histologic findings in these cases were very different, revealing complicated atherosclerotic lesions with evidence of plaque rupture, plaque hemorrhage, superimposed partially occluding thrombus, or recanalized occlusive thrombus (Fig. 2). This investigation served to emphasize that there were qualitative differences in the angiographic appearance of coronary stenoses which might have important clinical and prognostic implications.

In 1985, Ambrose and colleagues first reported the clinical correlates of these qualitative differences in the angiographic appearance of coronary stenoses (10). They demonstrated that patients with stable angina generally had uncomplicated coronary stenoses that were concentric with smooth luminal borders (Fig. 3), or

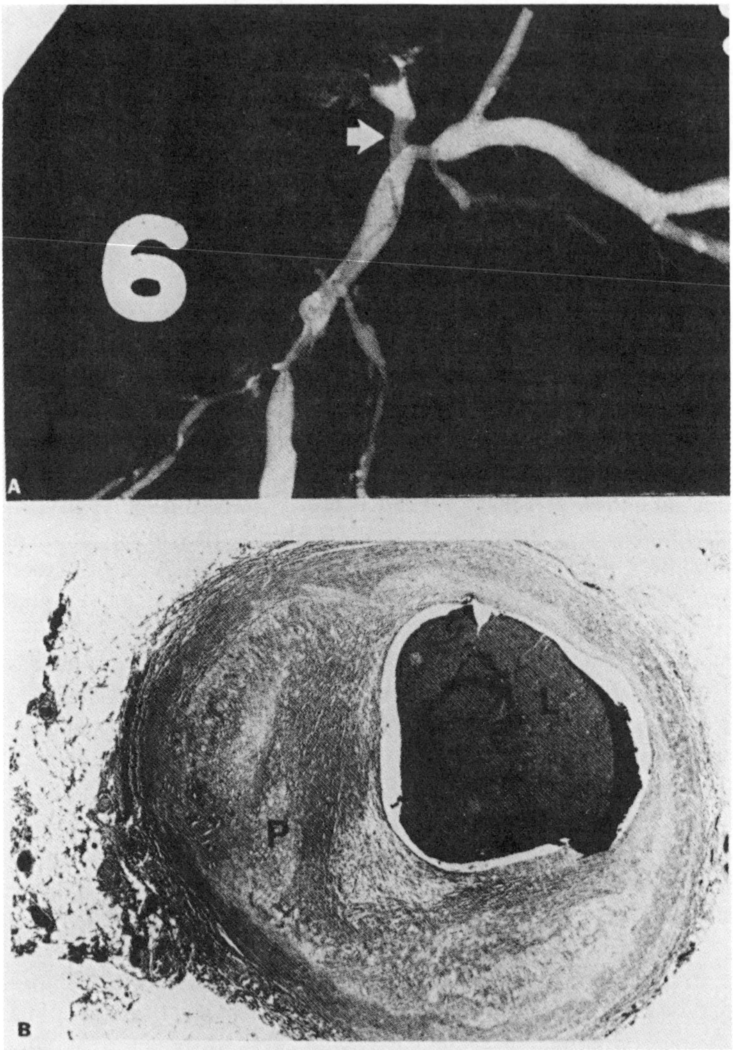

Figure 1 (A) Post-mortem angiogram of a type 1 stenosis of the left main coronary artery (arrow). There is an hourglass narrowing with smooth borders and no intraluminal filling defects. (B) The corresponding histologic section reveals an eccentric lumen (L) resulting from the presence of fibrous, fatty, atherosclerotic plaque (P) and is typical of uncomplicated lesions. Hematoxylin-eosin stain, original magnification X30. (From Ref. 9 with permission.)

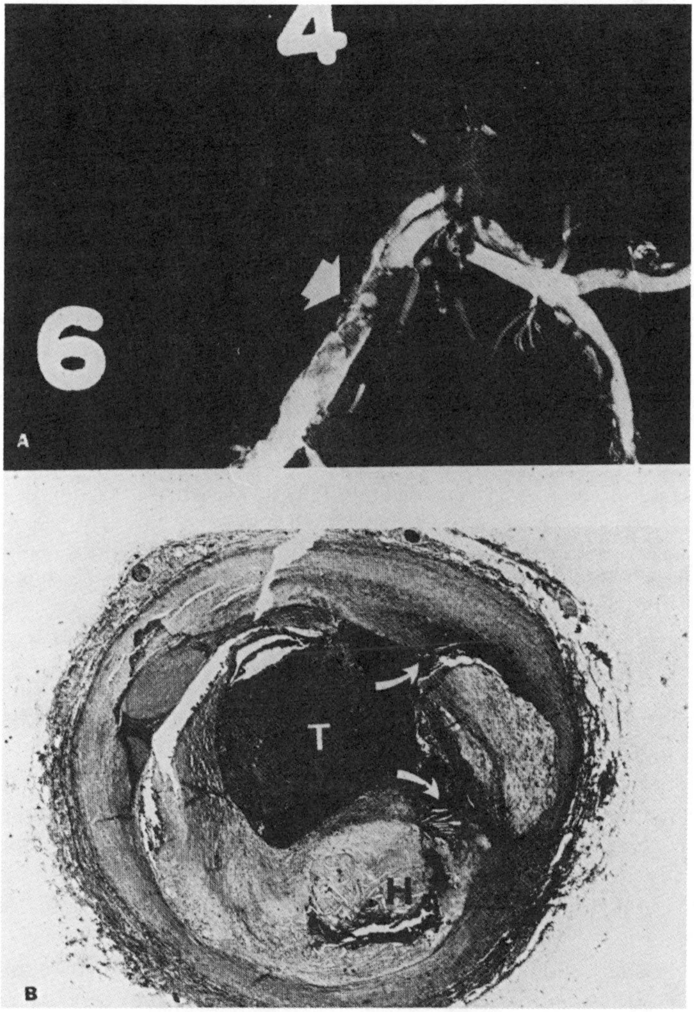

Figure 2 (A) Post-mortem angiogram of a type II stenosis of the proximal left anterior descending artery (arrow). The borders of the lesion are markedly irregular and there are numerous intraluminal lucencies in the area distal to the narrowing. (B) The corresponding histologic section shows a complicated atherosclerotic plaque with plaque rupture (arrows), intraplaque hemorrhage (H), and an intraluminal thrombus (T) that occludes the lumen almost totally. Hematoxylin-eosin stain, original magnification X30. (From Ref. 9 with permission.)

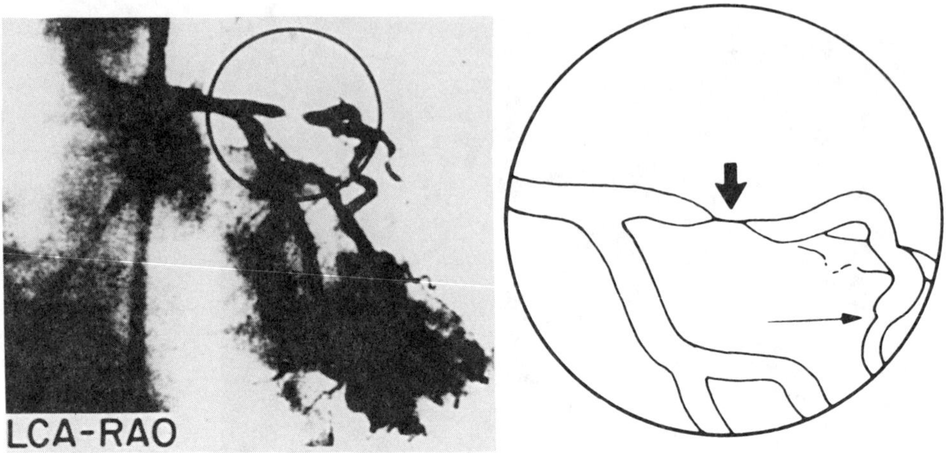

Figure 3 Representative left coronary angiogram (LCA) and schematic diagram of a concentric coronary stenosis. There is a severe stenosis of the proximal left anterior descending artery as seen in the right anterior oblique (RAO) projection. The **thick arrow** indicates the concentric lesion; the **thin arrow** indicates the distal left anterior descending artery. (From Ref. 10 with permission.)

eccentric, with a broad base and a smooth lumen (type I eccentric lesions, [Fig. 4]). Conversely, patients with unstable angina more often had stenoses which had a complex angiographic appearance. Such complex stenoses were usually eccentric and characterized by a narrow neck, overhanging edges, and irregular borders (type II eccentric lesions [Table 2, fig. 5]). Although this investigation did not specifically address the incidence of coronary thrombus in unstable angina, the authors did postulate that the type II eccentric lesion might represent the angiographic correlate of the ruptured, complicated atherosclerotic plaque as described by Levin and Fallon (9). The authors also suggested that such "complications" of previously stable atherosclerotic lesions might be a common cause of progression of coronary artery disease, which had previously been documented to occur in unstable angina (11). Several other investigations have now confirmed that patients with unstable angina have a higher incidence of coronary stenoses which display complex angiographic morphology (12–14).

Using quantitative angiography, Wilson et al. objectively characterized the qualitative differences in stenoses which had been described by Ambrose and colleagues (15). An ulceration index was developed by measuring serial arterial diameters within each lesion using computerized quantitative angiographic techniques. The ulceration index of coronary stenoses in patients with unstable angina was significantly different from that seen in lesions observed in patients

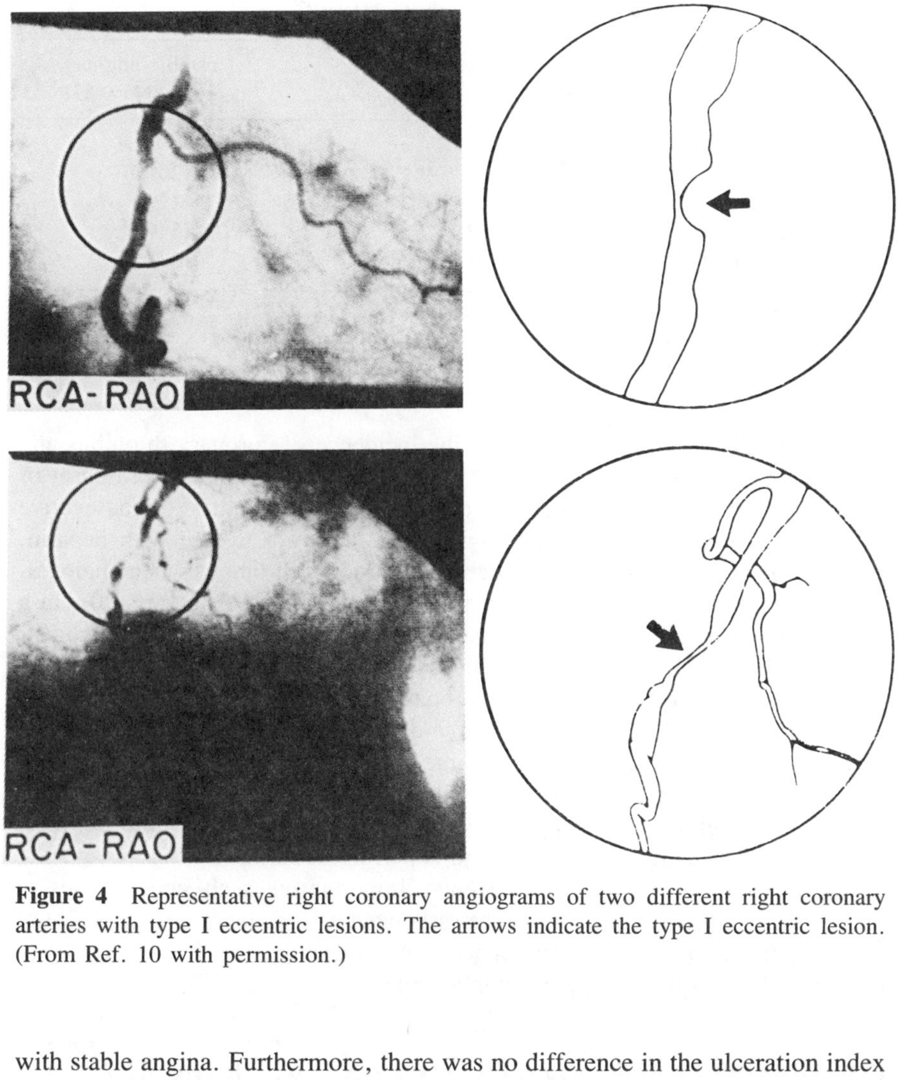

Figure 4 Representative right coronary angiograms of two different right coronary arteries with type I eccentric lesions. The arrows indicate the type I eccentric lesion. (From Ref. 10 with permission.)

with stable angina. Furthermore, there was no difference in the ulceration index found in vessels causing unstable angina when compared to that found in residual stenoses of infarct-related arteries in patients who had undergone successful thrombolysis for acute myocardial infarction.

The relationship between coronary thrombus formation and unstable angina has been demonstrated in several investigations. A review of previous angiographic studies reveals a wide variation in the detection rate of intracoronary thrombi with the incidence ranging from 6 to 52% (16–19). In the majority of cases thrombus is associated with stenoses characterized by complex angiograph-

Table 2 Angiographic Morphology of Coronary Artery Obstructions

	Stable angina pectoris (N = 47)	Unstable angina pectoris (N = 63)
No. of vessels	55	92
Concentric	26(47%)**	24(26%)
Type I eccentric	19(35%)*	16(17%)
Type II eccentric	4(7%)	50(54%)***
Multiple irregularities	6(11%)*	2(2%)

*$p < 0.05$; **$p < 0.01$; ***$p < 0.001$ by student's *t*-test.
Source: Ref. 10 with permission.

ic morphology. The large variation in the incidence of coronary thrombus and unstable angina most likely represents the variable time interval from onset of symptoms to the time of angiography (14). In a prospective trial of consecutive patients presenting with unstable angina who were not treated with heparin, Williams et al. reported a 27% incidence of coronary thrombus when angiography was carried out a mean of 5 days after the onset of symptoms (20). In a second investigation from the same institution (14), a high incidence of coronary thrombus was found in patients with intractable, rest angina, and also the presence of coronary thrombus and coronary stenoses of complex morphology were both found to be strongly predictive of in-hospital cardiac events (defined as death, myocardial infarction, and the need for urgent revascularization). Although this represents the only prospective analysis of the clinical implications of complex angiographic morphology, it does confirm the common clinical observation that complex stenoses with superimposed thrombus are frequently associated with adverse clinical events. Importantly, such complex lesion morphology has also been shown to be associated with an increased incidence of acute complications during percutaneous balloon angioplasty, creating a dilemma with obvious managment implications.

CARDIAC CATHETERIZATION IN UNSTABLE ANGINA

Some cardiologists believe that the patient with unstable angina who responds well to medical therapy does not require routine cardiac catheterization. These physicians maintain that catheterization should only be carried out in the patient who has continued symptoms despite adequate medical therapy or if noninvasive assessments suggest the presence of left main or severe, three-vessel coronary artery disease. However, it is standard practice in many centers, including our own, to catheterize most patients with unstable angina prior to their discharge

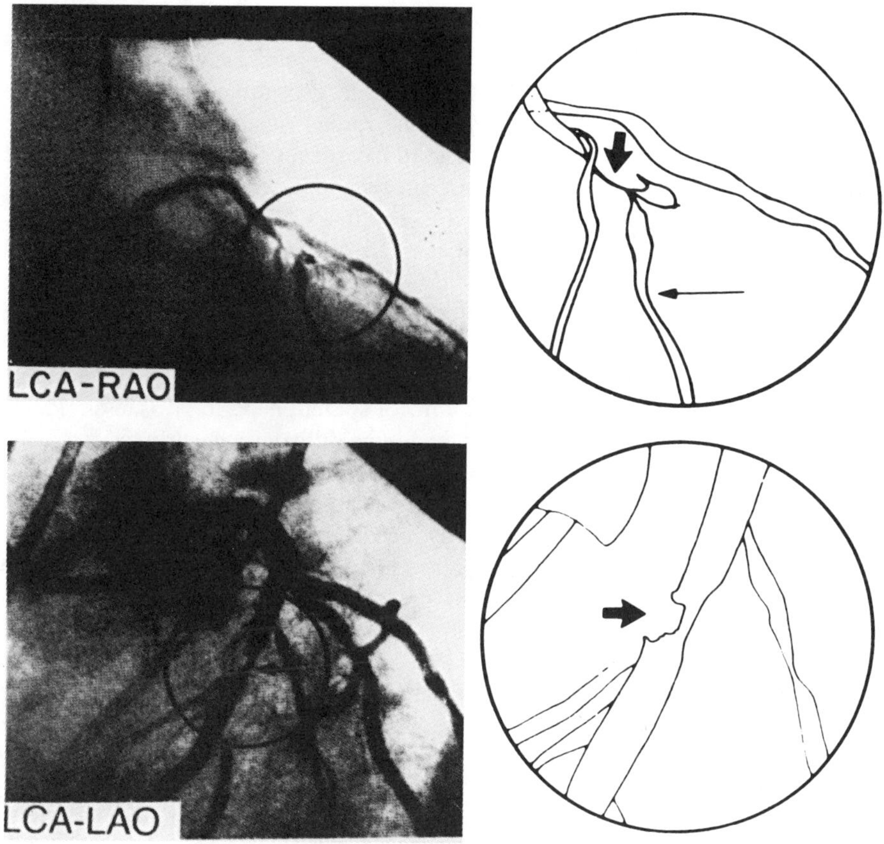

Figure 5 Representative left coronary angiograms (LCA) and schematic diagrams of two different left anterior descending arteries with type II eccentric lesions. The **thick arrows** indicate the lesions; the **thin arrow** indicates the distal left anterior descending artery. LAO = left anterior oblique projection; RAO = right anterior oblique projection. (From Ref. 10 with permission.)

from hospital, unless there are obvious contraindications to possible angioplasty or bypass surgery. This approach provides the consultant with knowledge of the coronary anatomy and left ventricular function early on in the course of unstable angina. In turn, this allows for more definitive risk stratification of the patient, thus guiding the therapeutic approach. Patients with left main coronary artery disease and severe three-vessel coronary artery disease will be identified and arrangements can be made for urgent or semiurgent coronary artery bypass surgery. Patients with discrete single- or double-vessel coronary disease, who are candidates for percutaneous transluminal angioplasty, will also be identified. A small number of patients with no obstructive coronary disease will be found, who may or may not have spasm identified with an ergonovine challenge. These patients have an excellent prognosis, and no further investigation is necessary. Finally, occasional patients will be found to have severe, diffuse distal coronary artery disease which is unsuitable for either angioplasty or bypass grafting.

The patient with unstable angina who continues to have symptoms despite medical management requires urgent cardiac catheterization. It is extremely important to optimize ongoing medical therapy in preparation for cardiac catheterization. The angiographic procedure has the potential to precipitate ischemia along with hemodynamic compromise, and thus attention to optimal stabilization of the patient cannot be overemphasized. Patients with unstable angina should generally receive 5000 units of sodium heparin prior to angiography. In those very unstable patients receiving full dose heparin prior to the procedure, the infusion should not be discontinued but should be maintained up to the time of catheterization. Judicious use of sedation is important, as is attention to signs of heart failure or rhythm disturbance. If there are multiple, recurring episodes of pain despite aggresive therapy, or if there there is evidence of hemodynamic instability, it is our practice to initiate intra-aortic balloon counterpulsation prior to catheterization. This usually allows the patient to be stabilized and minimizes the risk of further ischemia or hemodynamic compromise during the catheterization. Obviously the decision to insert an intra-aortic balloon pump (IABP) prior to angiography must be individualized. However, in general, if evidence of ongoing ischemia cannot be reversed prior to proceeding with catheterization, IABP insertion is warranted.

Once the patient has been stabilized, left heart catheterization can usually be carried out safely. Although either the brachial or femoral approach can be used, the femoral approach offers the advantages of immediate vascular access for intra-aortic balloon counterpulsation and technical ease in the performance of percutaneous transluminal balloon angioplasty. The disadvantage of this approach is the relative lack of control afforded by preformed catheters, which may be detrimental in the setting of critical left main stenoses. If there has been any evidence of either congestive heart failure or hemodynamic compromise, right heart catheterization should be performed prior to angiography, thus allowing cardiac filling pressures to be optimized and monitored throughout the procedure. Since ionic contrast agents can cause both negative inotropic and lusitropic myocardial effects, bradycardia, prolongation of the QT interval, and significant systemic hypotension, we generally use nonionic contrast media in the very unstable patient. In comparison with standard ionic and high-osmolar contrast agents, the newer agents have significantly fewer electrical and myocardial depressant effects (21). Regardless of the type of contrast material employed, it is important to limit both the number and amount of contrast injections in an effort to prevent provocation of further ischemia. If selective coronary angiography is completed and the patient remains pain-free, then left ventriculography can also be performed safely. However, if coronary angiography reveals important disease of the left main coronary artery or if there is evidence of ongoing ischemia, then left ventriculography should be avoided and ventricular function can be assessed using two-dimensional echocardiography. Finally, it is important to recognize that management of the unstable patient does not stop with the completion of a coronary angiogram. Although patients who have been very unstable will generally respond to intra-aortic balloon counterpulsation, they still require definitive therapy. Thus decisions must be made concerning the need for bypass surgery of percutaneous transluminal angioplasty soon after angiography has been completed. It is the responsibility of the angiographer to ensure that the appropriate communication is undertaken and that prompt decisions concerning further management are made.

Complications of Cardiac Catheterization in Unstable Angina

Large prospective studies of the complications of cardiac catheterization have been reported by the CASS investigators and the Society for Cardiac Angiography (22,23). The overall complication rate in these investigations was approximately 1.8%, with an incidence of myocardial infarction and procedure related mortality of approximately 0.2% and 0.1%, respectively. The presence of unstable angina represents an independent risk factor for procedure-related myocardial infarction and mortality. Other important risk factors for myocardial infarction and death as a consequence of cardiac catheterization include left main and multivessel coronary artery disease, left ventricular dysfunction, and recent myocardial infarction.

Significant left main coronary stenosis represents a particularly important risk factor for death as a consequence of cardiac catheterization. Previous reports have suggested that left main coronary artery stenosis carries a procedure-related mortality rate of up to 15% (24,25). Although present-day mortality rates do not appear to be this high, left main stenosis was associated with a death rate several times higher than the overall mortality rate in the report of the Society for Cardiac Angiography (23). Furthermore, the presence of left main stenosis in the setting of unstable angina appears to place the patients at an even greater risk of both death and procedure-related myocardial infarction.

INTRA-AORTIC BALLOON COUNTERPULSATION IN UNSTABLE ANGINA

Intra-aortic balloon counterpulsation is an effective method for the management of ischemia in patients with unstable angina (27). Importantly, this procedure carries the risk of serious morbidity and thus its indications need to be clearly defined.

The IABP was first introduced in 1967 as a method of providing circulatory assistance for patients suffering from cardiogenic shock (28). Initially, both insertion and removal of the balloon required surgical cutdown on the femoral artery. By 1979, percutaneous insertion techniques had been developed, allowing the balloon to be introduced at the bedside or in the catheterization laboratory (29). This advance led to broader use of the IABP and its common application by the cardiologist. As use of the IABP increased, so did reports concerning its complications. An understanding of the nature and frequency of such complications, and the patients most likely to suffer them, is an important component of the decision to use the IABP in any given clinical situation.

A wide variety of complications of the IABP have been reported (28–33). The majority of these complications are vascular and include bleeding, hematoma formation, pseudoaneurysm development, arteriovenous fistulae, aortic dissection, embolic phenomena (both thrombotic and atheromatous), along with visceral and extremity ischemia. Infectious complications are not uncommon and include both local wound infections and systemic sepsis. Neurologic complications include ischemic neuritis, spinal cord ischemia, and cerebral embolic phenomena, all of which are quite uncommon. Although many of these complications are reversible following balloon removal and appropriate therapy, they are occasionally fatal (particularly in the case of aortic dissection) or lead to extremity amputation. The complication rate associated with IABP insertion varies widely in the literature. In some small series no complications are reported (29), whereas in others complication rates approaching 50% have been described (32). An analysis of most trials would suggest that significant complications occur in 10–20% of cases (27–33). Vascular complications account for most of the serious morbidity with the need for vascular surgery reported to be approximately 3–4% and a requirement for amputation in about 1%. Aortic dissection appears to occur in less than 1% of patients, but it is the most common cause of death directly attributable to balloon insertion. Most trials reporting the complication rates of IABP insertion reviewed the clinical experience with this technique more than 10 years ago. At that time there was a suggestion that the percutaneous insertion technique was associated with a higher rate of vascular complications than the surgical approach to balloon placement (31). At the present time the surgical approach is only rarely applied, and it is likely that the complication rate of the percutaneous technique is lower than it was 10 years ago. Nevertheless, it is clear that certain patients are at extremely high risk of vascular complications. This is particularly true of female patients undergoing IABP insertion, where it seems that the smaller caliber of the ileofemoral system leads to a much higher risk of vascular trauma and subsequent extremity ischemia (31,32). The presence of peripheral vascular disease also presents a major risk for subsequent vascular complications (31,32). Peripheral vascular disease is the most common cause of primary balloon insertion failure, which is reported to occur in 5–10% of patients in most series. Importantly, balloon insertion failure itself is frequently associated with vascular complications. A history of diabetes or hypertension have also been demonstrated to be independent risk factors for IABP complications (32). Interestingly, age has not been found to be an independent risk factor for IABP complications (31,32).

There has never been a randomized trial of the efficacy of intra-aortic balloon counterpulsation in the setting of unstable angina. Although there is general agreement that the IABP is extremely effective in the management of certain patients with unstable ischemic syndromes, the substantial complication rate must always be kept in mind when making the decision to proceed with balloon insertion. The following clinical situations represent circumstances where most physicians involved in cardiovascular care would consider IABP insertion appropriate.

1. The patient with unstable angina who has symptoms which are refractory to medical management may be considered a candidate for coronary artery bypass surgery or percutaneous transluminal angioplasty. In patients who have not yet been catheterized, the IABP is effective in relieving ischemia and in facilitating emergency angiography. For those in whom ischemia recurs following diagnostic catheterization , the IABP will relieve ischemia and provide hemodynamic stability while arrangements are made for coronary artery bypass surgery or percutaneous transluminal angioplasty.
2. The patient with a recent history of unstable angina who is found at diagnostic catheterization to have severe left main coronary artery disease is at high risk for myocardial infarction and death. These patients are best served by urgent surgery, however, at many centers prophylactic IABP insertion is carried out. This approach is mandatory if the catheterization is complicated by further ischemia and if immediate surgery is not logistically feasible.
3. Finally, prophylactic insertion of an IABP is advocated by many surgeons prior to cardiac surgery in the patient with unstable angina complicated by severe left ventricular dysfunction. This approach is felt to optimize perfusion to viable myocardium during the immediate preoperative period and reduce the risk of acute pump failure.

SUMMARY

Modern management of unstable angina can provide prompt and effective relief of ischemic symptoms in the majority of patients. Medical, surgical, and percutaneous transluminal approaches have improved significantly over the past decade, providing the physician with a number of therapeutic options. Cardiac catheterization can be performed safely in the majority of patients with unstable ischemic syndromes and provides important diagnostic, prognostic, and therapeutic information. Although intra-aortic balloon counterpulsation carries the risk of serious morbidity, in the appropriately selected patient it can provide effective relief and/or prophylaxis of ischemia.

REFERENCES

1. Alison HW, Russell RO, Mantle JA, Kouchoukos NT, Moraski RE, Rackley CE. Coronary anatomy and arteriography in patients with unstable angina pectoris. Am J Cardiol 1978; 41:204–9.
2. Conti CR, Brawley RK, Griffith LSC, Pitt B, O'Neal Humphries J, Gott VL, Ross RS. Unstable angina pectoris: morbidity and mortality in 57 consecutive patients evaluated angiographically. Am J Cardiol 1973; 32:745–50.
3. Ouyang P, Brinker JA, Mellits ED, Weisfeldt ML, Gerstenblith G. Variables predictive of successful medical therapy in patients with unstable angina: selection by multivariate analysis from clinical, electrocardiographic, and angiographic evaluations. Circulation 1984; 70:367–76.
4. Plotnick GD, Fisher ML, Carliner NH, Becker LC. Cardiac catheterization in patients with unstable angina. Recent onset vs crescendo pattern. JAMA 1980; 244:574–6.
5. Victor MF, Likoff MJ, Mintz GS, Likoff W. Unstable angina pectoris of new onset: a prospective clinical and arteriographic study of 75 patients. Am J Cardiol 1981; 47:228–32.
6. DeWood MA, Spores J, Notske R, Mouses LT, Burroughs R, Golden MS, Lang HT. Prevalence of total coronary occlusion during the early hours after transmural myocardial infarction. N Engl J Med 1980; 303:897–902.
7. Friedman M, Van den Bovenkamp GJ. Pathogenesis of a coronary thrombus. Am J Pathol 1966; 48:19–44.
8. Chandler AB. Mechanisms and frequency of thrombosis in the coronary circulation. Thrombus Res 1974; 4(Supp 1):3–23
9. Levin DC, Fallon JT. Significance of the angiographic morphology of localized coronary stenoses: histopathologic correlations. Circulation 1982; 66:316–20.
10. Ambrose JA, Winters SL, Stern A, Eng A, Teichholz LE, Gorlin R, Fuster V. Angiographic morphology and the pathogenesis of unstable angina pectoris. J Am Coll Cardiol 1985; 5:609–16.
11. Moise A, Theroux P, Taeymans Y, Descoings B, Lesperance J, Waters DD, Pelletier GB, Bourassa MG. Unstable angina and progression of coronary atherosclerosis. N Engl J Med 1983; 309:685–9.
12. Rehr R, Disciascio G, Vetrovec G, Cowley M. Angiographic morphology of coronary artery stenoses in prolonged rest angina: evidence of intracoronary thrombosis. J Am Coll Cardiol 1989; 14:1429–37.
13. Ambrose JA, Winters SL, Arora RR, Eng A, Riccio A, Gorlin R, Fuster V. Angiographic evolution of coronary artery morphology in unstable angina. J Am Coll Cardiol 1986; 7:472–8.

14. Freeman MR, Williams AE, Chisholm RJ, Armstrong PW. Intracoronary thrombus and complex morphology in unstable angina. Circulation 1989; 80:17–23.
15. Wilson RF, Holida MD, White CW. Quantitative angiographic morphology of coronary stenoses leading to myocardial infarction or unstable angina. Circulation 1986; 73:286–93.
16. Zack PM, Ischinger T, Aker UT, Dincer B, Kennedy HL: The occurrence of angiographically detected intracoronary thrombus in patients with unstable angina pectoris. Am Heart J 1984; 108:1408–12.
17. Bresnahan DR, Davis JL, Holmes DR, Smith HC. Angiographic occurrence and clinical correlates of intraluminal coronary artery thrombus: role of unstable angina. J Am Coll Cardiol 1985; 6:285–9.
18. Vetrovec GW, Cowley MJ, Overton H, Richardson DW. Intracoronary thrombus in syndromes of unstable myocardial ischemia. Am Heart J 1981; 102:1202–8.
19. Capone GJ, Nelson W, Meyer B, Meister SG. Frequency of filling defects by angiography in angina pectoris at rest. Am J Cardiol 1985; 56:403–6.
20. Williams AE, Freeman MR, Chisholm RJ, Patt NL, Armstrong PW. Angiographic morphology in unstable angina pectoris. Am J Cardiol 1988; 62:1024–7.
21. Gertz EW, Wisnewski JA, Chiu D, Akin JR, Hu C. Clinical superiority of a new nonionic contrast agent (iopamidol) for cardiac angiography. J Am Coll Cardiol 1985; 5:250–8.
22. Davis K, Kennedy JW, Kemp HG Jr, Judkins MP, Gosselin AJ, Killip T. Complications of coronary arteriography from the collaborative study of coronary artery surgery (CASS) Circulation 1979; 59:1105–12.
23. Kennedy JW, Registry Committee of the Society for Cardiac Angiography. Complications associated with cardiac catheterization and angiography. Cathet Cardiovasc Diagn 1982; 8:5–11.
24. Wolfson S, Grant D, Ross AM, Cohen LS. Risk of death related to coronary arteriography: role of left coronary arterial lesions. Am J Cardiol 1976; 37:210–16.
25. Bourassa MG, Noble J. Complication rate of coronary arteriography: a review of 5250 cases studied by percutaneous femoral technique. Circulation 1976; 53:106–14.
26. Cohen MV, Cohn PF, Hermann MV, Gorlin R. Diagnosis and prognosis of left main coronary artery obstruction. Circulation 1972; 46(Supp 1):57–65.
27. Gold HK, Leinbach RC, Sanders CA, Buckley MJ, Mundth ED, Austen WG. Intra-aortic balloon pumping for control of recurrent myocardial ischemia. Circulation 1973; 47:1197–203.
28. Kantrowitz A, Tjonneland, Freed PS, Phillips SJ, Butner AN, Sherman JL. Initial clinical experience with intraaortic balloon pumping in cardiogenic shock. JAMA 1968; 203:113–18.
29. Bregman D, Nichols AB, Weiss MB, Powers ER, Martin EC, Casarella WJ. Percutaneous intraaortic balloon insertion. Am J Cardiol 1980; 46:261–4.
30. Weintraub RM, Aroesty JM, Paulin S, Levine FH, Markis JE, LaRaia PJ, Cohen SI, Kurland GF. Medically refractory unstable angina pectoris. 1. Long-term follow-up of patients undergoing intra-aortic balloon counterpulsion and operation. Am J Cardiol 1979; 43:877–82.

31. Gottlieb SO, Brinker JA, Borkon AM, Kallman CH, Potter A, Gott VL, Baughman KL. Identification of patients at high risk for complications of intraaortic balloon counterpulsation: a multivariate risk factor analysis. Am J Cardiol 1984; 53:1135–9.
32. Kantrowitz A, Wasfie T, Freed PS, Rubenfire M, Wajszczuk W, Schork MA. Intraaortic balloon pumping/1967 through 1982: analysis of complications in 733 patients. Am J Cardiol 1986; 57:976–83.
33. Goldberger M, Tabak SW, Shah PK. Clinical experience with intra-aortic balloon counterpulsation in 112 consecutive patients. Am Heart J 1985; 111:497–502.

7

Holter Monitoring of ST-Segment Activity

Peter H. Stone

Brigham and Women's Hospital and Harvard Medical School
Boston, Massachusetts

INTRODUCTION

The pathophysiologic process of myocardial ischemia includes a cascade of manifestations which occur in a generally predictable sequence: shifting of metabolic substrates for energy metabolism, prolonged myocardial relaxation, impaired myocardial contraction, ST-segment deviation, and ultimately, but not necessarily, the perception of ischemic pain or angina pectoris. Methods exist to assess each of these metabolic or hemodynamic disturbances, such as position emission tomography, high fidelity intracardiac pressure recording, or radionuclide or contrast left ventriculography, but these techniques are not suitable for prolonged monitoring to identify the high risk patient with an acute ischemic syndrome, nor are they appropriate to detect the presence of clinical instability or intermittent ischemic jeopardy. Use of the patient's perception of continued anginal symptoms, associated with reversible ST-segment deviation, as a gauge to reflect the presence of ongoing ischemia has been the traditional means to guide the urgency of escalating medical or revascularization therapy (1,2), but symptoms alone may not provide a sufficiently accurate index of disease activity.

In recent years, prolonged ambulatory ECG (AECG or Holter) monitoring for periods of 24 to 72 hours has been used to evaluate the presence of ischemia in a variety of syndromes of coronary disease and has revealed that episodes of reversible ST-segment deviation are common in all clinical syndromes of coronary disease (stable coronary disease, unstable angina, Prinzmental's variant angina, and the early convalescent phase following a myocardial infarction) and that the majority of ischemic episodes identified by AECG monitoring are asymptomatic or "silent" (3,4). Confirmation that these episodes of ST-segment deviation represent true episodes of ischemia, and not ECG artifacts, is substantiated by studies correlating reversible ST-segment deviation with reversible filling defects using radionuclide perfusion imaging (5,6), transient elevations of intracardiac filling pressures (7), and transient wall motion abnormalities using ambulatory radionuclide ventriculography (8,9). If episodes of recurrent asymptomatic ischemia are present in patients with unstable angina and are associated with an adverse cardiac prognosis, then perhaps their presence should be specifically sought with AECG monitoring and the results of such monitoring should be used to help guide management decisions. The purpose of this chapter is to review the use of AECG monitoring in patients with unstable angina pectoris to determine its value and role in the diagnosis and management of this acute ischemic syndrome.

INCIDENCE OF ST-SEGMENT DEVIATION IN PATIENTS WITH UNSTABLE ANGINA

Based on the presence of anginal symptoms alone, early experience treating unstable angina with bed rest, supplemental oxygen, nitrate preparations, and beta-adrenergic blockers indicated that more than 95% of patients became symptom-free with an aggressive medical regimen (10). Symptom control was even further improved with the addition of a calcium channel blocker, particularly nifedipine, to the medical regimen (11–13). With the advent of AECG monitoring in the early and mid-1980s, however, it became clear that a large number of patients exhibited refractory episodes of asymptomatic or silent ischemia, which persisted despite adequate control of symptoms with an intense medical regimen (Table 1). Although the medical regimens and the timing of initiation of AECG monitoring were not uniform in these small studies, it is remarkable that in the era of treatment with a combination regimen of nitrates, beta-blockers, and calcium channel blockers, approximately 50–70% of patients exhibited transient episodes of asymptomatic ST-segment deviation (Table 1). In recent years the incidence of episodes of asymptomatic ischemia has been dramatically reduced since heparin and aspirin have become routinely added to the previous regimens (22–24) (Table 1), reflecting the fact, discussed in greater detail below, that unstable angina is often due to a ruptured intracoronary plaque and consequent formation of a subtotally occlusive thrombus. Although all of the studies involving full heparinization and aspirin utilize small sample sizes, and some have only been presented in abstract form (24,25), the incidence of asymptomatic ischemia is generally reported to be only approximately 4–16% in patients treated with platelet-active or antithrombotic therapy (Table 1). This reduced incidence of

Table 1 Incidence of Episodic ST-Segment Deviation in Patients with Unstable Angina

Ref.	*n*	Time Holter initiated	Duration of recording	Medication at time of recording	% Patients with episodes of ST deviation
Conventional treatment					
14	42	1st 24 hr	24	Propranolol, nitrates	59
		2nd 24 hr			57
		3rd 24 hr			72
15	88	On admission to CCU	27	Nitrates	19
16	70	On admission to CCU	48	Nitrates, BB, CCBAs	53
17	49	Hospital discharge	24	Nitrates, BB, CCBAs	59
18	88	4 days after maximal treatment	Not specified	CCBAs, nitrates, SQ low dose heparin	55
19	38	As soon as diagnosis made	60	Nitrates, CCBs, BB, IV heparin	42
20	135	6.5 hr after rest angina	24	Nitrates 59%, CCBs 59%, BB 41%, ASA 12%	66
21	232	<6 hr after admission	40	Not provided	22
Conventional treatment + heparin/ASA					
22	40	On admission	8	Nitrates, BB, CCBAs, ASA, heparin	16
23	66	<24 hr after admission	41	Nitrates, BB, CCBAs, ASA, heparin	11
24	27	Not specified	26	Heparin plus conventional therapy	4

BB = beta-blockers; CCBAs = calcium channel blocking agents; ASA = aspirin.

Table 2 Frequency Distribution of Direction of ST-Segment Deviation in Patients with Unstable Angina

Ref.	No. patients	No. patients with ST-deviation (percent of total)	Percent of patients with: ST ↓ (%)	ST ↑ (%)	ST ↓ and ↑ (%)
14	42	28 (67%)	79	14	7
19	38	16 (42%)	38	44	19
20	135	89 (66%)	62	20	18

asymptomatic ischemia by aspirin and heparin parallels the reduction in anginal symptoms observed in the same population treated with similar therapy (26).

Episodes of rest ischemia in patients with unstable angina are often due to intermittent complete occlusion of a coronary artery by thrombus, with resultant transmural ischemia (27–29) without a preceding increase in myocardial O_2 demand (30,31). Consistent with this known pathophysiology, AECG monitoring has revealed that a large number of patients with unstable angina exhibit episodes of reversible ST-segment elevation, occurring in patients either as an isolated phenomenon or co-existently with episodes of ST-segment depression (Table 2). Similar to the previous hemodynamic studies during rest angina in the coronary care unit (30,31), these asymptomatic episodes detected by AECG monitoring are generally not preceded by an important increase in heart rate (20,32) (i.e., a surrogate for myocardial O_2 demand). The distribution of direction of ST-segment deviation and the pattern of heart rate activity observed in patients with unstable angina contrasts sharply with the observations in patients with stable angina, in which the large majority of ischemic episodes are due to increases in heart rate and blood pressure (33,34) and essentially all are associated with ST-segment depression.

INFLUENCE OF TIME OF INITIATION OF AECG RECORDING ON INCIDENCE OF ASYMPTOMATIC ISCHEMIA

The hospital course of patients with unstable angina is often characterized by episodes of angina occurring either at rest or with minimal activity at the time of admission, with symptoms resolving in the majority shortly after admission following initiation of bed rest and anti-ischemia medication (10,12,26). This phenomenon of unstable symptoms early in the hospital course followed by clinical stability is mirrored in the angioscopic observations of the coronary arteries in patients with unstable angina (35): Patients with unstable angina and recent rest angina exhibit a ruptured plaque and superimposed intraluminal thrombus, while patients who have stabilized without recent rest pain exhibit a more smooth and glistening intraluminal surface without thrombus, presumably due to reendothelialization of the recent thrombus.

One would anticipate that the incidence of episodes of asymptomatic ischemia identified by continuous AECG monitoring would parallel the same pattern as observed with symptomatic episodes, with frequent episodes present on admission followed by rapid reduction of episodes once hospital therapy is progressively titrated. However, the incremental benefit of progressive escalation of anti-ischemia medication has not been systematically studied. Previous studies document that propranolol, diltiazem, nifedipine, and verapamil are each effective in reducing episodes of rest angina in patients with unstable angina, but few of the studies utilized continuous ECG monitoring or directly addressed the phenomenon of asymptomatic ischemia (3,36). In fact, as seen in Table 1, the incidence of ischemic episodes seems more dependent on the type of anti-ischemic medication used than the time of recording during hospital stay. In the era before treatment with aspirin and/or heparin, the incidence of ischemia was approximately 60% in patients monitored within the first few hours of hospitalization (14,16,20) and a very similar incidence in patients monitored many days later, at a time of medical stability or prior to hospital discharge (17,18). In contrast, the incidence of ischemic episodes appears to be only 10–15% in patients treated with aspirin and heparin (22,23). Meaningful information concerning the temporal occurrence of ischemic episodes in unstable angina is not available from these studies, however, because the number of patients studied in each investigation is small; AECG monitoring was performed only once in each study, and none of the studies performed serial monitoring; the duration of recording per patient was highly variable, and hence the detection rate of the presence of ischemia was not comparable (37); and because the heterogeneity of the diagnostic criteria of "unstable angina" may preclude generalizing the observation from one study population to the observations from another. At this time a more complete characterization of the time course of ischemic episodes in unstable angina is unknown.

ANATOMIC AND PATHOPHYSIOLOGIC CORRELATES OF ASYMPTOMATIC ISCHEMIA IN PATIENTS WITH UNSTABLE ANGINA

Since the appreciation that the clinical syndrome of unstable angina is largely due to the development of a ruptured atherosclerotic plaque and the formation of a subtotal thrombus formation (38–40), especially in those patients with recent rest angina (35), a number of investigators have explored the relationship between the incidence of asymptomatic ischemia and the angiographic extent of coronary disease and the estimation of the presence of intracoronary thrombus. Langer et al. (20) observed that 76% of patients with episodes of transient ST-segment deviation had multivessel coronary disease and 18% had left main disease, compared to 54% ($p < 0.01$) and 4% ($p < 0.05$), respectively, in the patients without such episodes. Similarly, Pozzati et al. (18) reported that the 38 patients with episodes of transient ischemia not only had more severe coronary stenoses compared to the 36 patients without such episodes (89% vs. 54% luminal diameter obstruction, $p < 0.0001$), but also more frequently exhibited complex lesion morphology characterized by an overhanging edge or irregular lesion borders (79% vs. 28%, $p < 0.001$). Langer and colleagues (41) further evaluated their 135 patients with unstable angina (and rest angina) who underwent 24-hour AECG within a mean of 6.5 hours of their qualifying episode of angina and coronary angiography (performed a mean 4.2 days after admission) and observed that the 86 patients with angiographic evidence of thrombus had more frequent and severe persisting episodes of ischemia compared to the 49 patients without thrombus. Episodes of transient ST-segment deviation were found in 80% of patients with thrombus compared to 58% of those without thrombus ($p < 0.025$); the frequency of ischemic episodes were greater in those with thrombus (6.1 vs. 3.5, $p < 0.01$); and the cumulative duration of ischemia was longer (110 vs. 60 minutes, $p < 0.05$). Of those patients who had episodes of ischemia by AECG monitoring, there was no difference in the frequency of asymptomatic vs. symptomatic episodes (92% in those with thrombus and 93% of those without thrombus, pNS), nor in the magnitude of ST-segment deviation (1.8 vs. 1.7 mm, pNS).

The importance of the pathophysiologic role of intracoronary thrombus in unstable angina is underscored by the more recent studies of AECG monitoring in which aspirin or heparin is included in the anti-ischemia regimen, as noted above (Table 1). Furthermore, a recent report confirms the dramatic effect of heparin on the incidence of documented refractory episodes of asymptomatic ischemia. Serneri and coworkers (42) randomized 97 patients with either ≥3 episodes of reversible ST-segment deviation or 1 anginal attack lasting ≥20 minutes despite isosorbide dinitrate, nifedipine, and metoprolol to a variety of anticoagulant or antithrombotic regimens: heparin infusion ($n = 21$), heparin by intermittent bolus ($n = 18$), aspirin 325 mg/day ($n = 19$), and t-PA infusion (1.75 mg/kg) followed by heparin and aspirin ($n = 20$). They observed that the heparin infusion reduced episodes of angina 94% ($p < 0.001$), asymptomatic ischemia by 71% ($p < 0.001$), total ischemic episodes by 78% ($p < 0.001$), and total ischemic duration by 81% ($p < 0.001$). In contrast, they found that the heparin administered as an intermittent bolus, aspirin, and t-PA had nonsignificant reduction in these endpoints. Wallis et al. (25), however, noted in a preliminary report that the incidence of transient ischemia was similar in 20 patients treated with a continuous administration of heparin to increase the activated PTT to 2× control compared to 26 patients similarly treated but without heparin. Theroux and coworkers have not reported the results of AECG monitoring, but noted that either aspirin, heparin, or the combination dramatically reduced the episodes of angina compared to placebo (26). In a very small number of patients, Nicklas and coauthors (22) also observed in a randomized clinical trial of t-PA (150 mg/8 hr) vs. placebo in 40 patients with rest angina that 4 patients assigned to t-PA had transient ischemic episodes prior to administration of the study drug and none had episodes after receiving the drug, whereas the one patient assigned to placebo who had episodes of ischemia before the study drug continued to have episodes after the infusion.

Most of the previous studies are extremely limited by utilization of small sample size, heterogeneity of diagnostic criteria of "unstable angina," and insufficient data concerning clinical, angiographic, and AECG characteristics. Two large, ongoing, multicenter clinical trials (Thrombolysis in Myocardial Ischemia [T3] and tPA in Unstable Angina Study [UNSA]) will be utilizing AECG monitoring in a total of almost 3000 patients with unstable angina and non–Q-wave myocardial infarction to more completely investigate the relationships between clinical, angiographic, and AECG characteristics, and to determine the clinical significance of asymptomatic ischemic events.

PROGNOSTIC SIGNIFICANCE OF THE PRESENCE OF EPISODES OF TRANSIENT ISCHEMIA

From the earliest description of the presence of episodes of asymptomatic ischemia, their adverse prognostic significance has been appreciated (Table 3). Although episodes of symptomatic ischemia (angina) frequently coexist in patients who manifest episodes of asymptomatic ischemia, the episodes of asymptomatic ischemia occur many times more frequently than the episodes of angina (16,17,19,20,23,42) and hence provide a more powerful and discriminating gauge to assess ongoing ischemia and, consequently, cardiac risk. Some studies suggest that the episodes of asymptomatic ischemia are less severe than the episodes of symptomatic ischemia, as evidenced by a shorter duration of ischemia and a smaller magnitude of ST-segment deviation (20). Nevertheless, in a 2-year follow-up of 70 patients with unstable angina, Gottlieb and colleagues (43) found that asymptomatic ischemia detected by AECG monitoring was the most important ($p < 0.001$) predictor of an unfavorable outcome (death, infarction, or need for revascularization), followed by the presence of chest pain occurring during the initial 2 study days ($p < 0.01$). The relative risk for an unfavorable outcome was 5 if asymptomatic ischemia was detected, 3 if chest pain was reported, and 15 if both variables were present (Fig. 1). No other demographic, clinical, or anatomic variables were found to be significant predictors of an adverse 2-year outcome in the presence of these two variables.

Table 3 Prognostic Significance of Episodes of Asymptomatic Ischemia

			Outcomes (%)							
			Death		MI			Severe angina/Need for Revascularization		
Ref.	n	Duration of follow-up (months)	With SI	No SI	With SI		No SI	With SI		No SI
15	88	3	3	6	18	*	4	18	*	7
16	70	1	0	0	16	**	3	27	*	9
43	70	24	5	0	27	**	3	30	*	9
18	88	12	13	0	15	*	10	48	*	25
23	66	13.3	14	3	29	*	10	100	**	42
					"Unfavorable outcome"					
					With SI		No SI			
17	52	6			SI $\geq$ 60 min; 94 SI $<$ 60 min; 70	***	5			
19	38	1			48	*	20			
20	135	In-hosp			48	**	20			
21	232	6.75			44	*	15			

* $p < 0.05$; ** $p < 0.01$; *** $p < 0.001$.
SI = silent ischemia during ambulatory ECG monitoring. "Unfavorable outcome" is defined variably as the occurrence of death, myocardial infarction, recurrent unstable angina, or revascularization procedure.

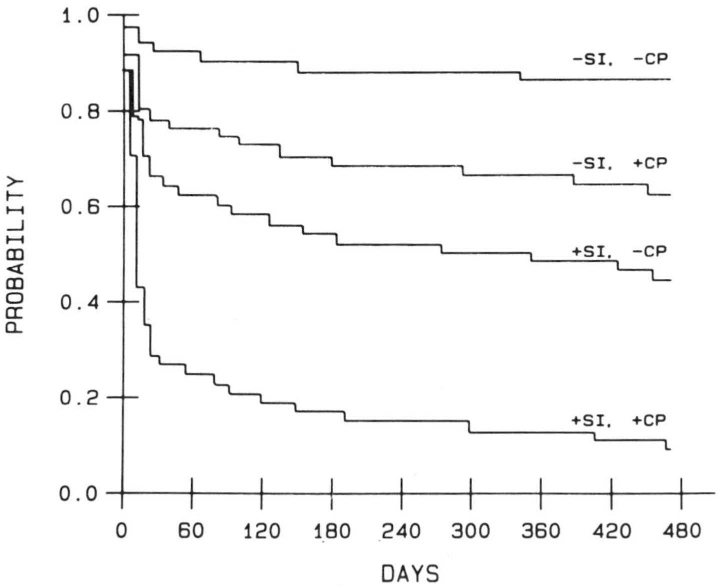

Figure 1 Relative risk curves derived from Cox's hazard function analysis demonstrating the risk for death, myocardial infarction, or revascularization for recurrent symptoms and illustrating the effects of the silent ischemia (SI) and recurrent chest pain (CP) variables on adverse outcome. There is a fivefold relative risk for outcomes associated with silent ischemia and a threefold relative risk associated with chest pain during the initial 2 days. When both variables are present, the relative risk for experiencing an adverse outcome is increased by a factor of 15. (From Ref. 43 with permission.)

Although a small sample size was utilized, Wilcox et al. (23) found that the presence of transient ischemia during monitoring initiated within 24 hours of hospitalization for unstable angina was 92% specific for the development of either death or nonfatal MI, but quite insensitive (25%). The only other variable more accurate for predicting a major event in their study was the presence of recurrent rest pain during hospitalization, which had a 100% sensitivity and a 49% specificity.

In some of the studies, the incidence of death is infrequent and the endpoints of death, myocardial infarction, and need for revascularization is combined as a single endpoint of "unfavorable" outcome (17,19,20,21). However, use of such an endpoint may be hazardous and even inappropriate since selection of patients for revascularization is extremely subjective on the part of both physician and patient, may be more or less routine in certain institutions or with certain physicians, and may even be influenced by knowledge of the AECG in some observational studies. Nevertheless, in almost all studies the presence of ≥1

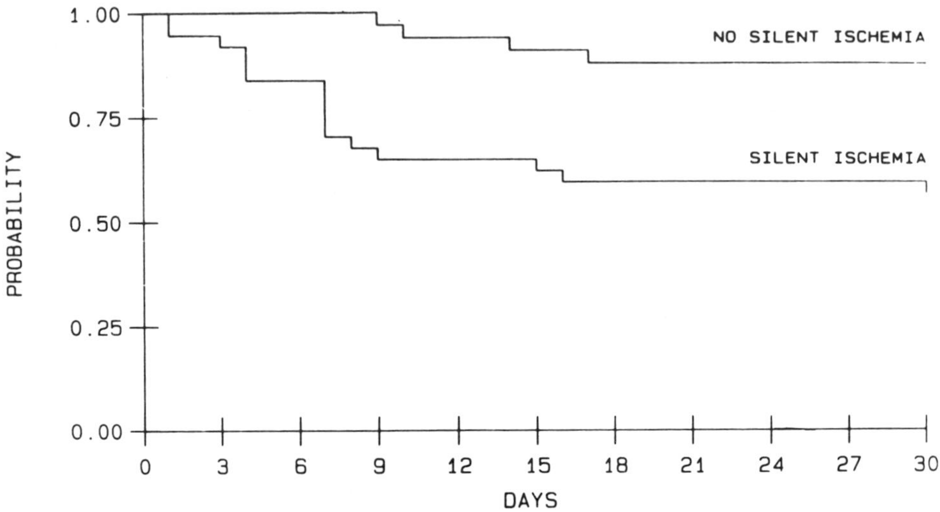

Figure 2 Kaplan-Meier curves comparing the cumulative probabilities of not experiencing myocardial infarction or revascularization for recurrent angina during a period of 30 days for the 37 patients with silent ischemia (Group 1) and 33 patients without it (Group 2), as detected by continuous electrocardiographic monitoring ($p < 0.002$). (From Ref. 16 with permission.)

episodes of ST-segment deviation confers significantly adverse prognostic impact on both early (<1 month) (16,19,20) and later (>1 month) follow-up (15,17,18,21,23,43).

Furthermore, there appears to be a progressively more adverse effect based on the cumulative duration of observed ischemia, although the only available studies are those prior to the era of using aspirin and/or heparin therapy (16,17,20). Gottlieb and coworkers (16) observed by multivariate analysis that the presence of transient asymptomatic ischemia on a 48-hour AECG was the best predictor of the development of MI or revascularization for recurrent symptomatic angina within 1 month follow-up ($p < 0.002$) compared to 14 other variables tested (Fig. 2), and that those patients with ≥60 min of asymptomatic ischemia per 24 hours had a worse prognosis than those with episodes of ischemia, but cumulative duration <60 min/24 hr ($p = 0.04$) (Fig. 3). Similarly, during a 3- to 6-month follow-up, Nademanee and colleagues (17) found that of 23 patients without evidence of transient ischemia on an AECG recorded after anginal symptoms were controlled with maximal medical therapy, only 1 patient died. In contrast, of 11 patients with a cumulative duration of ischemia <60 min/24 hr, 3 required revascularization for recurrent severe angina; and of 18

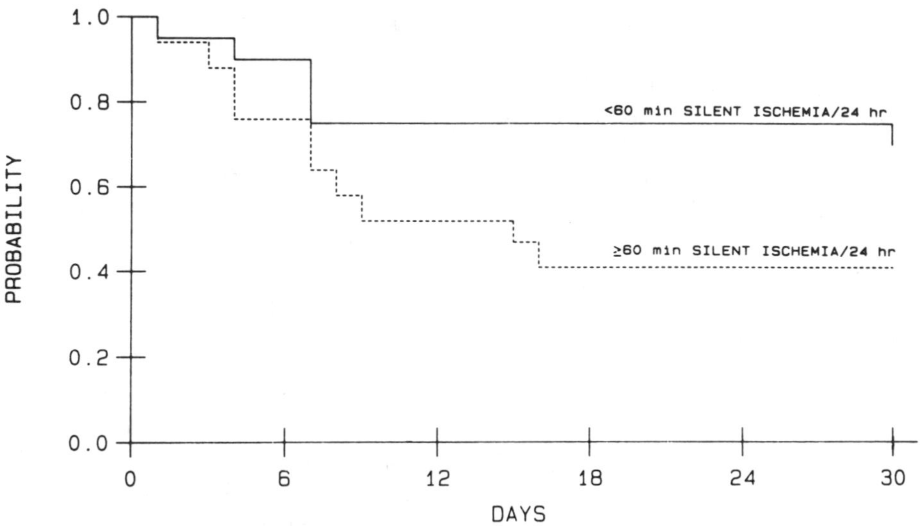

Figure 3 Kaplan-Meier curves showing the cumulative probabilities of not experiencing myocardial infarction or revascularization for recurrent angina during a period of 30 days in the patients with silent ischemia, comparing the patients with less than 60 minutes of silent ischemia per 24 hours and those with more than 60 minutes per 24 hours during the 2 days of electrocardiographic monitoring ($p = 0.04$). (From Ref. 16 with permission.)

patients with cumulative ischemia ≥60 min/24 hr, 5 patients (28%) had an MI, 2 of which were fatal, and 12 (43%) required coronary revascularization for recurrent angina. A "favorable" clinical outcome free of a cardiac event was present in 95% of patients without transient ischemia, 70% of patients with asymptomatic ischemia <60 min/24 hr, and in only 6% of patients with ischemia ≥60 min/24 hr.

PROGNOSTIC SIGNIFICANCE OF TRANSIENT ISCHEMIC EPISODES VS. EXERCISE TEST PERFORMANCE

In patients with stable angina there have been a number of studies correlating the presence and severity of asymptomatic ischemia during AECG monitoring to exercise test performance (44,45), but the experience in unstable angina is extremely limited, due in large part to the relatively infrequent use of the exercise test to stratify risk in patients with unstable angina. In a preliminary report, Freedman et al. (46) observed that of 32 patients with either unstable angina (n = 24) or a small MI (n = 8), 13 (41%) had episodes of transient ischemia on AECG monitoring recorded for 35 ± 8 hr and that 17 patients (53%) had a positive exercise test. There was a strong relationship between ischemia detected by AECG monitoring and by exercise testing: 71% of patients with a positive exercise test had a positive AECG recording, while only 7% of patients with a negative exercise test had an abnormal AECG ($p = 0.001$). Patients with a positive AECG tended to have a shorter mean exercise time compared to patients with a negative AECG (9.1 ± 5 min vs. 11.7 ± 5 min, $p = 0.07$), and a lower exercise capacity: 71% of patients with a maximum workload <4 METS had a positive AECG vs. 32% of patients with a maximum workload ≥4 METS ($p = 0.06$).

Marmur and colleagues (47) compared the 6-month prognostic significance of the results of 24-hr AECG monitoring initiated 7 ± 5 hr after the qualifying episode of angina to an exercise thallium test using the standard Bruce protocol 5 ± 2 days after the episode of angina. At the time of follow-up, 14 patients (26%) experienced an "unfavorable" outcome: 1 died, 2 experienced a nonfatal MI, and 11 were readmitted with unstable angina. Although on AECG monitoring 30 patients (56%) had evidence of asymptomatic ischemia, there was a similar frequency of transient ischemia in those with a favorable outcome (22 of 40 patients [55%]) and in those with an unfavorable outcome (8 of 14 patients [55%], *p* NS). Similarly there was no significant association between the duration of ST-segment deviation and the probability of an adverse outcome. The ST-segment response during exercise was not useful to predict outcome, but those patients with a favorable outcome had a greater double product at peak exercise and were receiving fewer medications than those patients who experienced an unfavorable outcome. In contrast to the lack of prognostic insight from AECG monitoring and ST segment activity during exercise, the results from exercise thallium scintigraphy were particularly useful to predict outcome. Patients with a favorable outcome had a thallium defect size of 7 ± 15% compared to 20 ± 22% defect size in those patients with an unfavorable outcome ($p = 0.03$). The prognostic effect was present only in the differences in the *reversible* defect, and not defects due to previous myocardial infarction. Using a multiple logistic regression analysis, the presence of previous infarction was the only independent significant predictor of a cardiac event within 6 months ($p = 0.018$). However, in the 38 patients without a previous infarction, the size of the reversible thallium defect was the only predictor ($p = 0.028$). It is certainly possible that the value of the AECG is underrepresented in this very small study because it includes only patients who had both an AECG on admission and an exercise treadmill test 5 days later. The AECG may identify patients at risk for early in-hospital cardiac events (20) occurring prior to the time of stability when the exercise test could be performed. The events predicted by the AECG may already have occurred by the time of the exercise test, so that the later events would not be predicted. Furthermore, the AECG may be of value to predict cardiac events in those patients not candidates for exercise test procedures.

SUMMARY AND CONCLUSIONS

The available studies concerning AECG monitoring in patients with unstable angina are flawed by being very small and by the fact that medical therapy has dramatically changed since the use of aspirin and/or heparin has become commonplace. Episodes of ambulatory asymptomatic ischemia appear to have been very common when medical regimens included nitrates, beta-blockers, and calcium blockers, but appear to be much reduced since aspirin and heparin have been included in the regimen. Patients with episodes of ischemia appear to be at high risk for developing an adverse cardiac event, although this has not been explored in patients treated with aspirin or heparin. Studies comparing the prognostic significance of the AECG with that of the exercise test with or without thallium scintigraphy, as well as with other clinical or angiographic variables, are needed. A number of large-scale clinical trials are current in progress, such as the Thrombolysis in Myocardial Ischemia (T3) and the tPA in Unstable Angina Trial (UNSA), which will more clearly identify the current incidence of asymptomatic ischemia detected by AECG monitoring in patients with unstable angina, and will also provide insight concerning the prognostic value of AECG monitoring.

ACKNOWLEDGMENT

I am grateful to Mary Gillan for help in the preparation of the manuscript.

REFERENCES

1. Gazes PC, Mobley EM Jr, Faris HM Jr, Duncan RC, Humphries GB. Pre-infarction (unstable) angina—a prospective study: ten year follow-up. Prognostic significance of electrocardiographic changes. Circulation 1973; 48:331–7.
2. Mulcahy R, Awadhi AHA, deBuitlear M, Tobin G, Johnson H, Contoy R. Natural history and prognosis of unstable angina. Am Heart J 1985; 109:753–8.
3. Stone PH. Mechanisms of silent myocardial ischemia: implications for selection of optimal therapy in Kellerman JJ, Braunwald E (eds). Silent myocardial ischemia: a critical appraisal. Adv Cardiol 1990; 37:328–48.
4. Ouyang P, Chandra NC, Gottlieb SO. Frequency and importance of silent myocardial ischemia identified with ambulatory electrocardiographic monitoring in the early in-hospital period after acute myocardial infarction. Am J Cardiol 1990; 65:267–70.
5. Deanfield JE, Selwyn AP, Chierchia S, Maseri A, Ribiero P, Krikler S, Morgan M. Myocardial ischemia during daily life in patients with stable angina: its relation to symptoms and heart rate changes. Lancet 1983; 2:753.
6. Deanfield JE, Shea M, Ribiero P, deLandsheere CM, Wilson RA, Horlock P, Selwyn AP. Transient ST segment depression as a marker of myocardial ischemia during daily life. Am J Cardiol 1984; 54:1195.

7. Levy RD, Shapiro LM, Wright C, Mockus LJ, Fox KM. The hemodynamic significance of asymptomatic ST segment depression assessed by ambulatory pulmonary artery pressure monitoring. Br Heart J 1986; 56:526–30.
8. Wilson RA, Sullivan PJ, Moore RA, et al. An ambulatory ventricular function monitor: validation and preliminary clinical results. Am J Cardiol 1983; 52:601–6.
9. LaVeau PJ, Rozanski A, Krantz DS, et al. Transient left ventricular dysfunction during provocative mental stress in patients with coronary artery disease. Am Heart J 1989; 118:1–8.
10. Russell RO Jr, Moraski RE, Kouchoukos N, et al. Unstable angina pectoris: national cooperative study group to compare surgical and medical therapy. II. In-hospital experience and initial follow-up results in patients with one, two, and three vessel disease. Am J Cardiol 1978; 42:839–48.
11. Gerstenblith G, Ouyang P, Achuff SC, et al. Nifedipine in unstable angina: a double blind randomized trial. N Engl J Med 1982; 306:885–9.
12. Muller JE, Turi ZG, Pearle DL, Schneider JF, Serfas DH, Morrison J, Stone PH, Rude RE, Rosner B, Sobel BE, Tate C, Scheiner E, Roberts R, Hennekens CH, Braunwald E. Nifedipine versus conventional therapy for unstable angina pectoris: a randomized double-blind comparison. Circulation 1984; 69:728–39.
13. Holland Interuniversity Nifedipine/Metoprolol Trial (HINT) Research Group. Early treatment of unstable angina in the coronary care unit: a randomized, double-blind, placebo-controlled comparison of recurrent ischemia in patients treated with nifedipine or metoprolol or both. Br Heart J 1986; 56:400–13.
14. Mooss AN, Aronow WS, Sketch M, Mohiuddin SM, Ryschon K. Serial ambulatory monitoring in patients with unstable angina pectoris. Clin Cardiol 1983; 6:435–9.
15. Johnson SM, Mauritson DR, Winniford MD, et al. Continuous electrocardiographic monitoring in patients with unstable angina pectoris: identification of high-risk subgroup with severe coronary disease, variant agina, and/or impaired early prognosis. Am Heart J 1982; 103:4–16.
16. Gottlieb SO, Weisfeldt ML, Ouyang P, Mellits ED, Gerstenblith G. Silent ischemia as a marker for early unfavorable outcomes in patients with unstable angina. N Engl J Med 1986; 314:1214–9.
17. Nademanee K, Intarachot V, Josephenson MA, Rieders D, Mody FV, Singh BN. Prognostic significance of silent myocardial ischemia in patients with unstable angina. J Am Coll Cardiol 1987; 10:1–9.
18. Pozzati A, Bugiardini R, Borghi A, Ottani F, Morgagni G, Puddu P. Prognostic significance of myocardial ischemia refractory to maximal medical therapy in unstable angina. Abstract. Circulation 1988; 78 (Suppl II):421.
19. VonArnim T, Gerbig HW, Krawietz W, Hofling B. Prognostic implications of transient-predominantly silent-ischemia in patients with unstable angina pectoris. Eur Heart J 1988; 9:435–40.
20. Langer A, Freeman MR, Armstrong PW. ST-segment shift in unstable angina: pathophysiology and association with coronary anatomy and hospital outcome. J Am Coll Cardiol 1989; 13:1495–502.
21. Phadke K, Mulcahy D, Parameshwar J, McCrae A, Keegan J, Wright C, Sparrow J, Blackwood R, Fox K. Early continuous ECG monitoring predicts unfavorable short

term outcome in patients with unstable angina but not in acute myocardial infarction. Abstract. J Am Coll Cardiol 1991; 63A.
22. Nicklas JM, Topol EJ, Kander N, O'Neill WW, Walton JA, Ellis SG, Gorman L, Pitt B. Randomized, double-blind, placebo-controlled trial of tissue plasminogen activator in unstable angina. J Am Coll Cardiol 1989; 13:434–41.
23. Wilcox I, Freedman SB, Kelly DT, Harris PJ. Clinical significance of silent ischemia in unstable angina pectoris. Am J Cardiol 1990; 65:1313–16.
24. Ouyang P, Chandra NC, Schulman SP, Gottlieb SO. Effect of heparin discontinuation on silent ischemia in patients with unstable angina. Abstract. J Am Coll Cardiol 1991: 17:312A.
25. Wallis DE, O'Connor C, Hakki AH, and the Multicenter Unstable Angina Group. Continuous heparin in unstable angina: effects on silent ischemia. Abstract. Circulation 1988; 78(Suppl II):98.
26. Theroux P, Ouimet H, McCans J, Latour J-G, Joly P, Levy G, Pelletier E, Juneau M, Stasiak J, deGuise P, Pelletier G, Rinzler D, Waters DD. Aspirin, heparin, or both to treat acute unstable angina. N Engl J Med 1988; 319:1105–11.
27. Folts JD, Crowell EB Jr, Rowe GG. Platelet aggregation in partially obstructed vessels and its elimination with aspirin. Circulation 1976; 54:365–70.
28. Muller JE, Tofler GH, Stone PH. Circadian variation and triggers of onset of acute myocardial infarction. Circulation 1989; 79:733–43.
29. Davies MJ. A macro and micro view of coronary vascular insult in ischemic heart disease. Circulation 1990; 82(Suppl II):38–46.
30. Figueras J. Mechanism of rest and nocturnal angina: observations during continuous hemodynamic and electrocardiographic monitoring-circulation. 1979; 59:955–68.
31. Chierchia S, Bruneli C, Simonetti I, Lazzari M, Maseri A. Sequence of events in angina at rest: primary reduction in coronary flow. Circulation 1980; 61:759–68.
32. Nademanee K, Intarachot V, Singh PN, Josephson MA, Singh BN. Characteristics and clinical significance of silent myocardial ischemia in unstable angina. Am J Cardiol 1986; 58:26B–33B.
33. Deedwania PC, Nelson JR. Pathophysiology of silent myocardial ischemia during daily life: hemodynamic evaluation of simultaneous electrocardiographic and blood pressure monitoring. Circulation 1990; 82:1296–304.
34. Andrews TC, Toyosaki N, Glasser SP, MacCallum G, West TW, Gibson RS, Shook T, Raby K, Fenton T, Stone PH and the ASIS Study Group. Heart rate activity preceding episodes of ambulatory ischemia: pathophysiologic and therapeutic implications. Abstract. J Am Coll Cardiol 1991; 17:223A.
35. Sherman CT, Litvack F, Grundfest W, Lee M, Hickey A, Chaux A, Kass R, Blanche C, Matloff J, Morgenstern L, Ganz W, Swan HJC, Forrester J. Coronary angioscopy in patients with unstable angina pectoris. N Engl J Med 1986; 315:913–9.
36. Stone PH. Calcium antagonists for Prinzmetal's variant agina, unstable angina and silent myocardial ischemia: therapeutic tool and probe for identification of pathophysiologic mechanisms. Am J Cardiol 1987; 59:101B–115B.
37. Tzvoni D, Gavish A, Benhorin J, Banai K, Keren A, Stern S. Day-to-day variability of myocardial ischemic episodes in coronary artery disease. Am J. Cardiol 1987; 60:1003–5.

38. Davies MJ, Thomas AC. Placque fissuring—the cause of acute myocardial infarction, sudden ischemic death and crescendo angina. Br Heart J 1985; 53:363–73.
39. Falk E. Unstable angina with fatal outcome: dynamic coronary thrombosis leading to infarction and/or sudden death. Autopsy evidence of recurrent mural thrombosis with peripheral embolization culminating in total vascular occlusion. Circulation 1985; 71:699–708.
40. Fuster V, Badimon L, Cohen M, Ambrose JA, Chesebro J. Insights into the pathogenesis of acute ischemic syndromes. Circulation 1988; 77:1213–20.
41. Langer A, Freeman MR, Armstrong PM. Relationship of angiographic detected intracoronary thrombus and silent myocardial ischemia in unstable angina pectoris. Am J Cardiol 1990; 66:1381–2.
42. Serneri GGN, Gensini GF, Poggesi L, Trotta F, Modesti PA, Boddi M, Ieri A, Margheri M, Casolo GC, Bini M, Rostagno C, Carnovali M, Abbate R. Effect of heparin, aspirin, or alteplase in reduction of myocardial ischemia in fractory unstable angina. Lancet 1990; 335:615–8.
43. Gottlieb SO, Weisfeldt ML, Ouyang P, Mellits ED, Gerstenblith G. Silent ischemia predicts infarction and death during 2 year follow-up of unstable angina. J Am Coll Cardiol 1987; 10:756–60.
44. Campbell S, Barry J, Rocco MB, Nabel EG, Mead-Walters K, Rebecca GS, Selwyn AP. Features of the exercise test that reflect the activity of ischemic heart disease out of hospital. Circulation 1986; 74:72–80.
45. Deedwania PC, Carbajal EV. Exercise test predictors of ambulatory silent ischemia during daily life in stable angina pectoris. Am J Cardiol 1990; 66:1151–6.
46. Freedman SB, Wilcox I, Doyle SJ, McCredie R, Harris PJ, Kelly DT. Silent ischemia on ambulatory recordings after unstable angina or small MI: Relationship to results of stress testing. Abstract. Circulation 1988; 78(Suppl II):469.
47. Marmur JD, Freeman MR, Langer A, Armstrong PW. Prognosis in medically stabilized unstable angina: early Holter ST-segment monitoring compared with predischarge exercise thallium imaging. Ann Intern Med 1990; 113:575–9.

8

Risk Stratification in Unstable Angina
Role of Exercise Electrocardiography, Thallium Scintigraphy, Dipyridamole Imaging, and Evaluation of Left Ventricular Function

Alan C. Braverman*

Brigham and Women's Hospital and Harvard Medical School
Boston, Massachusetts

INTRODUCTION

Unstable angina pectoris is a common medical problem associated with a significant risk of subsequent cardiac events such as cardiac death, nonfatal myocardial infarction, and the requirement for coronary revascularization. Patients admitted to hospital with unstable angina have an early mortality rate of 3–5% (1–5) and a 7–14% risk of nonfatal myocardial infarction (1–4,6,7). Follow-up studies have documented a one-year mortality rate of 5–12% (7–9) and a nonfatal myocardial infarction rate of 6–14% (1,8,9). A significant percentage of patients are readmitted within a 12-month period for recurrent unstable angina (5,8–11).

Given the frequency of unfavorable cardiac events following the onset of unstable angina, many have attempted to stratify these patients using noninvasive methods into low-risk and high-risk groups similar to the risk stratification used following acute myocardial infarction. The clinical history (2,12), resting electrocardiogram (2,3,5,6,12,13), exercise electrocardiogram (5,6,10,11,14–16), resting thallium perfusion scintigram (17–19), exercise thallium perfusion scintigram (5,20,21), echocardiogram (22), and ambulatory Holter monitor (3,5,23) have all been used for prognostication in patients presenting with unstable angina.

New modalities useful in the diagnosis of coronary artery disease such as dipyridamole thallium scintigraphy (24–26), dipyridamole echocardiography

* *Present affiliation*: Washington University Medical Center, St. Louis, Missouri.

(27), exercise echocardiography (28–30), and technetium-99m isonitrile myocardial imaging (31) have been developed and may also have a role in determining outcome after stabilization in patients with unstable angina.

The extent and severity of coronary artery disease (4,5,13) and the degree of left ventricular dysfunction (2,4) play an important role in determining prognosis and assessing potential benefits from revascularization in unstable angina patients (32). While percutaneous transluminal coronary angioplasty may be an attractive approach for managing many patients with unstable angina, a major, randomized, controlled trial comparing medical therapy to coronary angioplasty has not been completed in this population. While many patients with unstable angina have preserved left ventricular function and will stabilize on aggressive medical therapy, the Veterans Administration Cooperative Study for the treatment of patients with unstable angina showed a survival advantage for surgical revascularization rather than medical therapy only in patients with severe three-vessel coronary artery disease or a reduced ejection fraction (32). Thus, cardiac catheterization and coronary angiography may not be necessary in those patients deemed to be at low risk for subsequent cardiac events, but is mandatory if substantial left ventricular dysfunction or a suspicion of multivessel disease exists.

This chapter will review the salient features of the various noninvasive tests used to assess myocardial ischemia in patients with coronary artery disease with special emphasis on prognostic indicators. In addition, the data available on the risk stratification of the patient with unstable angina who stabilizes after hospitalization on medical therapy will be reviewed.

NONINVASIVE METHODS TO ASSESS CORONARY ISCHEMIA

Unstable angina is often defined as the new onset or rapid acceleration of a previously established anginal syndrome and includes rest pain or prolonged ischemic chest pain. While ongoing unstable angina can be considered an absolute contraindication to exercise stress testing, patients who stabilize on medical therapy may safely undergo subsequent exercise testing. Many studies have demonstrated that submaximal or maximal exercise testing can be safely performed within 3–5 days after stabilization of unstable angina patients (5,6,10,11,14–16,20,21).

In those patients with typical symptoms of angina pectoris, the prevalence of angiographically documented coronary artery disease approaches 85–95% (33), and therefore the majority of patients presenting with unstable angina will have angiographically important coronary disease. Exercise testing in this population is of little utility in the diagnosis of coronary disease, but is very useful to ascertain whether individual patients are at high risk or low risk for future adverse cardiac events. This is especially important since plaque fissure and thrombus formation appear to mediate many episodes of unstable angina, and, with thrombus resolution, the underlying coronary stenosis may not necessarily lead to inducible ischemia on exercise testing (5).

When considering the importance of angiographically documented coronary disease, it is important to remember that the anatomy of the coronary vessels does not predict the functional significance of the lesions present. Certain patients with three-vessel coronary artery disease are well-collateralized and have minor inducible ischemia with a good exercise capacity, while others may have single-vessel coronary artery disease with large segments of reversible ischemia, a large amount of myocardium at risk, and a poor exercise capacity.

In addition, the underlying left ventricular function is more important prognostically than the exercise electrocardiographic response or angiographic results in patients with coronary artery disease (33,34). For the same degree of coronary artery disease, a clinical history of prior myocardial infarction or congestive heart failure or the objective evidence of left ventricular dysfunction (by echocardiogram or radionuclide ventriculogram) carries a poorer prognosis (32).

Exercise Electrocardiography

The exercise electrocardiogram can contribute important information about the prognosis of patients with coronary artery disease (33) (Table 1). Electrocardiographic markers for severe coronary artery disease and a poorer prognosis include marked (>2 mm) ST-segment depression, downsloping ST-segment depression, ST-segment depression occurring at a low workload (either early in the exercise test or at a heart rate less than 120/minute), multiple lead ST-segment depression, and ST-segment depression persisting several minutes into recovery (33) (Table 2).

Nonelectrocardiographic indicators of a poorer prognosis include poor exercise capacity (inability to complete stage I of a maximal exercise protocol), exercise-induced hypotension, and chronotropic incompetence (Table 3). While these markedly abnormal exercise test responses have a relatively high specificity for critical coronary artery disease (three vessel or left main coronary artery disease), they are not very sensitive (35). Exercise duration or capacity also has important independent prognostic implications. Patients who are able to complete a maximal exercise test achieving predicted heart rate and blood pressure responses can have an excellent prognosis, even though they manifest exercise-induced ST-segment depression (35,36).

Whether the presence of angina during an exercise test adds independent prognostic information above and beyond the ST-segment response or the exercise duration is somewhat controversial. Dagenais et al. reported that patients with a painless, strongly positive exercise electrocardiogram have rates of

Table 1 Prognosis in Patients According to Exercise Test Results

	Follow-up (% alive)	
	12 months	48 months
All patients evaluated for chest pain		
Exercise ECG		
Normal	99	94
Ischemic ST-segments	92	80
Equivocal	96	88
Exercise duration and/or heart rate achieved		
Stage IV or higher and/or heart rate 160/min or more	99	95
Stage I and/or heart rate 120/min or less	85	78
CAD documented angiographically		
Exercise ECG		
Normal	92	90
Ischemic ST-segments	92	77
Equivocal	91	74
Exercise duration and/or heart rate achieved		
Stage IV or higher and/or heart rate 160/min or more	99	90
Stage I and/or heart rate 120/min or less	84	58

CAD = coronary artery disease; ECG = electrocardiogram.
Source: Ref. 33.

Table 2 Exercise Test Responses Considered Predictive for Severe Multivessel and/or Left Main Coronary Artery Disease

Electrocardiographic
ST-segment response
Downsloping
Elevation[a]
ST-segment depression exceeding 2.5 mm
Serious ventricular dysrhythmias occurring at low (120–130/min) heart rates
Early onset (first 3 min) of ischemic ST-segment depression or elevation
Prolonged duration (≥8 min) in the postexercise recovery period of ischemic ST-segment depression
Nonelectrocardiographic
Low achieved heart rate (≤120/min)
Hypotension[b] (≥ 10 mmHg in systolic pressure at any time during the test)
Rise in diastolic blood pressure (≥110–120 mmHg)
Low achieved rate-pressure product (≤15,000)
Inability to exercise beyond 3 min

[a]ST elevation in leads showing a Q wave of prior transmural myocardial infarction is not an ischemic response but rather reflects an underlying wall motion disorder.
[b]In the absence of antihypertensive medications or hypovolemia.
Source: Ref. 33.

Table 3 Prognostically Important Variables in Patients with Coronary Artery Disease Undergoing Exercise Testing

Cardiomegaly on chest X-ray films
Prior myocardial infarction
History of congestive heart failure
Positive exercise ECG
Achieved heart rate of less than 120/min
Depressed ejection fraction at rest or during exercise
Achieved systolic blood pressure of 130 mmHg or less
Effort hypotension
Inability to complete stage I on standard Bruce protocol
Male sex
Age

ECG = electrocardiogram.
Source: Ref. 33.

death (sudden cardiac, nonsudden cardiac, and noncardiac death) similar to patients with induced angina, and their survival rate also varies according to exercise duration achieved (37).

False-negative exercise tests are most commonly due to inadequate exercise workload. If a patient is unable to achieve 85% of a predicted heart rate for age, the test should be considered nondiagnostic. In addition, anti-anginal medications such as beta blockers may blunt the exercise heart rate and blood pressure response and confound the test results by delaying the onset of exercise induced ischemia.

Exercise Thallium-201 Scintigraphy

The use of exercise thallium-201 scintigraphy increases the sensitivity and specificity for detecting coronary artery disease over exercise electrocardiography (33,38). The major utility of thallium-201 scintigraphy is when the resting electrocardiogram reveals abnormalities such as left ventricular hypertrophy, left bundle branch block, digitalis-effect, and ST-T wave abnormalities that preclude accurate assessment of the ST-segment response to exercise. In addition, in patients with poor exercise capacity, thallium-201 scintigraphy may have a greater sensitivity for detecting coronary ischemia than exercise electrocardiography alone (38).

Thallium-201 scintigraphy may also have a role in improving detection of the patient with severe coronary artery disease (38,39). Scintigraphic markers of extensive coronary artery disease include a diffuse, slow washout of thallium from the myocardium (38), transient ischemic dilation of the left ventricle (39), and increased thallium uptake by the lungs (40). While these findings are very specific for severe coronary artery disease, they are not very sensitive.

Several studies have been performed to assess the ability of exercise thallium-201 scintigraphy to predict future cardiac events (38,41). Using multivariate analyses, the total number and extent of reversible thallium defects and the severity of hypoperfusion are all independent predictors of future unfavorable cardiac events (38,41).

Since planar thallium-201 scintigraphy is based on qualitative visual assessment, computer algorithms have been developed for the quantitative analysis of thallium abnormalities in specific myocardial regions. Quantitative analysis improves the reproducibility of thallium scintigraphic studies, but not necessarily the accuracy (38). In addition, Detrano et al. have shown that the use of quantitative computer analysis improves the sensitivity of coronary disease detection at the expense of a lower specificity (42).

Planar thallium-201 imaging has several technical limitations such as spatial overlap of distinct myocardial regions, poor lesion contrast, and variable attenuation by overlying structures such as chest muscles and breast tissue. Single photon emission computed tomography (SPECT) uses a rotational camera for tomographic images in order to increase the accuracy of thallium-201 scintigraphy (43). Compared to planar imaging, single photon emission computed tomography is reported to improve the accuracy for detecting individual arterial defects, multivessel coronary artery disease, and the extent of myocardium at risk (43).

Exercise Echocardiography

Exercise echocardiography has also been utilized to evaluate patients with suspected coronary artery disease (28–30). During exercise, the development of regional wall motion abnormalities are relatively specific for significant coronary stenosis and correlate highly with thallium-201 scintigraphic perfusion defects (30). In experienced centers, adequate images can be obtained in greater than 85% of patients suspected of having coronary artery disease (29). In single-vessel coronary artery disease, a wall motion abnormality develops in a single coronary perfusion distribution. In multivessel coronary artery disease, wall motion abnormalities develop in two or more distinct coronary distributions (28). In a comparison of exercise electrocardiography and exercise echocardiography among patients with normal wall motion at rest, Ryan et al. found exercise echocardiography to be highly specific for coronary artery disease (28). Among patients with single-vessel disease, exercise echocardiography was significantly more sensitive than exercise electrocardiography. However, in patients with multivessel coronary disease, the two tests had similar sensitivities (28).

This technique may have similar efficacy as exercise thallium-201 scintigraphy in the patient with an abnormal resting electrocardiogram that precludes interpretation with exercise (30). The extent of segmental wall motion abnormality that develops during exercise would be expected to correlate with the amount of myocardium at risk, thus allowing prognostication. Further evaluation of exercise echocardiography is necessary to determine its reproducibility and ability to define low-risk and high-risk subsets in patients with coronary artery disease.

Exercise Radionuclide Angiography

As previously noted, left ventricular dysfunction at rest adds important prognostic information for the patient with coronary artery disease. Exercise-induced left ventricular dysfunction as measured by radionuclide angiography also identifies a subset of patients at higher risk for subsequent mortality and increased angina requiring coronary revascularization (44). Bonow et al. demonstrated that a subgroup of patients with three-vessel coronary artery disease and exercise-induced ST-segment depression and a decrease in ejection fraction during exercise had a significantly higher mortality rate than those with an unchanged or increased ejection fraction with exercise (44). However, the contribution of the abnormal decrease in ejection fraction with exercise to the increased cardiac events independent of the exercise capacity and ST-segment depression is unknown. Radionuclide angiography is limited by the many false-positive abnormal ejection fraction responses to exercise seen with hypertension, abnormal ventricular compliance, altered loading conditions, increasing age, and use of beta-blockers.

Dipyridamole-Thallium Scintigraphy

Many patients referred for exercise testing to evaluate coronary ischemia are unable to exercise adequately due to comorbid illnesses such as peripheral vascular disease or orthopedic problems. In such patients, pharmacologic coronary vasodilation using dipyridamole causes regional differences in myocardial perfusion which may be detected by thallium-201 imaging, echocardiographic wall motion abnormalities, or radionuclide ventriculography. Dipyridamole imaging studies are contraindicated in patients with severe bronchospastic pulmonary disease, which can be exacerbated by this agent. Aminophylline antagonizes the effects of dipyridamole on vascular smooth muscle and may be used to reverse coronary ischemia induced by dipyridamole.

Oral dipyridamole thallium imaging using 300 mg of dipyridamole has been shown to unmask redistribution indicating hypoperfusion of viable myocardium (24,25,45). Homma et al. found that 91% of patients with coronary artery disease had redistribution abnormalities on thallium scintigraphy after oral dipyridamole (24). Quantitative thallium-201 single photon emission computed tomography after oral dipyridamole also has high sensitivity and specificity for diagnosing coronary artery disease and identifying multivessel disease (25). However, oral dipyridamole requires 30–60 minutes to produce coronary vasodilation, which may persist for up to 60 minutes (45). This requires a greater physician and laboratory time commitment, making this route of administration less attractive.

Intravenous dipyridamole-thallium imaging has a sensitivity and specificity approaching 80–90% for detecting coronary artery disease without the time requirement of oral dipyridamole (45). Side effects of administration of intravenous dipyridamole include angina (30% of patients), hypotension (20% of patients), and need for reversal by administration of aminophylline (15% of patients) (26). This technique has been especially useful in risk stratification prior to peripheral vascular surgery (46) and has been reported to predict future cardiac events in asymptomatic patients with coronary artery disease (47).

Intravenous dipyridamole utilized with echocardiography has been shown to be a safe, sensitive, and highly specific method for the detection of angiographically important coronary artery disease (27). The development of wall motion abnormalities during dipyridamole stress has also been reported to be an independent predictor of future cardiac events such as cardiac death, nonfatal myocardial infarction, and need for coronary revascularization (27). Further investigation with dipyridamole echocardiography is warranted to determine its prognostic value in patients with coronary disease.

Technetium-99 Methoxyisobutyl Isonitrile (MIBI) Imaging

Technetium-99 methoxyisobutyl isonitrile (MIBI) is a new radionuclide perfusion imaging agent which may have a direct application in patients with unstable angina. Technetium-99m isonitrile has properties of both a perfusion agent and a myocardial viability agent (31). This agent differs from thallium in that it does not redistribute, allowing for acute injection and subsequent imaging up to 6 hours later (31). Unlike thallium-201 scintigraphy, technetium-99m isonitrile may be injected during acute coronary ischemia to assess the degree of perfusion abnormalities without the requirement of immediate imaging of the unstable patient. This technique may have applicability in the prognostic statification of patients with unstable angina, but requires further investigation.

RISK STRATIFICATION AFTER STABILIZATION OF UNSTABLE ANGINA

Patients admitted with unstable angina are at relatively high risk for unfavorable cardiac events during hospitalization and over the months following discharge. However, the majority of patients will stabilize on medical therapy during hospitalization, while severe, multivessel coronary artery disease (4,5,13) and the presence of left ventricular dysfunction (2,4,32) may predict an adverse long-term prognosis in patients with unstable angina. Cardiac catheterization is not feasible in all patients and is not necessary in those patients at low risk for subsequent cardiac events. A noninvasive approach to identify both low- and high-risk patients is desirable.

Initial evaluation of the patient with unstable angina who stabilizes on medical therapy should include an assessment of left ventricular function. Echocardiography is probably the commonest and cheapest test but radionuclide ventriculography is also used to assess ventricular function. The patient with depressed left ventricular function, usually from prior myocardial infarction, has a poorer long-term prognosis and may also have multivessel coronary artery disease (2,4,20,32). Thus, patients presenting with unstable angina who are found to have left ventricular dysfunction and are considered revascularization candidates (either bypass surgery or coronary angioplasty) should undergo coronary angiography to define the coronary anatomy without further noninvasive testing. The Verterans Administration Cooperative Study has demonstrated that surgical revascularization improves long-term survival in unstable angina patients with three-vessel coronary artery disease or impaired ejection fraction (32).

Clinical Characteristics

The natural history of patients with unstable angina treated medically was carefully documented in the era before coronary artery bypass surgery was freely available (2,12). Clinical characteristics on presentation can be used to stratify patients into different risk categories for future cardiac events. Frequent episodes of angina in the hospital (2,12,13,26), a prior history of stable angina (12), ischemic ST-segment changes during chest pain (12), or evidence of global ST-segment depression with pain (12,13,26) and prior myocardial infarction (2,12) identified those patients at highest risk for acute myocardial infarction and death during follow-up (12,13,26). Long-term mortality was also increased in older patients and those with overt evidence of ventricular dysfunction such as cardiomegaly or pulmonary venous congestion on chest X-ray (2).

However, using the patient's clinical characteristics and baseline electrocardiogram alone results in much overlap between patients deemed to be at low risk and those at high risk for subsequent cardiac events. Attempts to accurately predict cardiac events for the individual patient on clinical grounds alone can be very difficult. This has led to the use of Holter electrocardiographic monitoring and exercise stress testing to stratify patients with unstable angina.

Holter Electrocardiographic Monitoring

Ischemic ST-segment shifts on Holter electrocardiographic monitors have recently been identified as important prognostic indicators in patients with unstable angina pectoris (3,23). Gottlieb et al. performed continuous electrocardiographic monitoring for ST-segment shifts during the first 2 days of hospitalization in 70 patients admitted with unstable angina (23). The presence of painless ST-segment depression (transient ST-segment deviations of 1 mm or more from baseline, 0.08 second after the J-point, that lasted for at least one minute) during continuous monitoring identified patients at highest risk for myocardial infarction and the requirement for revascularization procedures due to recurrent ischemia during a 1-month follow-up period (23). In addition, patients with greater than 60 minutes of ST-segment shift during a 24-hour period had a significantly worse outcome than those with a shorter cumulative duration of ST-segment shift. Stepwize Cox hazard analysis revealed that silent ischemia was a more powerful predictor than recurrent chest pain of subsequent adverse cardiac events. In this study, the vast majority of ST-segment shifts were painless. Symptomatic ischemia had a high specificity (94%) but a low sensitivity (25%) for identifying the patients with unfavorable outcomes, while painless ST-segment shift had a specificity of 58% and sensitivity of 80% (23).

Langer et al. examined the ST-segment shift on the admission electrocardiogram and ST-segment shift on continuous Holter electrocardiographic monitor in 135 patients with unstable angina (3). Patients with an ST-segment shift on the admission electrocardiogram had a significantly higher rate of subsequent unfavorable outcomes (cardiac death, myocardial infarction, or coronary revascularization), multivessel coronary artery disease, and left main coronary artery stenosis compared to patients with no ST-segment changes. In this study, 89% of patients had ST-segment shifts on continuous Holter monitoring, and the vast majority were painless (92%) (3). Using a multiple regression analysis, the coronary anatomy was the best predictor of an unfavorable outcome, but when this was accounted for the absolute duration of ST-segment shift on continuous monitoring was the best predictor of an unfavorable outcome. While the admission electrocardiogram was less sensitive than Holter ST-segment monitoring in identifying patients with an unfavorable outcome (63% vs. 83%), if patients presented with ST-segment shift on the admission electrocardiogram, Holter monitor recording did not improve the sensitivity for predicting an unfavorable outcome.

Exercise Electrocardiography

With the advent and widespread use of exercise stress testing after myocardial infarction as a method for subsequent risk stratification, this technology was soon applied to the patient with unstable angina. Many authors have found that following 3–5 days of pain-free stabilization in-hospital, both submaximal and maximal exercise protocols can be safely performed in patients presenting with unstable angina (5,6,10,11,14–16, 20).

Recurrent Angina

Nixon et al. evaluated 61 patients presenting with unstable angina who stabilized on medical therapy (14). Submaximal bicycle ergometry to a maximum heart rate of 120/minute was performed within 3–7 days of admission without any adverse events. Either chest pain or ST-segment depression occurring during exercise predicted those patients most likely to develop severe, recurrent angina during follow-up. No data on subsequent adverse events such as myocardial infarction or death were reported in this study.

Unfavorable Outcome

Submaximal treadmill exercise electrocardiography using a modified Naughton protocol was performed in 125 patients using a 12-lead electrocardiogram 3–5 days following stabilization of unstable angina by Butman et al. (10). Angina or ≥1 mm ST-segment depression developed in 48% of patients during exercise testing, and during a one-year follow-up period, 87% of these patients had an "unfavorable outcome," defined as severe angina, recurrent unstable angina, requirement for revascularization, acute myocardial infarction, or cardiac death (Table 4, Fig. 1). Every patient with **both** angina and ST-segment depression had an unfavorable outcome. Only 29% of the patients with a negative exercise test had a cardiac event in the one-year follow-up period (10). In this series, the sensitivity and specificity of the submaximal exercise test in predicting outcome was 73% and 85%, respectively (10). This study suggested that patients with angina or ST-segment deviations (or especially both) during submaximal exercise testing should undergo cardiac catheterization with a view to revasculariza-

Table 4 Relationship Between Treadmill Test Results and Cardiac Events During Follow-Up

	Positive test (n = 60)	Negative test (n = 65)
Favorable outcome	8 (13%)	46 (71%)
Unfavorable outcome***	52 (87%)	19 (29%)
Class III or IV angina**	17 (28%)	2 (3%)
Unstable angina*	9 (15%)	3 (5%)
Coronary artery bypass surgery*	22 (37%)	11 (17%)
Acute myocardial infarction	3 (5%)	2 (3%)
Cardiac death	1 (2%)	1 (2%)

Favorable outcome = New York Heart Association class I or II angina at follow-up. *$p < 0.01$; **$p < 0.01$; ***<0.001. n = number of patients.
Source: Ref. 10.

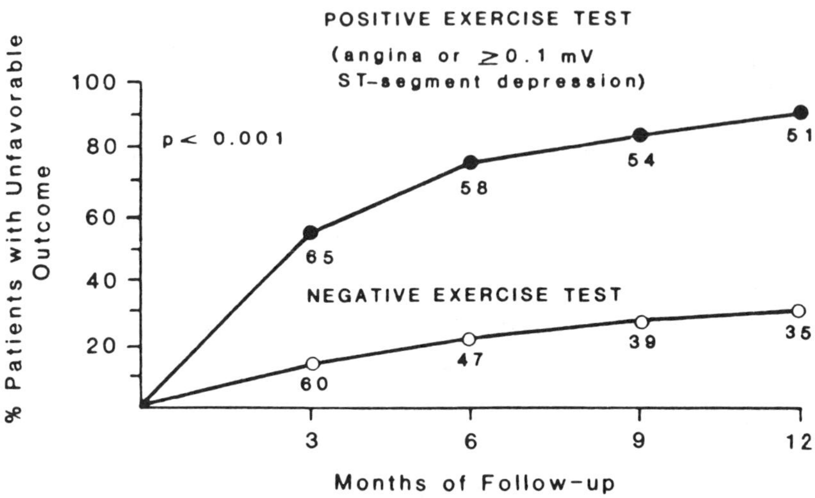

Figure 1 Cumulative incidence of unfavorable events in the 60 patients with a negative exercise test (open circles) and the 65 patients with a positive exercise test (solid circles) during the 12-month follow-up period. The numbers below the circles represent the number of patients remaining in each group at each follow-up interval. Unfavorable outcome = New York Heart Association class III or IV angina, unstable angina, acute myocardial infarction, coronary bypass artery surgery, or cardiac death during follow-up. (From Ref. 10.)

tion. Patients with a negative test can appropriately be treated medically and followed carefully.

The same authors have found that the sensitivity of the submaximal exercise test in detecting multivessel coronary artery disease was 65% and specificity was 89%, with a predictive value of a positive test of 92% and predictive value of a negative submaximal test of 57% (11). These data applied to "3-lead" rather than 12-lead electrocardiograms, and the predictive value of a "negative test" was lower in patients taking beta-blockers. These data suggest that patients who initially have a negative submaximal exercise test should later undergo symptom-limited maximal exercise testing (off beta-blockers) if multivessel coronary artery disease needs to be excluded with greater confidence.

Thallium Scintigraphy

Thallium scintigraphy can increase the sensitivity for detecting coronary artery disease and has been useful in determining prognosis in patients with coronary ischemia (38). Because a small but significant number of patients who have an unremarkable exercise electrocardiogram after stabilization of unstable angina will have a subsequent unfavorable cardiac event (10), thallium scintigraphy has been recently used to aid in risk stratification (5,20,21). The use of thallium-201 scintigraphy in patients with unstable angina is not a new concept.

Resting Scintigraphy

Resting thallium-201 scintigraphy has been used in patients presenting with unstable angina (17–19). Early scanning (within 6–11 hours of rest pain) has been used in an attempt to predict coronary anatomy, left ventricular wall motion, and hospital outcome. In unstable angina patients, without a history of prior myocardial infarction, a resting thallium defect may suggest that need for early revascularization is greater (18) but in patients with a history of prior infarction is not predictive of the need for revascularization or adverse events (18). In patients with known severe coronary artery disease and unstable angina, the size of the perfusion defect and the degree of left ventricular dysfunction are directly related (17). Those patients with large perfusion defects have worse ventricular function. In patients with unstable angina the combination of ischemic electrocardiographic changes and a positive resting thallium scan is associated with a complicated course (continuing angina, the occurrence of myocardial infarction or the need for revascularization) (19). Patients with large resting thallium defects alone were also more likely to have a complicated hospital course (19).

Exercise Scintigraphy

Exercise thallium scintigraphy is complementary to exercise electrocardiography in predicting the degree of coronary artery disease present. Freeman et al. prospectively studied 67 patients with unstable angina who responded to medical therapy to assess the value of exercise electrocardiography and thallium scintigraphy in determining the extent and severity of coronary artery disease (20). Symptom-limited exercise thallium scintigraphy was safely performed 3–6 days after admission. There was no significant difference in clinical, exercise electrocardiographic, or thallium scintigraphic variables between patients without significant obstructive coronary artery disease and those with single vessel disease. However, patients with three-vessel coronary artery disease had a significantly shorter exercise duration, lower peak exercise heart rate, lower peak systolic blood pressure response, and greater frequency of chest pain than those with ≤ 1 vessel coronary artery disease (20). A thallium defect size greater than one myocardial segment was a better predictor and had a higher specificity for multivessel coronary artery disease than ischemic electrocardiographic changes. The combination of exercise duration of less than 6 minutes or a thallium defect size of greater than one segment was present in 100% of patients with multivessel disease (20). Using multiple regression analysis, the size of the exercise thallium defect was the best indcpendent predictor of the extent of coronary artery disease, with exercise heart rate and presence of chest pain during exercise also predicting the severity of coronary artery disease. Therefore, after stabilization of unstable angina, symptom-limited exercise thallium scintigraphy, and electrocardiography can also be safely performed and has a higher sensitivity (82%) for detecting multivessel coronary artery disease than in studies using submaximal 12-lead exercise electrocardiography alone (65%) (10).

Later thallium-exercise testing performed in patients admitted to hospital with chest pain (without confirmed myocardial infarction) can be used to stratify high- and low-risk patients (21). The findings of an abnormal exercise thallium scintigram (fixed or reversible thallium defect) or ischemic electrocardiographic changes correlated significantly with the risk of subsequent cardiac events (nonfatal myocardial infarction or cardiac death) over the next 1–2 years. An abnormal exercise electrocardiogram was associated with a subsequent 15% cardiac event rate, while a reversible thallium defect was associated with a 17% one-year event rate (21). Patients having both an abnormal exercise electrocardiogram and an abnormal thallium scintigram represented the highest risk group, having a 21% cardiac event rate during follow-up. Importantly, over 97% of patients with a normal exercise electrocardiogram or a normal thallium scintigram had an event-free follow-up. The patients with an uninterpretable exercise electrocardiogram (due to resting ST-segment abnormalities from left ventricular hypertrophy, left bundle branch block, etc.) had a 12% cardiac event, indicating the importance of thallium scintigraphy in this patient group (21).

Dipyridamole Thallium Scintigraphy

Dipyridamole thallium scintigraphy has a high sensitivity for detecting coronary artery disease and may be especially suited for patients unable to perform dynamic exercise testing (45). However, there is little available data on the prognostic utility of dipyridamole thallium scintigraphy after stabilization of unstable angina pectoris.

Younis and coworkers performed intravenous dipyridamole thallium scintigraphy in 77 patients following an acute coronary event (44 with unstable angina) to evaluate this test (26). During follow-up evaluation, 10 patients had a nonfatal myocardial infarction or cardiac death, and each of these patients had either reversible, or, combined fixed and reversible, thallium defects. Using multiple logistic regression analysis, only a reversible thallium defect and the severity of coronary artery disease were significant predictors of subsequent cardiac events (recurrent angina, revascularization, nonfatal myocardial infarction, and cardiac death) (26).

Therefore, in this study, the presence of a reversible thallium defect identified those patients at higher risk for multivessel coronary disease and a worse prognosis. Importantly, none of the 14 patients in this series with a normal intravenous dipyridamole thallium scan had a major cardiac event during follow-up (26).

Comparison of Holter Electrocardiographic Monitoring, Exercise Electrocardiography, Thallium Scintigraphy, and Cardiac Catheterization

Prognostic information in patients presenting with unstable angina has been provided by continuous electrocardiographic ST-segment monitoring (3,23), exercise electrocardiography (6,10,11,14–16), and thallium scintigraphy (20,21). The relative value of each method has been compared. A prospective comparison of 24-hour Holter monitoring, quantitative exercise thallium tomography, and cardiac catheterization in 54 unstable angina patients who stabilized on medical therapy was performed and the relative value of each test in predicting subsequent cardiac events (recurrent unstable angina, nonfatal myocardial infarction, and cardiac death) was determined (5). Patients identified as having a favorable outcome had a higher maximum rate-pressure product during exercise, smaller-sized reversible thallium perfusion defect, and less severe coronary artery disease (5). (Table 5). Using a multiple regression analysis model, a history of a prior myocardial infarction was the most powerful predictor of outcome. In patients without prior myocardial infarction ($n = 38$), the size of the reversible thallium perfusion defect was the only predictor of unfavorable outcome and was superior to coronary angiography (Fig. 2).

Table 5 Exercise Testing in Patients with Unstable Angina

Variable	Patients with favorable outcome ($n = 40$)	Patients with unfavorable outcome ($n = 14$)	P-value (95% CI of Difference)
Exercise duration, min	8.0 ± 3.7	7.9 ± 3.2	0.94
Maximum ST depression, mm	0.6 ± 0.9	1.0 ± 1.0	0.16
Maximum heart rate, beats/min	144 ± 24	117 ± 27	0.001 (11 to 42)
Maximum systolic blood pressure, mmHg	169 ± 29	150 ± 39	0.064 (–11 to 39)
Maximum rate-pressure product, $\times 10^3$	24 ± 6	18 ± 7	0.0025 (2.4 to 10.5)
Calcium antagonists[a], *n*	24	13	0.0416
Beta-blockers[a], *n*	13	8	0.123
Nitrates[a], *n*	37	14	0.56

When appropriate, data are presented as mean ± SD.
[a]At the time of testing.
Source: Ref. 5.

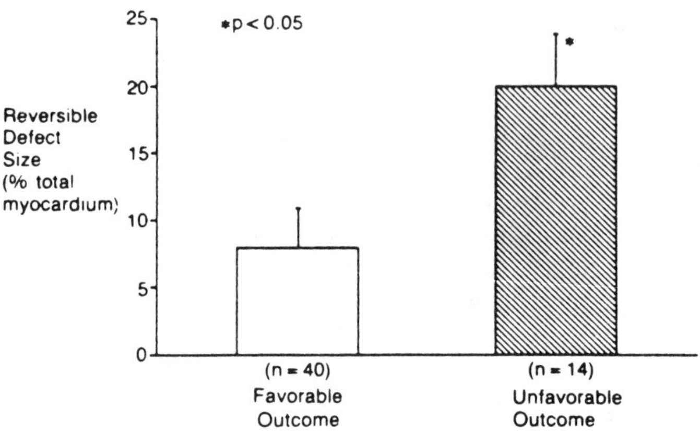

Figure 2 Reversible defect size expressed as percentage of total myocardium according to outcome at 6 months (mean ± SE). (From Ref. 5.)

These authors concluded that Holter monitoring of unstable angina patients for ST-segment shifts early after admission may predict in-hospital cardiac events, but is less useful in identifying patients who are destined to have an unfavorable outcome following discharge (3,5). Holter monitoring early after admission and exercise thallium scintigraphy for the patient who stabilizes on medical therapy may be an appropriate management strategy (5). Because of the frequent occurrence of unfavorable cardiac events in patients with prior myocardial infarction presenting with unstable angina, it is recommended that early coronary arteriography be strongly considered in this group.

SUMMARY

Patients presenting with unstable angina pectoris have a relatively high incidence of subsequent unfavorable cardiac events such as recurrent unstable angina, requirement for revascularization, nonfatal myocardial infarction, and cardiac death. High-risk patients include the subset with such clinical features as recurrent ischemia in-hospital, widespread ST-segment shifts during ischemia and evidence of prior myocardial infarction or congestive heart failure, i.e., left ventricular dysfunction. These patients should be considered for early coronary angiography and revascularization procedures in an attempt to improve long-term outcome. The patients without these high-risk features on admission who stabilize in-hospital on an aggressive anti-ischemic medical regimen present a difficult problem. While many of these patients will be event-free with a good

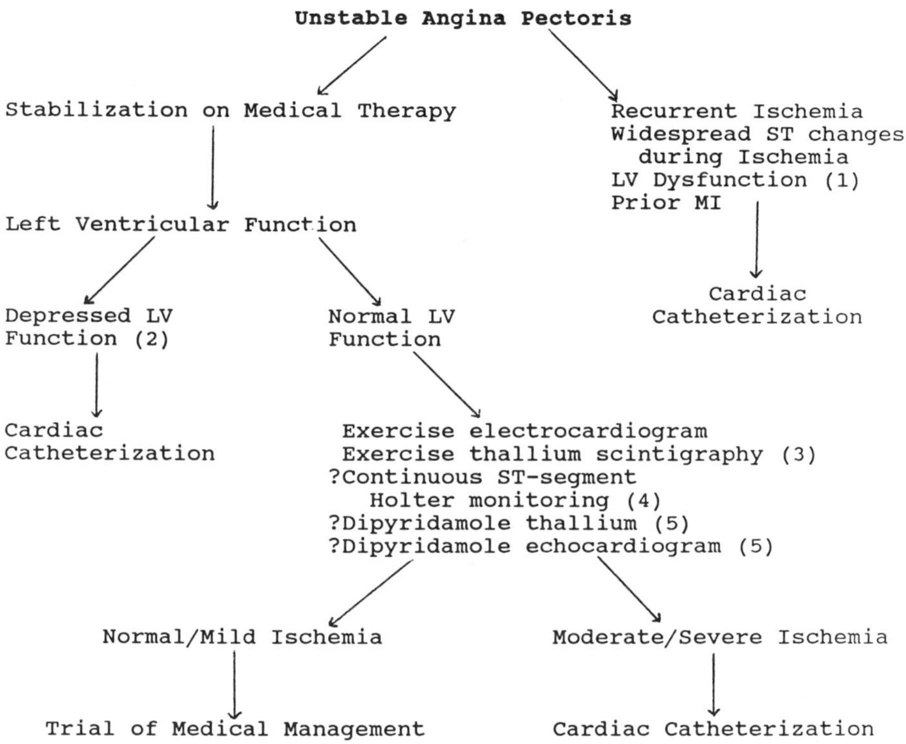

Figure 3 Decision tree for patients presenting with unstable angina. (1) Clinical findings of rales, S3 gallop, or cardiomegaly or pulmonary vascular redistribution on chest X-ray. (2) Left ventricular ejection fraction ≤50% by echocardiogram or radionuclide ventriculogram. (3) Thallium scintigraphy especially useful for patients with resting electrocardiographic abnormalities which preclude interpretation of the exercise electrocardiogram. (4) Early continuous ST-segment monitoring may predict patients at risk for in-hospital adverse cardiac events. (5) Dipyridamole imaging with thallium scintigraphy or echocardiography may be useful in patients unable to exercise.

prognosis, others will have a subsequent unfavorable cardiac event during short-term follow-up.

Cardiac catheterization is neither feasible nor necessary in all patients presenting with unstable angina. While coronary anatomy is important in determining prognosis, assessment of left ventricular function and coronary ischemia are often better predictors of subsequent outcome.

Submaximal symptom-limited exercise testing has been shown to be safe following stabilization of the patient with unstable angina. Noninvasive dynamic testing has shown that unstable angina patients with normal left ventricular function who have no inducible ischemia on exercise electrocardiography generally have a very favorable prognosis (5,11,20,21). Further identification of those patients at very low risk for cardiac events is also provided by normal exercise thallium scintigraphy. In the patient with a normal exercise electrocardiogram or normal exercise thallium scintigraphy after stabilization of unstable angina, routine early cardiac catheterization is not necessary. Careful observation on medical therapy in this low-risk subset should prove adequate for the greatest majority of patients.

Patients with inducible ischemia during dynamic testing should undergo coronary arteriography to define coronary anatomy in an attempt to further stratify patients into different risk subsets and determine benefits of revascularization with percutaneous balloon angioplasty or coronary artery bypass grafting (Fig. 3). Further investigation is required to determine the additive benefits of technetium-99m isonitrile imaging, intravenous dipyridamole thallium scintigraphy, dipyridamole echocardiography, and exercise echocardiography in unstable angina patients.

REFERENCES

1. National Cooperative Study Group. Unstable angina pectoris: national cooperative study group to compare surgical and medical therapy. II. In-hospital experience and initial follow-up results in patients with one, two, and three vessel disease. Am J Cardiol 1978; 42:839–48.
2. Heng MK, Norris RM, Singh BN, Partridge JB. Prognosis in unstable angina. Br Heart J 1976; 38:921–5.
3. Langer A, Freeman MR, Armstrong PW. ST segment shift in unstable angina: pathophysiology and association with coronary anatomy and hospital outcome. J Am Coll Cardiol 1989; 13:1495–1502.
4. Plotnick GD, Conti CR. Unstable angina: angiography, short- and long-term morbidity, mortality and symptomatic status of medically treated patients. Am J Med 1977; 63:870–3.
5. Marmur JD, Freeman MR, Langer AL, Armstrong PW. Prognosis in medically stabilized unstable angina: early Holter ST-segment monitoring compared with predischarge exercise thallium tomography. Ann Int Med 1990; 113:575–9.
6. Swahn E, Areskog M, Berglung U, Walfridsson H, Wallentin L. Predictive importance of clinical findings and a predischarge exercise test in patients with suspected unstable coronary artery disease. Am J Cardiol 1987; 59:208–14.
7. Lewis HD, Davis JW, Archibald DG, Steinke WE, Smitherman TC, Doherty JE, Schnaper HW, LeWinter MM, Linares E, Pouget JM, Sabharwal SC, Chesler E, DeMots H. Protective effects of aspirin against myocardial infarction and death in men with unstable angina. Results of a Veterans Administration cooperative study. New Engl J Med 1983; 309:396–403.
8. Wilcox I, Freedman SB, McCredie RJ, Carter GS, Kelly DT, Harris PJ. Risk of adverse outcome in patients admitted to the coronary care unit with suspected unstable angina pectoris. Am J Cardiol 1989; 64:845–8.

9. Mulcahy R, Awadhi A, Buitleor M, Tobin G, Johnson H, Contoy R. Natural history and prognosis of unstable angina. Am Heart J 1985; 109:753–8.
10. Butman SM, Olson HG, Gardin JM, Piters KM, Hullett M, Butman LK. Submaximal exercise testing after stabilization of unstable angina pectoris. J Am Coll Cardiol 1984; 4:667–73.
11. Butman SM, Olson HG, Butman LK. Early exercise testing after stabilization of unstable angina: correlation with coronary angiographic findings and subsequent cardiac events. Am Heart J 1986; 111:11–18.
12. Gazes PC, Mobley EM, Faris HM, Duncan RC, Humphries GB. Preinfarction (unstable) angina, a prospective study, ten year follow-up. Prognostic significance of electrocardiographic changes. Circulation 1973; 48:331–7.
13. Ouyang P, Brinker JA, Mellits ED, Weisfeldt ML, Gerstenblith G. Variables predictive of successful medical therapy in patients with unstable angina: selection by multivariate analysis from clinical, electrocardiographic, and angiographic evaluations. Circulation 1984; 70:367–76.
14. Nixon JV, Hillert MC, Shapiro W, Smitherman TC. Submaximal exercise testing after unstable angina. Am Heart J 1980; 99:772–8.
15. Swahn E, Areskog M, Wallentin L. Prognostic importance of early exercise testing in men with suspected unstable coronary artery disease. Eur Heart J 1987; 8:861–9.
16. Severi S, Orsini E, Marraccini P, Michelassi C, L'Abbate A. The basal electrocardiogram and the exercise test in assessing prognosis in patients with unstable angina. Eur Heart J 1988; 9:441–6.
17. Hakki AH, Iskandrian AS, Kane SA, Amenta A. Thallium-201 myocardial scintigraphy and left ventricular function at rest in patients with rest angina pectoris. Am Heart J 1984; 108:326–32.
18. Freeman MR, Williams AE, Chisholm RJ, Patt NL, Greyson ND, Armstrong PW. Role of resting thallium-201 perfusion in predicting coronary anatomy, left ventricular wall motion, and hospital outcome in unstable angina pectoris. Am Heart J 1989; 117:306–14.
19. Wackers FJ, Lie KI, Liem KL, Sokole EB, Samson G, van der Schoot JB, Durrer D. Thallium-201 scintigraphy in unstable angina pectoris. Circulation 1978; 57:738–42.
20. Freeman MR, Chisholm RJ, Armstrong PW. Usefulness of exercise electrocardiography and thallium scintigraphy in unstable angina pectoris in predicting the extent and severity of coronary artery disease. Am J Cardiol 1988; 62:1164–70.
21. Madsen JK, Stubgaard M, Utne HE, Hansen JF, van Duijvenkijk K, Reiber JHC, Christofferssen K. Prognosis and thallium-201 scintigraphy in patients admitted with chest pain without confirmed acute myocardial infarction. Br Heart J 1988; 59:184–9.
22. Nixon JV, Brown CN, Smitherman TC. Identification of transient and persistent segmental wall motion abnormalities in patients with unstable angina by two-dimensional echocardiography. Circulation 1982; 65:1497–503.
23. Gottlieb SO, Weisfeldt ML, Ouyang P, Mellits ED, Gerstenblith G. Silent ischemia as a marker for early unfavorable outcomes in patients with unstable angina. New Engl J Med 1986; 314:1214–9.

24. Homma S, Callahan RJ, Ameer B, McKusick KA, Strauss HW, Okada RD, Boucher CA. Usefulness of oral dipyridamole suspension for stress thallium imaging without exercise in the detection of coronary artery disease. Am J Cardiol 1986; 57:503–8.
25. Borges-Neto S, Magmarian JJ, Jain A, Roberts R, Verani MS. Quantitative thallium-201 single photon emission computed tomography after oral dipyridamole for assessing the presence, anatomic location and severity of coronary artery disease. J Am Coll Cardiol 1988; 11:962–9.
26. Younis LT, Byers S, Shaw L, Barth G, Goodgold H, Chaitman BR. Prognostic value of intravenous dipyridamole thallium scintigraphy after an acute myocardial ischemic event. Am J Cardiol 1989; 64:161–6.
27. Picano E, Severi S, Michelassi C, Lattanzi F, Masini M, Orsini E, Distante A, L'Abbate A. Prognostic importance of dipyridamole-echocardiography test in coronary artery disease. Circulation 1989; 80:450–7.
28. Ryan T, Vasey CG, Presti CF, O'Donnell JA, Feigenbaum H, Armstrong WF. Exercise echocardiography: detection of coronary artery disease in patients with normal left ventricular wall motion at rest. J Am Coll Cardiol 1988; 11:993–9.
29. Armstrong WF. Exercise echocardiography: ready, willing and able. J Am Coll Cardiol 1988; 11:1359–61.
30. Armstrong WF, O'Donnell J, Dillon JC, McHenry PL, Morris SM, Feigenbaum H. Complementary value of two-dimensional exercise echocardiography to routine treadmill exercise testing. Ann Int Med 1986; 105:829–35.
31. Machac J. Technetium-99m isonitrile; a perfusion or a viability agent? J Am Coll Cardiol 1989; 14:1685–8.
32. Parisi AF, Khuri S, Deupree RH, Sharma GVRK, Scott SM, Luichi RJ. Medical compared with surgical management of unstable angina. 5-year mortality and morbidity in the Veterans Administration study. Circulation 1989; 80:1176–89.
33. Goldschlager N, Sox HC. The diagnosis and prognostic value of the treadmill exercise test in the evaluation of chest pain, in patients with recent myocardial infarction, and in asymptomatic individuals. Am Heart J 1988; 116:523–35.
34. Detrano R, Froelicher VF. Exercise testing: uses and limitations considering studies. Prog Cardiovasc Dis 1988; 31:173–204.
35. Weiner DA, Ryan TJ, McCabe CH, Chaitman BR, Sheffield LT, Ferguson JC, Fisher LD, Tristani F. Prognostic importance of clinical profile and exercise test in medically treated patients with coronary artery disease. J Am Coll Cardiol 1984; 3:772–9.
36. Bogaty P, Degenais GR, Cantin B, Alain P, Rouleau JR. Prognosis in patients with a strongly positive exercise electrocardiogram. Am J Cardiol 1989; 64:1284–8.
37. Dagenais GR, Rouleau JR, Hochart P, Magrina J, Cantin B, Dumesnil JG. Survival with painless strongly positive exercise electrocardiogram. Am J Cardiol 1988; 62:892–5.
38. Kotler TS, Diamond GA. Exercise thallium-201 scintigraphy in the diagnosis and prognosis of coronary artery disease. Ann Int Med 1990; 113:684–702.
39. Weiss AT, Berman DS, Lew AS, Nielsen J, Potkin B, Swan HJC, Waxman A, Maddahi J. Transient ischemic dilatation of the left ventricle on stress thallium-201 scintigraphy: a marker of severe and extensive coronary artery disease. J Am Coll Cardiol 1987; 9:752–9.

40. Boucher CA, Zir LM, Beller GA, Okada RD, McKusick KA, Strauss HW, Pohost GM. Increased lung uptake of thallium-201 during exercise myocardial imaging: clinical, hemodynamic, and angiographic implications in patients with coronary artery disease. Am J Cardiol 1980; 46:189–96.
41. Iskandrian AS, Hakki AH, Kane-Marsch S. Prognostic implications of exercise thallium-201 scintigraphy in patients with suspected or known coronary artery disease. Am Heart J 1985; 110:135–43.
42. Detrano R, Janos A, Lyons KP, Marcondes G, Abbassi N, Froelicher VF. Factors affecting sensitivity and specificity of a diagnostic test: the exercise thallium scintigram. Am J Med 1988; 84:699–710.
43. Fintel DJ, Links JM, Brinker JA, Frank TL, Parker M, Becker LC. Improved diagnostic performance of exercise thallium-201 single photon emission computed tomography over planar imaging in the diagnosis of coronary artery disease: a receiver operating characteristic analysis. J Am Coll Cardiol 1989; 13:600–12.
44. Bonow RO, Kent KM, Rosing DR, Lan KKG, Lakatos E, Borer JS, Bacharach SL, Green MV, Epstein SE. Exercise-induced ischemia in mildly symptomatic patients with coronary artery disease and preserved left ventricular function. New Engl J Med 1984; 311:1339–45.
45. Iskandrian AS, Heo J, Askenase A, Segal BL, Auerbach N. Dipyridamole cardiac imaging. Am Heart J 1988; 115:432–43.
46. Boucher CA, Brewster DC, Darling RC, Okada RD, Strauss HW, Pohost GM. Determination of cardiac risk by dipyridamole thallium imaging before peripheral vascular surgery. New Engl J Med 1985; 312:389–94.
47. Younis CT, Byers S, Shaw L, Barth G, Goodgold H, Chaitman BR. Prognostic importance of silent myocardial ischemia detected by intravenous dipyridamole thallium myocardial imaging in asymptomatic patients with coronary artery disease. J Am Coll Cardiol 1989; 14:1635–41.

9

General Management Strategy in Patients with Unstable Angina

John D. Rutherford

Brigham and Women's Hospital and Harvard Medical School
Boston, Massachusetts

As for all forms of coronary artery disease, the ultimate prognosis of the patient is largely determined by the cumulative amount of myocardial damage that has accrued. Impaired ventricular function is the most important adverse determinant of prognosis in patients who survive myocardial infarction (1) and in patients with chronic stable angina (2), and this relationship also appears true for patients presenting with unstable angina pectoris. Patients with unstable angina who have evidence of moderate to severe left ventricular dysfunction appear to have a survival advantage when treated with aggressive revascularization therapy compared with a standard medical regimen especially when they have multivessel coronary artery disease (3,4). Therefore, soon after the patient has presented with unstable angina, it is important to make an assessment of left ventricular function. This is usually easily achieved with two-dimensional echocardiography. In patients with normal left ventricular function who stabilize on a standard medical regimen, subsequent risk stratification will be performed by some form of stress testing (see Chapter 8). Patients who have moderate or severe degrees of ventricular dysfunction are likely to have a worse prognosis if they are treated conservatively, and early coronary angiography will usually be contemplated with a view to revascularization if appropriate. In these patients, if significant left main coronary artery disease or severe multivessel coronary artery disease is discovered, revascularization will almost always be recommended (see Chapters 12–14). Other factors will also influence the choice of conservative or aggressive management plans:

1. Patients who continue to have rest angina despite maximally tolerated doses of all three categories of oral therapy (beta-blockers, nitrates, and calcium antagonists), aspirin, intravenous heparin, and intravenous nitroglycerin will almost always go forward for revascularization by either PTCA or coronary surgery.

2. Patients with rest pain despite a full medical regimen are more likely to have evidence for intracoronary clot at the time of angiography. If intracoronary clot is clearly present, the chance of successful percutaneous transluminal coronary angioplasty is diminished in the affected vessel and many cardiologists will consider continuing full anticoagulation with heparin (or, perhaps, intracoronary lytic therapy) for hours or days in an attempt to dissolve the clot and allow for a more successful definitive revascularization procedure. Obviously, this course of action can only be adopted if the patient remains relatively stable.

3. If revascularization is being contemplated, especially by coronary artery surgery, certain factors will adversely effect prognosis. Female patients will have a higher operative mortality and less successful revascularization because their smaller coronary arterial size is less amenable to successful revascularization. Elderly females are often the highest risk candidates. Evidence of renal dysfunction, pulmonary dysfunction, or lack of adequate venous conduits will also influence the decision to adopt an aggressive or conservative approach. Patients who have previously had revascularization surgery will have a higher operative mortality and less complete revascularization, although most will achieve symptomatic relief.

4. Patients with postinfarction unstable angina (unstable angina occurring within several weeks of a documented acute myocardial infarction) can pose difficult management decisions. The general strategy will often be determined by the amount of left ventricular (or right ventricular) damage the patient has accumulated prior to the onset of unstable angina. For patients with evidence of major left ventricular damage (extensive Q-wave infarction, severe ventricular dysfunction, gallop rhythms, or left ventricular failure) in whom the risks of revascularization are high, physicians will usually aim initially for a conservative approach. Such patients will be treated with an aggressive medical regimen including intravenous nitroglycerin, heparin, and beta-blockers if possible, possibly calcium antagonists, and, if despite these measures unstable symptoms persist, intra-aortic balloon will be contemplated with a view to angiography and revascularization albeit at relatively high risk. In patients with evidence of relatively minor left ventricular damage (i.e., patients with non–Q-wave infarction or modest enzyme releases), left ventricular function will be assessed, coronary angiography will usually be performed, and revascularization considered at relatively modest risk. Again, the presence of intracoronary clot may lead to treatment with aspirin or heparin for several days before coronary angioplasty is performed in the affected vessel.

The choice of medical regimens will be discussed in Chapters 10 and 11, and the pros and cons of percutaneous transluminal coronary angioplasty and cardiac surgery will be discussed in Chapters 12, 13, and 14.

REFERENCES

1. Multicenter Post-infarction Research Group. Risk stratification and survival after myocardial infarction. N Engl J Med 1983; 309:331–6.
2. Varnauskas E, the European Coronary Study Group. Survival, myocardial infarction and employment status in a prospective, randomized study of coronary bypass surgery. Circulation 1985; 72[Supp V]: 90–101.
3. Luchi RJ, Scott SM, Deupree RH, the Principal Investigators and their associates of the Veterans Administration Cooperative Study No. 28. Comparison of medical and surgical treatment for unstable angina pectoris. N Engl J Med 1987; 316:977–84.
4. Scott SM, Luchi RJ Deupree RH, Veterans Administration Unstable Angina Cooperative Study Group. Veterans Administration Cooperative Study for treatment of patients with unstable angina. Results in patients with abnormal ventricular function. Circulation 1988; (Supp I): 113–21.

10

The Use of Anticoagulant, Antiplatelet, and Thrombolytic Therapy in the Treatment of Unstable Angina

John D. Rutherford

Brigham and Women's Hospital and Harvard Medical School
Boston, Massachusetts

INTRODUCTION

The coronary artery lesion associated with unstable angina tends to be eccentric and irregular rather than being symmetric and smooth-bordered, and may be associated with filling defects on coronary angiography, which are assumed to be caused by coronary thrombi (1–4) and may form in response to activation of platelets (5) or alterations in the clotting system. Both pathologic (6,7) and angiographic (1–3,8–13) studies have suggested the presence of coronary artery thrombus in patients with unstable angina. Thrombus has also been observed in the coronary arteries at coronary angioscopy in patients undergoing cardiac surgery for unstable angina pectoris (14). Biochemical data have also implicated thrombus formation in the pathogenesis of unstable angina (5,12).

In patients presenting early after the onset of angina at rest, coronary arteriography has shown a relatively high incidence of thrombus or complex lesions (13), and subsequent adverse cardiac events (death, myocardial infarction, and urgent revascularization) appear more frequent in patients with coronary thrombus (73%), complex coronary morphology (55%), or multivessel disease (58%) than in patients without these angiographic features, in whom the respective rates were 17, 31, and 7%. Seventy-five percent of patients requiring urgent angiography for continuing angina late after hospital admission had coronary thrombi (13). Coronary thrombus appears to be a strong angiographic predictor of subsequent adverse cardiac events. Since recent episodes of rest angina can be associated with nonocclusive thrombi (14), and because of the potential importance of platelet activation and thrombus formation in the pathogenesis and clinical outcome of unstable angina, management strategies that include (a) anticoagulant drugs, (b) antiplatelet drugs, and, more recently, (c) thrombolytic therapy have been used.

ANTICOAGULANT THERAPY

A number of clinical studies have suggested that early therapy with heparin (at times associated with subsequent oral anticoagulant therapy) may have a salutary effect in patients with "preinfarction" or unstable angina (15–19). Heparin exerts its anticoagulant activity by binding to and activating antithrombin III, which neutralizes thrombin (20).

A study of patients with preinfarction angina by Wood et al. (1961), was terminated prematurely because it was felt that patients treated with anticoagulants had a substantially better outcome (16). One hundred patients were given anticoagulants (severe cases were given heparin IM for the first 24 hr, then either phenindione, ethyl biscoumacetate, or nicoumalone for a minimum of 6 weeks), and 50 patients were treated more conservatively. The last 30 control patients constituted a subgroup who were not considered good candidates for anticoagulants (i.e., a history of peptic ulcer, bruising, or physician prejudice), thus unbalancing the randomization process. Only 3% of the patients given anticoagulants had myocardial infarction within the next 2 months, compared with 22% of the control patients. The minimum mortality in the respective groups was 6 and 30%. The results of this study influenced subsequent clinical practice and were supported by a study performed in India by Vakil (1962) (17). He randomized 190 patients with preinfarction angina to anticoagulants (IM or IV heparin, followed by oral anticoagulants for a minimum of 3 months) and 156 patients to a conservative regimen. The overall myocardial infarction rate over 3 months was 41% with a mortality of 16%. The patients treated with anticoagulants had a myocardial infarction rate of 36% and a 3-month mortality of 9.5%, compared with respective rates of 49 and 24% in the patients managed conservatively.

In a randomized, prospective trial of anticoagulants, reported in 1986, 102 patients with unstable angina (treated with analgesics or beta-blockers sparingly and randomized to anticoagulants with heparin 10,000 U intravenously every 6 hr for 48 hr with warfarin started on admission and continued for 6 months), there appeared to be less recurrent unstable angina and fewer deaths in the treated patients than in the control group (21).

Telford and Wilson (18) showed a marked reduction in mortality and myocardial infarction rate in patients assigned to either heparin and atenolol or heparin alone, compared with patients assigned to atenolol alone or placebo. The results

Table 1 Endpoints in Unstable Angina Trial

Treatment		AMI	Refractory Angina
Placebo	$N = 118$	14	27
Aspirin	$N = 121$	4 ($p = 0.012$)	20 ($p = 0.217$)
Heparin	$N = 118$	1 ($p < 0.001$)	10 ($p = 0.002$)
Aspirin and heparin	$N = 122$	2 ($p = 0.001$)	13 ($p = 0.011$)

Source: Ref. 22.

of this study are difficult to interpret because, of the 400 patients initially randomized, incorrect recruitment led to subsequent withdrawal of 186 patients.

Theroux et al. (22) have shown, in a double-blind trial of patients with unstable angina, that heparin alone (1000 U/hr), aspirin alone (325 mg twice daily), and their combination are effective in reducing subsequent in-hospital cardiac events. Myocardial infarction occurred in 12% of patients given placebo, compared with 3% ($p = 0.01$) of patients given aspirin, 0.8% of patients given heparin ($p = 0.001$), and 1.6% of patients given aspirin plus heparin ($p = 0.003$, Table 1). Recurrent angina occurred less frequently in the heparin-treated group, but the small sample size precluded direct comparison of the relative efficacy of aspirin versus heparin therapy on this endpoint or on fatal events. Although heparin and aspirin each appeared to have a salutary effect on subsequent morbid events in patients with unstable angina, neither agent taken as the sole therapy appeared better than the other.

ANTIPLATELET THERAPY

Aspirin Therapy

Aspirin inhibits adenosine diphosphate (ADP)-induced platelet aggregation and the collagen-induced release of adenosine triphosphate (ATP), serotonin, and platelet antiheparin activity (platelet factor 4), as well as immediately and irreversibly acetylating the cyclooxygenase in platelets (23). The inhibition of this latter enzyme prevents formation of thromboxane A_2 (24), and platelets are unable to synthesize new enzymes to replace the inactivated enzyme so that platelet function is not restored until new platelets enter the circulation. Therefore, the inhibitory effects of aspirin on platelet aggregation occur immediately and continue to be detected 4–7 days after a single oral dose. In contrast, aspirin inhibition of the cyclooxygenase in the cells of the vessel wall is reversible because these cells can synthesize new enzyme.

The use of aspirin therapy in patients with unstable angina has been examined in several large trials: the study by Theroux et al. (22), the Veterans Administration Cooperative Study (25), and the Canadian Multicenter Trial (26) and the RISC Study (27). In the Veterans Administration Cooperative Study (25), 1266 men with unstable angina were randomly assigned to placebo or 324 mg of aspirin in buffered solution (Alka Seltzer), to be taken daily for 3 months. During the treatment period, death or acute myocardial infarction occurred in 10.1% of placebo-treated and 5.0% of aspirin-treated patients ($p = 0.0005$). Follow-up at one year showed persistence of the beneficial effects of 3 months of aspirin therapy. There was no evidence of gastrointestinal side effects from the study medicine.

In the Canadian Multicenter Trial (26), 555 patients with unstable angina were enrolled in a double-blind, placebo-controlled study and randomly assigned, within 8 days of hospitalization, to therapy with aspirin (325 mg four times daily), sulfinpyrazone (200 mg four times daily), both therapies, or neither therapy. Follow-up lasted 2 years. The combined incidence of cardiac death and nonfatal myocardial infarction was 8.6% in the groups given aspirin and 17.0% in the other groups, representing a risk reduction with aspirin of 51% ($p = 0.008$). Analysis by intention to treat yielded risk reductions with aspirin of 30% for the outcome of cardiac death or nonfatal acute myocardial infarction, 56% for cardiac death alone, and 43% for all deaths. Sulfinpyrazone had no observed benefit (Fig. 1).

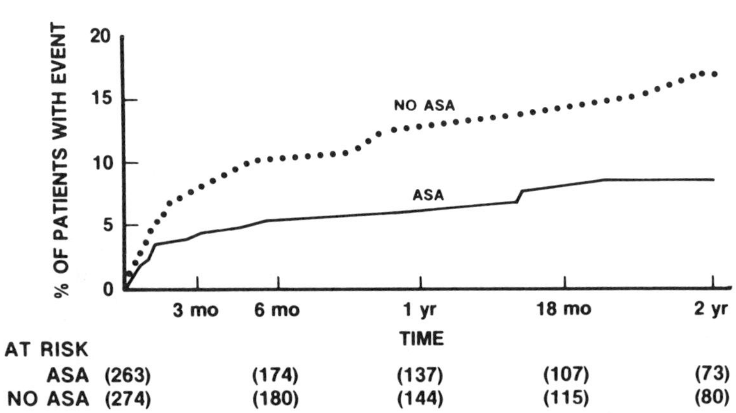

Figure 1 Influence of aspirin (325 mg four times daily) on the occurrence of cardiac death or nonfatal myocardial infarction in patients receiving aspirin (ASA) or no aspirin (NO ASA). The graph is a life table depiction of the cumulative risk and time of the first occurrence of an outcome event. The numbers of patients at risk are noted below the graph. The incidence of cardiac death or nonfatal myocardial infarction was 8.6% in the ASA groups and 17% in the other groups. (Reprinted with permission from Ref. 26.)

In the RISC Group study, 796 men with unstable coronary artery disease (unstable angina or non–Q-wave myocardial infarction) were randomized to placebo-controlled treatment with oral aspirin (75 mg per day) and/or 5 days of intermittent intravenous heparin (27). Endpoints were death or nonfatal myocardial infarction analyzed by the intention-to-treat principle. This study showed that aspirin (75 mg per day) reduced the myocardial infarction and death rate in such patients at 1–3 months after presentation and that the combination of aspirin and heparin might be more effective during initial hospitalization.

Each major study indicates that administration of aspirin to patients with unstable angina will reduce subsequent morbid and fatal events, both acutely and in the long term.

Ticlopidine Therapy

Ticlopidine, an antiplatelet agent which, unlike aspirin, does not block cyclooxygenase but seems to interfere with the fibrinogen receptor and the ADP-mediated platelet activation mechanism reduces non-fatal myocardial infarction and vascular death in patients with unstable angina when compared to conventional therapy (28). Since this agent is expensive, can cause neutropenia (approximately 1% of patients) and can elevate serum cholesterol (by approximately 10%) its definitive role remains unclear (29).

THROMBOLYTIC THERAPY

The presence of intracoronary thrombus appears to be a strong angiographic predictor of subsequent recurrence of angina (4,13), myocardial infarction (4–13), the need for urgent coronary artery revascularization, or death (13). Therefore coronary anatomy has been analyzed in a number of trials of unstable angina before and after thrombolytic therapy (2,4,8,9,10,30), and quantitative analyses of changes in the morphology of coronary artery narrowings have been undertaken (1–9,14) (Fig. 2). To determine how often intracoronary thrombus is present during spontaneous ischemic attacks in patients with rest angina, Gotoh et al. (4) performed coronary angiography in 37 such patients. All patients had significant stenoses (>50% diameter narrowing) of at least one major coronary artery. In addition, 57% had intracoronary thrombus present in major coronary arteries, 38% had fixed narrowings without evidence of intracoronary thrombus, and 5% exhibited coronary spasm. Twenty of the 21 patients with intracoronary thrombus improved after thrombolytic therapy with intracoronary urokinase. Patients with intracoronary thrombus had a high frequency (71%) of recurrent symptoms even after successful thrombolysis, in contrast to a much lower recurrence rate (36%) among patients without intracoronary thrombus. Myocardial infarction within 4 weeks after cathcterization was observed more frequently

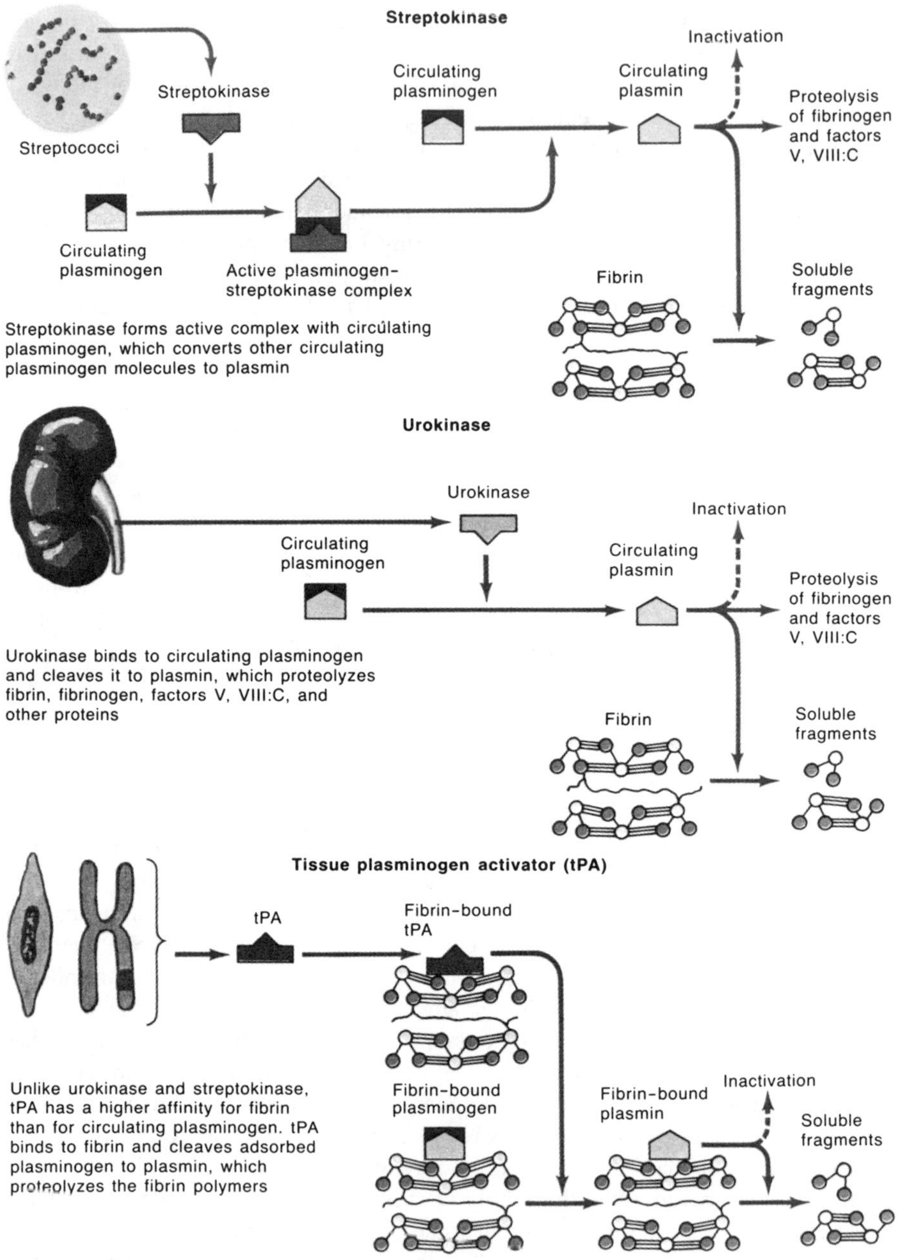

Figure 2 Mode of action of different forms of lytic therapy. (From Ref. 35 with permission.)

in patients with intracoronary thrombus (24%) than in those without thrombus (7%).

Thrombolytic therapy may be associated with a decrease in angiographic evidence of intracoronary thrombus (9) and also favorably alter the myocardial ischemia threshold in patients with unstable angina (30). De Zwaan et al. (9) showed that thrombolytic therapy (intracoronary SK or IV rt-PA) administered to 41 patients a mean of 19 hr after their last episode of angina led to fewer patients with angiographic evidence of intracoronary thrombus. Before thrombolytic therapy was instituted, 68% of patients had evidence of intracoronary thrombus, compared with 39% after therapy. Thrombolytic therapy did not appear as effective in patients with very tight stenoses (>90% diameter narrowing). There is also a suggestion that thrombolytic therapy may reduce the amount of provocable ischemia in patients with rest angina. In 40 patients with rest angina, Topol et al. (30) reported a significant increase in pacing thresholds to angina after rt-PA infusion without a comparable decrease in coronary stenosis. Three patients who received rt-PA had marked angiographic resolution of the culprit lesion and no longer exhibited pacing-induced ischemia.

Thus, unstable angina is often associated with intracoronary thrombosis, which appears to be a marker for subsequent adverse clinical events. However, even in the absence of overt changes in coronary anatomy, thrombolytic therapy may raise the ischemic threshold in patients with unstable angina, for unclear reasons.

The clinical efficacy of thrombolytic therapy has been examined in several small randomized studies. Gold et al. (31) reported short-term clinical improvement following thrombolytic therapy in patients with continuing unstable angina after 12–48 hr of standard therapy. Coronary angiography was not performed before thrombolytic therapy was administered. Twenty-four patients were randomly assigned to placebo or rt-PA (12-hr infusion of 1.75 mg/kg) and followed for a mean of 7 days. In patients treated with placebo, unstable angina persisted in 6/11 (54%) and coronary arteriography showed intracoronary thrombus in 8/11 (73%), compared with persistent unstable angina in 1/12 of the rt-PA treated group (8%) and no evidence of intracoronary thrombus in 11 patients. Benefit late after thrombolytic therapy has also been claimed. Ardissino et al. showed that a combination of rt-PA and heparin was more likely to keep patients with unstable angina free of ischemia than the use of heparin alone (32). Lawrence et al. (33) randomized patients with unstable angina to either IV streptokinase (SK) for 24 hr followed by warfarin during the next 6 months, or warfarin alone (20 patients in each group). None of the patients underwent coronary arteriography. After 6 months of follow-up, there were eight fatal or morbid events (four acute myocardial infarctions, four sudden deaths) in the patients treated with warfarin alone, compared with a single sudden death in the group treated with SK initially followed by warfarin.

The published studies testing the efficacy of thrombolytic therapy in patients with unstable angina do not have sufficient power to demonstrate a statistical difference. It has been estimated that the incidence of myocardial infarction or refractory angina over a 7-day period after the onset of unstable angina in patients managed with heparin is approximately 2 and 10%, respectively (34). Trials in larger patient populations with more endpoints are required to establish whether thrombolytic therapy is clinically beneficial in patients with unstable angina. Two such trials are in progress, the UNSA and TIMI III trials.

The UNSA (unstable angina) trial is a multicenter, randomized, double-blind study in which patients receive IV rt-PA or placebo within 12 hr of the onset of symptoms. Coronary arteriography is discouraged unless medical therapy fails. All patients can receive standard medical therapy, including sedation, beta-blockers, calcium antagonists, nitrates, bed rest, oxygen, aspirin, and heparin. The primary composite endpoint of unsatisfactory outcome at 4 days and 6 weeks after randomization includes death, documented myocardial infarction, angina associated with ECG changes, and cumulative evidence of ischemia during Holter monitoring. The incidence of stroke or other hemorrhagic events is also being studied. This trial is designed to establish whether thrombolytic therapy will have a salutary effect on clinical outcome in patients with unstable angina rather than the influence of thrombolytic therapy on coronary anatomy.

The NHLBI-funded Thrombolysis in Myocardial Ischemia Trial (TIMI-III) is conducting two randomized, blinded studies in patients with unstable angina and non–Q-wave myocardial infarction. The studies are designed to answer whether rt-PA produces improvement in angiographically determined myocardial perfusion or stenosis and what is the optimal initial and follow-up management strategy for patients with unstable angina. The first question asks whether rt-PA is superior to the addition of placebo to conventional therapy (including heparin and aspirin) and the second asks during follow-up whether there is a need for routine angiography, followed, if the anatomy is suitable, by revascularization. Success of therapy will be judged from the number of patients who do not experience death, myocardial infarction, disabling stroke, or failure of therapy (defined as significant recurrent ischemic pain at rest, or unsatisfactory results on Holter monitoring or ETT with thallium). The sample will be of sufficient size (2300 patients) to establish clearly the risks versus benefits of rt-PA therapy, as well as the value of angiography followed by revascularization.

In summary, few patients presenting with unstable angina currently are given thrombolytic therapy. Usual initial measures include bed rest, sedation, beta-blockers, calcium antagonists, nitrates, aspirin, and heparin. In the majority of patients, intensive medical therapy will alleviate symptoms, and on a case-by-case basis, physicians proceed either directly to coronary arteriography or to risk stratification with exercise testing. Some physicians manage unstable angina by proceeding promptly with revascularization and hope that this strategy will have a salutary affect on the natural history of the ischemic process. Whether this approach has advantages over a more conservative strategy is unknown, and several ongoing trials are addressing this important issue.

REFERENCES

1. Holmes D, Hartzler G, Smith H, Fuster V. Coronary artery thrombosis in patients with unstable angina. Br Heart J 1981; 45:411–16.
2. Vetrovec GW, Leinbach RC, Gold HK, Cowley MJ. Intracoronary thrombolysis in syndromes of unstable ischemia: angiographic and clinical results. Am Heart J 1982; 104:946–52.
3. Capone G, Wolf N, Meyer B, Meister S. Frequency of intracoronary filling defects by angiography in angina pectoris at rest. Am J Cardiol 1985; 56:403–6.
4. Gotoh K, Minamino T, Katoh O, Hamano Y, Fukui S, Hori M, et al. Pathophysiology and natural history: unstable angina. The role of intracoronary thrombus in unstable angina: angiographic assessment and thrombolytic therapy during ongoing anginal attacks. Circulation 1988; 77:526–34.
5. Fitzgerald D, Roy L, Catella F, Fitzgerald G. Platelet activation in unstable coronary disease. N Engl J Med 1986; 315:983–9.
6. Davies MJ, Thomas AC, Knapman PA, Hangartner JR. Intramyocardial platelet aggregation in patients with unstable angina suffering sudden ischemic cardiac death. Circulation 1986; 73:418–27.
7. Falk E. Unstable angina with fatal outcome: dynamic coronary thrombosis leading to infarction and/or sudden death. Autopsy evidence of recurrent mural thrombosis with peripheral embolization culminating in total vascular occlusion. Circulation 1985; 71:699–708.
8. Ambrose JA, Hjemdahl MC, Borrico S, Sherman W, Cohen M, Gorlin R, et al. Quantitative and qualitative effects of intracoronary streptokinase in unstable angina and non-Q wave infarction. J Am Coll Cardiol 1987; 9:1156–65.
9. de Zwaan C, Bar F, Janssen J, de Swart H, Vermeer F, Wellens H. Effects of thrombolytic therapy in unstable angina: clinical and angiographic results. J Am Coll Cardiol 1988; 12:301–9.
10. Mandelkorn JB, Wolf NM, Singh S, Shechter JA, Kersh RI, Rodgers DM, et al. Intracoronary thrombus in nontransmural myocardial infarction and in unstable angina pectoris. Am J Cardiol 1983; 52:1–6.
11. Bresnahan D, Davis D, Holmes D, Smith H. Angiographic occurrence and clinical correlates of intraluminal coronary artery thrombus: role of unstable angina. J Am Coll Cardiol. 1985; 6:285–9.
12. Kruskal J, Commerford P, Franks J, Kirsch R. Fibrin and fibrinogen-related antigens in patients with stable and unstable coronary artery disease. N Engl J Med 1987; 317:1361–5.
13. Freeman M, Williams A, Chisholm R, Armstrong P. Intracoronary thrombus and complex morphology in unstable angina: relation to timing of angiography and in-hospital cardiac events. Circulation 1989; 80:17–23.

14. Sherman CT, Litvack F, Grundfest W, Lee M, Hickey A, Chaux A, et al. Coronary angioscopy in patients with unstable angina pectoris. N Engl J Med 1986; 315:913–19.
15. Nichol E, Phillips W, Casten G. Virtue of prompt anticoagulant therapy in impending myocardial infarction: experience with 318 patients during a 10 year period. Ann Intern Med 1959; 50:1158–73.
16. Wood P. Acute and subacute coronary insufficiency. Br Med J 1961; 1:1779–82.
17. Vakil R. Preinfarction syndrome: management and followup. Am J Cardiol 1964; 14:55–63.
18. Telford A, Wilson C. Trial of heparin versus atenolol in prevention of myocardial infarction in intermediate coronary syndrome. Lancet 1981; 1:1225–8.
19. Mulcahy R, Al AAH, de BM, Tobin G, Johnson H, Contoy R. Natural history and prognosis of unstable angina. Am Heart J 1985; 109:753–8.
20. Hirsh J. Drug Therapy. Heparin. N Engl J Med 1991; 324:1565–74.
21. Williams DO, Kirby MG, McPherson K, Phear DN. Anticoagulant treatment of unstable angina. Br J Clin Pract 1986; 40:114–16.
22. Theroux P, Ouimet H, McCans J, Latour JG, Joly P, Levy G, et al. Aspirin, heparin, or both to treat acute unstable angina. N Engl J Med 1988; 319:1105–11.
23. Harker L, Fuster V. Pharmacology of platelet inhibitors. J Am Coll Cardiol 1986; 8:21B–32B.
24. Hjemdahl-Monsen CE, Lewis HD, Cairns J, Chesebro JH, Fuster V. Role of antithrombotic therapy in unstable angina, myocardial infarction and sudden death. J Am Coll Cardiol 1986; 8:67B–75B.
25. Lewis H, Davis J, Archibald D. Protective effects of aspirin against acute myocardial infarction and death in men with unstable angina: results of a Veterans Administration cooperative study. N Engl J Med 1983; 309:396–403.
26. Cairns JA, Gent M, Singer J, Finnie KJ, Froggatt GM, Holder DA, et al. Aspirin, sulfinpyrazone, or both in unstable angina: results of a Canadian multicenter trial. N Engl J Med 1985; 313:1369–75.
27. The RISC Group. Risk of myocardial infarction and death during treatment with low dose aspirin and intravenous heparin in men with unstable coronary artery disease.
28. Balsano F, Rizzon P, Violi F, Scrutinio D, Cimminiello F, Pasotti C, Rudelli G, the Studio della Ticlopidina nell'Angina Instabile Group. Antiplatelet treatment with ticlopidine in unstable angina. A controlled multicenter clinical trial. Circulation 1990; 82:17–26.
29. Fitzgerald G. Ticlopidine in unstable angina. A more expensive aspirin? Circulation 1990; 82:294–5.
30. Topol E, Nicklas J, Kander N, Walton J, Ellis S, Gormon L, et al. Coronary revascularization after intravenous tissue plasminogen activator for unstable angina pectoris: results of a randomized, double-blind placebo-controlled trial. Am J Cardiol 1988; 62:368–71.
31. Gold H, Johns J, Leinbach R, Yasuda T, Grossbard E, Zusman R, et al. A randomized, blinded, placebo-controlled trial of recombinant human tissue-type plasminogen activator in patients with unstable angina pectoris. Circulation 1987; 75:1192–9.

32. Ardissino D, Barberis P, De Servi S, Mussini A, Rolla A, Visani L, Specchia G. Recombinant tissue-type plasminiogen activator followed by heparin compared with heprin alone for refractory unstable angina pectoris. Am J Cardiol 1990; 66:910–14.
33. Lawrence J, Shepherd J, Bone I, Rogen A, Fulton W. Fibrinolytic therapy in unstable angina pectoris: a controlled clinical trial. Thromb Res 1980; 17:767–77.
34. Ambrose JA, Alexopoulos D. Thrombolysis in unstable angina: will the beneficial effects of thrombolytic therapy in myocardial infarction apply to patients with unstable angina? J Am Coll Cardiol 1989; 13:1666–71.
35. Moake JL, Levine JD. Thrombotic disorders. Clinical Symposia; 37:18, 1985.

11

Nitrates, Beta Adrenoceptor Blockers, and Calcium Antagonists

Michael J. Landzberg

Brigham and Women's Hospital
Boston, Massachusetts

Elliott M. Antman

Brigham and Women's Hospital and Harvard Medical School
Boston, Massachusetts

INTRODUCTION

Unstable angina is now recognized to be a heterogenous grouping of ischemic states, each varying in pathogenesis, presentation, and prognosis (1).

Myocardial ischemia, by definition, occurs when coronary blood flow is unable to meet the heart's metabolic demands. Decreased coronary blood flow, increased myocardial oxygen requirements, or a combination of the two may induce myocardial ischemia. The emergence of an unstable pattern of angina either may represent progression of native coronary artery disease, severe enough to cause a major limitation of coronary blood flow, or may signify the transformation of an atherosclerotic plaque from a "quiescent" state to an "active" one (2). Abnormal vasoreactivity, including localized vasoconstriction or even intense focal spasm (e.g., Prinzmetal's variant angina), may also contribute to the clinical picture of unstable angina.

The imbalance between oxygen supply and myocardial demand results in painful as well as clinically silent episodes of myocardial ischemia. These episodes of ischemia may not only cause immediate deterioration in ventricular function, but may induce prolonged postischemic changes in systolic and disastolic function, or "stunning," of the affected myocardium, lasting for hours to days postreperfusion (3). Patients with unstable angina may also suffer from a chronic "low flow" state of myocardial perfusion. To offset this decrease in myocardial oxygen supply, "down-regulation" of cardiac metabolism, or "hibernation," has been hypothesized. The chronic depression of ventricular function may return to normal after reperfusion of the affected myocardium (4).

The goals of treatment for patients with symptoms of unstable angina are many, and include clinical stabilization via a reduction in the frequency of ischemic episodes, improvement in ventricular systolic and diastolic function, and prevention of the progression of unstable angina to myocardial infarction or death. Treatment regimens focus on decreasing the major determinants of myocardial oxygen demand (heart rate, wall stress, and myocardial contractility) while concomitantly altering the determinants of oxygen supply (heart rate, left ventricular end-diastolic pressure, diastolic perfusion pressure of the coronary arteries, and coronary vascular tone and resistance).

In this chapter we will examine the rationale and benefits of pharmacotherapeutic interventions with nitrates, beta-blockers, and calcium antagonists in the treatment of unstable angina. There are relatively few large-scale randomized control trials analyzing the benefit of the use of these agents in patients with unstable angina and most trials have sampled small test populations, which, in many cases, have insufficient statistical power to allow definitive conclusions. Furthermore, medications often have not been tested in sufficiently varying dose regimens within given protocols to adequately explore the dose response relationship of drug effect. "Positive" results have often been published in the form of "subgroup analyses," different from the hypotheses intended to be tested by the main study protocol. While results of such subgroup analyses may be provocative, they should be interpreted with caution and are best viewed as the stimulus for further large-scale randomized trials. Our primary clinical information regarding the use of organic nitrates, beta-blocking agents, and calcium antagonists in the treatment of unstable angina is, therefore, limited in scope. Cinical practice remains largely based upon the pooled results of existing randomized trials (the most important of which we will examine here in greater detail) and collective anecdotal experience.

ORGANIC NITRATES

Nitroglycerin has been employed in the management of anginal syndromes since the late nineteenth century and enthusiasm for its use has waxed and waned over the past 40 years (5). The pendulum has clearly swung back in favor of nitrate therapy as a mainstay in the treatment of ischemic heart disease syndromes (6).

Pharmacology and Pathophysiology

Nitrates act as vasodilators in all vascular beds. With the recent understanding of the importance of endothelial function in the control of vascular tone (7), the primary mechanism of action of the organic nitrates has been further elucidated. Normal vascular endothelium responds to vasoactive mediators and various stimuli, including changes in blood flow, hypoxia, and shear stress, by secreting regulatory factors including endothelium-derived relaxing factors (EDRF) and endothelin. These substances act locally on vascular smooth muscle to produce vasodilatation or vasoconstriction, respectively. The endothelium-dependent relaxing factors stimulate soluble guanylate cyclase in vascular smooth muscle cells to convert magnesium-GTP to cyclic GMP (cGMP) (8,9). This second messenger, in turn, activates cGMP-dependent protein kinase, that dephosphorylates, among other proteins, the light chain of myosin and thereby leads to smooth muscle relaxation. Organic nitrates have been shown to similarly affect the endothelial-dependent relaxation pathway. Metabolically, these agents are sequentially reduced to nitric and nitrous acid, and subsequently converted to short-lived sulfhydryl-containing nitrosothiols that activate guanylate cyclase (10). During this process, intracellular thiols become oxidized. As will be discussed later, stores of sulfhydryl-containing donor molecules may become depleted with chronic nitrate administration, potentially limiting the effectiveness of these agents.

The cardiac benefits of nitrate therapy are best understood by separating their systemic effects from those occurring locally within the coronary circulation.

Systemic Effects of Organic Nitrates

In the systemic circulation, at relatively low concentrations, nitrates act primarily on the venous and arterial vascular beds, causing maximal venodilatation of both the small and large veins. As vascular capacitance rises, circulating blood volume is redistributed, and preload and afterload are reduced to both the right and left sides of the heart. This results in decreased ventricular volumes and reduced wall stress experienced by the contracting ventricles. These beneficial hemodynamic effects of nitrates have been confirmed in patients with unstable angina (11). In the nonresistance arterial beds, vasodilatation produces an increase in vascular conductance and compliance, and thereby increases luminal diameter. Significant decreases in systemic vascular resistance and blood pressure occur only with higher doses of nitrates. As nitrate concentrations rise, arteriolar resistance falls, altering both regional and systemic blood flow patterns. This action of nitrates may stimulate a baroreceptor-mediated response, and sympathetic tone may increase, causing undesired vasoconstriction and tachycardia.

Coronary Vascular Effects of Organic Nitrates

In the coronary bed, a balance of nitrate effects is reached. Initial vasodilatation leads to increased coronary blood flow, which may be offset by reflex sympathetic vasoconstriction. Improved left ventricular hemodynamics decreases myocardial energy expenditure and, in turn, causes a decrease in coronary blood flow through autoregulatory mechanisms. Nitrates may cause local vasodilation at sites of increased vascular tone or focal stenoses. In the ischemic myocardium, a

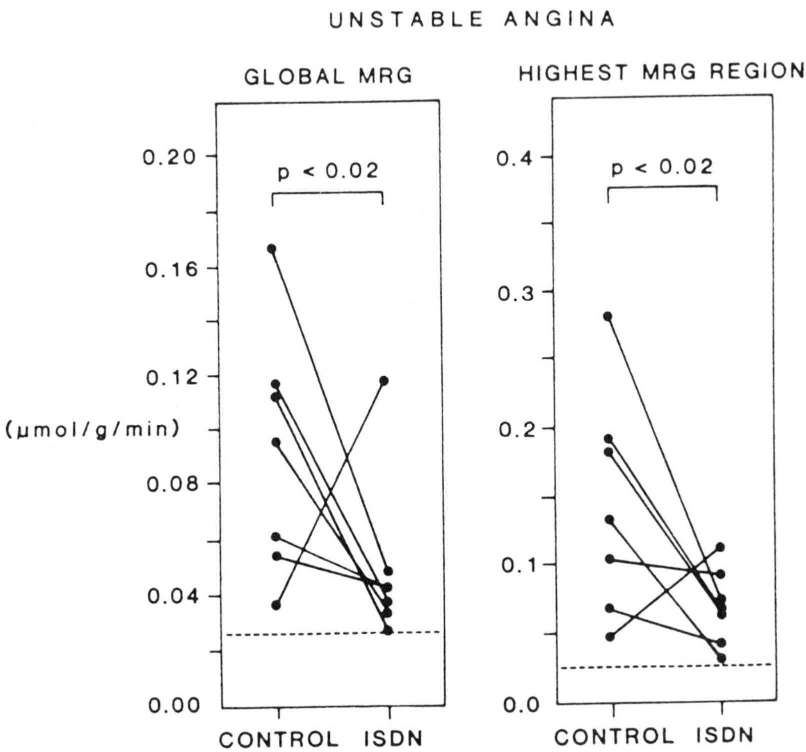

Figure 1 Myocardial metabolic rate for glucose (MRG) measured by positron emission tomography during control and isosorbide dinitrate treatment in patients with unstable angina. Global and regional glucose utilization is significantly lower with isosorbide dinitrate. (From Ref. 12 with permission.)

preferential shunting of flow to both subendocardium and ischemic regions may be produced by nitrate therapy, helping correct existing metabolic imbalances. Recent studies with positron emission tomography (PET) scanning in patients with unstable angina have confirmed both abnormal glucose metabolism in patients with this syndrome as well as the restoration, towards normal, of glucose utilization with the addition of nitroglycerin therapy (Fig. 1) (12). Enhanced coronary blood flow seen with nitroglycerin administration has been shown to improve postischemic contractile dysfunction in "stunned" myocardium, as well.

Clinical Trials with Organic Nitrates

The widespread availability of ever-increasing varieties and preparations of nitrates (oral, sublingual, transdermal, transmucosal, and intravenous forms) has

Table 1 Nitrate Pharmacokinetics and Recommended Dosages

Medication	Recommended Dosage (mg)	Onset of Action (min)	Peak Action (min)	Duration
Sublingual NTG	0.3–0.8	2–5	4–8	10–30 min
Sublingual ISDN	2.5–10	5–20	15–60	45–120 min[a]
Oral NTG spray	0.4	2–5	4–8	10–30 min
Buccal NTG	1–3	2–5	4–10	30–300 min
Oral ISDN	10–60	15–45	45–120	2–6 hr
Oral NTG	6.5–19.5	20–45	45–120	2–6 hr
NTG ointment (2 percent)	½–2 inches	15–60	30–120	3–8 hr
NTG discs (transdermal)	10–20 mg	30–60	60–180	Up to 24 hr[b]

NTG = nitroglycerin; ISDN = isosorbide dinitrate.
Higher doses may be needed, especially in congestive heart failure.
[a]Up to 3 to 4 hours in some studies.
[b]Clinical effects may not persist for 24 hours.
Source: From Abrams J. Nitrates. Med Clin North Am 1988; 72(1), with permission.

made these agents popular in the treatment of unstable angina (Table 1). Reliance on the use of nitrates is largely based upon anecdotal experience and inference drawn from these agents' therapeutic effects on patients with chronic stable exertional angina or from the results of small open-label clinical trials. Given the spontaneous variability in the occurrence of ischemic episodes in unstable angina, the usefulness of such information, derived from noncontrolled trials, is limited.

Intravenous preparations of nitrates, available since the late 1970s, have been favored in the intensive-care setting because of the ease of titration of dose, rapid onset of action, and rapid termination of vascular effects. In the early 1980s, a number of uncontrolled trials examined the use of intravenous nitrate preparations for patients with angina refractory to the prevailing conventional therapy. In the English literature, nine trials, with a combined population of 280 patients, using varying dosage regimens in different anginal settings, showed significant, and sometimes dramatic, reductions in anginal frequency with the use of intravenous nitrates. No other morbid or mortal endpoints were shown to be significantly reduced.

To date, only two randomized controlled trials have examined the role of intravenous nitroglycerin as monotherapy in the treatment of unstable angina. Distante et al. (13) enrolled 20 consecutive patients with progressive, uncontrolled vasospastic angina and known significant coronary artery disease in a prospective double-blind, double-crossover study of the use of intravenous nitrates. Intravenous nitrates were adminstered at doses of 0.25–5.0 mg/hr over 24-hr periods. Side effects were negligible. Electrocardiographically determined ischemic episodes, with or without pain, were significantly decreased during infusion of isosorbide dinitrate when compared both to control and to placebo values (less than 20 events/day during nitrate infusion versus approximately 100 events/day with control). Curfman and colleagues examined whether increasing circulating nitrate concentration by use of intravenous preparations was more effective than other modalities of nitrate therapy in decreasing ischemic episodes in patients with unstable angina (14). Forty consecutive patients with rest angina were prospectively randomized to receive intravenous nitroglycerin (10–200 μg/min) or a combination of oral isosorbide dinitrate (80–240 mg/day) and topical nitroglycerin ointment (0.5–2.0 inches of 2% paste every 6 hours) over a 72-hr period, in doses adjusted to produce comparable systemic effects (25% reduction in mean arterial pressure). Side effects were negligible. While both regimens significantly decreased the number of ischemic episodes/day, neither regimen showed a greater treatment benefit. A trend toward more consistent control of ischemic events during the first 24 hr of treatment was noted with the use of intravenous nitrates. However, it should be noted that the small population size involved in this study resulted in a lack of statistical power to show a significant difference in outcomes between the two treatment strategies.

Recommendations

Based upon extensive clinical experience in numerous centers, we recommend the use of organic nitrates for decreasing the number of ischemic events in patients with unstable angina. Existing randomized controlled trials have not shown a reduction in other morbid or mortal endpoints with nitrate therapy. This may represent either a true lack of benefit from nitrate therapy, or it may simply reflect insufficient statistical power of the trials attempting to show such a treatment effect (probably on the order of 10–20%). There is no clear benefit from the use of intravenous forms when compared to combinations of oral and topical nitrates. Intravenous nitroglycerin, however, has the advantage of rapid titration and a short biologic half-life (3 min). If side effects do occur, they will rapidly disappear with discontinuation of the medication. In addition, substantial evidence exists that intravenous nitrates reduce short-term mortality in patients following acute myocardial infarction (15). Its use, therefore, may be of benefit in those patients with unstable angina who progress to myocardial infarction.

Infusion rates can begin as low as 10–20 μg/min and can be rapidly titrated every 5–10 min on an individualized patient basis. Some clinical centers employ doses as high as 200–400 μg/min, safely, without pulmonary arterial monitoring if mean arterial pressure is reduced by no more than 15% of control values.

Side effects of intravenous nitrates are infrequent and may include headache, as well as reflex bradycardia (16), both of which terminate quickly with discontinuation of the drug. Cautious use of nitrates is recommended in the setting of preload-dependent states such as right ventricular infarction, hypovolemia, or constrictive or effusive pericardial disease.

A less frequently encountered side effect, seen with the administration of large dosages of nitrates for a prolonged treatment period, is methemoglobinemia. This occurs as a result of the ability of organic nitrates to oxidize hemoglobin's iron moiety from its ferrous (Fe^{2+}) to its ferric (Fe^{3+}) state. The primary manifestation of methemoglobinemia is cyanosis, occurring at methemoglobin levels greater than 5%. However, patients can remain asymptomatic until methemoglobin levels reach 30%, when progressive fatigue, nausea, headache, and tachypnea develop, ultimately progressing to central nervous system, respiratory, and cardiac failure, at methemoglobin levels greater than 55–70%. While an affected patient's blood can appear chocolate-colored when examined, a more reliable diagnosis can be made from arterial blood gas sampling and quantification of methemoglobin levels. Therapy for mild methemoglobinemia includes discontinuation of nitrate therapy, inspiration of 100% oxygen, and potential red blood cell transfusions. With levels of methemoglobin greater than 60%, or in the presence of cyanosis, methylene blue, in doses of 1–2 mg/kg may be administered. This agent serves as a cofactor accelerating the reduction of methemoglobin by NADH-methemoglobin reductase. Clinical responses can be seen within one hour of methylene blue administration (17).

Another uncommon side effect of high dose intravenous nitrate therapy is alcohol intoxication. Nitrates require dilution in sufficient concentrations of alcohol because of poor solubility in aqueous preparations. Commonly prescribed preparations consist of nitroglycerin dissolved in solutions ranging between 5 and 70% ethyl alcohol. Prolonged continuous infusions, therefore, can, on rare occasions, produce alcohol intoxication, manifesting itself initially as mild to moderate alterations in central nervous system function (18). This adverse reaction is reversible with discontinuation of intravenous nitrates and substitution with alternate modes of organic nitrate delivery.

Nitrate Tolerance

While speculated upon since the late 1800s (19), well-controlled studies in the early 1980s first established the rapid development of tolerance to the antianginal and anti-ischemic effects of long-acting and continuously administered nitrates in chronic stable anginal syndromes (5,6,20,21). After noting rising requirements of intravenous nitroglycerin for pain relief in many patients with rest angina, a similar state of nitrate tolerance in unstable anginal syndromes has been hypothesized.

Three mechanisms have been proposed to explain the development of tolerance to continuous or frequently administered nitroglycerin.

At steady state, nitroglycerin is continuously metabolized by target vascular tissues, establishing an arterial-venous concentration gradient for nitroglycerin. This gradient decreases with the development of tolerance, consistent with a decreased metabolic conversion of organic nitrates in target tissues. Depletion of *S*-nitrosothiol intermediates seen with the development of nitrate tolerance is accompanied by a decreased rate of activation of the enzyme guanylate cyclase (22) which is the result of decreased *S*-nitrosothiol production rather than alterations in guanylate cyclase activity (23). Depletion of sulfhydryl-containing donors may, therefore, ultimately be responsible for the development of nitrate tolerance (10,24).

Prolonged administration of nitroglycerin to patients has been noted to produce hemodilution (25). This ability of nitroglycerin to effect an increase in intravascular volume without a concomitant increase in total body weight has been recently confirmed, and suggests a nitroglycerin-induced fluid shift from extravascular to intravascular spaces (26). This increase in intravascular volume may limit the ability of nitroglycerin to decrease intraventricular volume, intracavitary pressure, and myocardial demand, and may therefore account for the development of tolerance to some of the effects of oral nitrates.

Organic vasodilators, including nitroglycerin, activate reflex mechanisms by stimulation of both the sympathetic adrenergic system and the renin-angiotensin axis. This "neurohumoral activation" causes paradoxical vasoconstriction and sodium retention and limits nitrate effectiveness (27). In patients with congestive heart failure, development of nitrate tolerance has been accompanied by reflex increases in plasma renin, body weight, and heart rate. These effects were eliminated after discontinuation of the offending nitrate regimen, concomitant with restoration of baseline nitrate responsiveness. In similar fashion, nitrate regimens that produced either partial or no tolerance were accompanied by partial or no neurohumoral activation (28). There remains debate as to the occurrence and relative importance of these reflex mechanisms in patients treated with nitroglycerin for coronary artery disease, without concomitant congestive heart failure (29,30).

Therapeutically, while a number of small-scale pilot studies have confirmed the potentiating effects of sulfhydryl donors, including *N*-acetylcysteine and methionine, on the systemic and coronary vasodilatory and hemodynamic actions of nitrate therapy, other studies have failed to show reversal of tolerance with these agents. When used chronically, *N*-acetylcysteine administration causes a high incidence of gastrointestinal side effects (31). Methionine is better tolerated, but has been less well studied. The sulfhydryl donors have been hypothesized to act either via the increased formation of *S*-nitrothiols, or as cofactors for the action of the enzyme, organic nitrate ester reductase, thus restoring the arterial and venodilating properties of nitroglycerin in the tolerant state. However, sulfhydryl cofactors may enhance the effects of nitroglycerin independent of the existence of a nitrate-tolerant state (32). It is more likely that some of the properties of oral nitrates are enhanced by tolerant-dependent, and some by tolerant-independent, actions of the sulfhydryl donors (26). Only one randomized, double-blinded, controlled study has examined the concomitant administration of *N*-acetylcysteine with nitroglycerin in patients with unstable angina. Horowitz and coworkers found no additional benefit by adding *N*-acetylcysteine to nitroglycerin therapy in the control of painful episodes in 46 patients with unstable angina who were unresponsive to standard treatment (33). However, the co-administration of *N*-acetylcysteine with nitroglycerin caused an unexpected significant reduction in the progression to myocardial infarction in these patients. The authors hypothesized a possible antiplatelet effect of *S*-nitroso *N*-acetylcysteine, a metabolite of the administered parent drug.

Reflex neurohumoral activation can be combated by the concomitant administration of sympathetic antagonists or renin-angiotensin inhibitors. Levy and colleagues showed that the co-administration of angiotensin converting enzyme inhibitors with nitroglycerin abolished the development of nitrate tolerance in normal volunteers (25). However, there are no studies of the potential benefits of angiotensin converting enzyme inhibition in the treatment of nitrate tolerance in patients with coronary ischemic syndromes.

The possibility of using diuretic therapy to counteract intravascular volume expansion, and thereby potentially limit nitrate tolerance, is currently under investigation (34).

BETA ADRENOCEPTOR BLOCKERS

Beta adrenoceptor blocking agents (beta-blockers) were introduced into clinical practice in the early 1960s and rapidly became one of the major pharmaceutical breakthroughs of the twentieth century. Their role in the management of chronic stable exertional angina and in the reduction of mortality and prevention of recurrence of myocardial infarction is now well established (35). However, the role of beta-blockers in limiting progression to infarction and prevention of death in the treatment of patients with unstable angina is less well studied.

Pharmacology and Pathophysiology

Norepinephrine and epinephrine function as the primary endogenous catecholamines, exerting their metabolic and physiologic influence via interactions with target cell surface receptors. Consequent to catechol-receptor binding, activation of a heterotrimeric G protein (G_S) occurs on the internal surface of the cell membrane, leading to dissociation of the alpha subunit from the beta-gamma subunit. Thc effector enzyme, adenyl cyclase, is activated by the free alpha subunit, causing increased production of cyclic adenosine monophosphate (cAMP) (36). This results in phosphorylation of the sodium channel (decreasing sodium ion conductance) and stimulates a protein kinase to phosphorylate calcium and potassium channels (increasing calcium and potassium ion conductance). Independent of cAMP, G_S can directly regulate calcium, potassium, and sodium channels, as well. The direct consequence of catecholamine-mediated myocyte stimulation, therefore, includes modulation of ion flux, resulting in elevation of the action potential plateau and shortening of the action potential. Heart rate is increased, as well, due to the cAMP-stimulated increase in the depolarization rate of the sinus node (37).

Epinephrine and norepinephrine exert relatively selective effects on various subtypes of receptors, which have been subclassified into alpha and beta types (38). These demarcations have been based upon the relative potencies of epinephrine and norepinephrine for stimulation of receptor-mediated physiologic responses in target tissues. Alpha receptors show slightly greater effect from norepinephrine than from epinephrine, which in turn has greater effect than similar concentrations, of isoproterenol, an adrenergic agonist. Beta receptors show increased effect from isoproterenol than epinephrine, which in turn has greater effect than equal concentrations of norepinephrine. These receptors have been further subclassified into alpha-1/alpha-2 and beta-1/beta-2 subtypes. The beta receptor subtyping was originally based upon relative potencies of norepinephrine and epinephrine, but it is now recognized to reflect the tissue location of these receptors, as well. Beta-1 receptors (located primarily in the heart) have equal response to norepinephrine and epinephrine, while beta-2 receptors (located primarily in vascular and bronchial smooth muscle, but also exhibited in cardiac muscle) have greater response to epinephrine than norepinephrine.

Beta-blocking agents differ in their secondary properties of intrinsic sympathomimetic activity, relative alpha/beta adrenoceptor selectivity, membrane stabilizing ability, and cardioselectivity. Their common class action resides in their ability to competitively inhibit catechol binding at beta adrenoceptor sites. This receptor blockade prevents the normal catechol receptor stimulation of adenyl cyclase and reduces production of cyclic AMP. As discussed above, this causes a reduction in the metabolic and physiologic processes normally governed by catechol stimulation on target tissues.

During acute myocardial ischemia, depletion of high energy phosphate stores or alterations in membrane phospholipid composition have been theorized to account for the observed externalization of beta adrenoceptors to the cell surface from an intracellular pool, with a concomitant change of these receptors from an "uncoupled" to a "coupled" state (39). This causes an increased density of beta adrenoceptors that are functionally coupled to the G_S regulatory protein, on the cell surface. Reperfusion rapidly reverses this receptor flux. During early myocardial ischemia, as well, enzyme specific sensitization of adenyl cyclase occurs, theoretically secondary to covalent modification of this enzyme (40). This increase in surface receptors and sensitization of adenyl cyclase leads to an augmented responsiveness of the myocardial adenyl cyclase system to catechol stimulation, with potential contribution to the development of malignant arrhythmias and further spreading of ischemia (41). With prolonged periods of ischemia, cell surface receptor density remains elevated. However, functional uncoupling of these receptors to the G_S regulatory protein, as well as reduction of the responsiveness of adenyl cyclase, occurs, leading to reduced responsiveness of the adenyl cyclase system to endogenous catecholamines (42). The relationship between the clinical benefit seen with the use of beta-blocking agents in acute ischemic syndromes and the functional changes in beta adrenoceptor density and function remains to be elucidated.

Blockade of beta-1 adrenergic receptors leads to reduction of resting and exercise-induced heart rate. Myocyte contraction is altered, as well, due to a reduction in the maximal velocity of fiber shortening and a decrease in isometric contractile force. This results in a decreased rate of rise (dP/dt) of left ventricular pressure. In ischemic myocardium, beta-blockers reduce catecholamine levels (43) and thereby decrease catechol-induced free fatty acid production. This metabolic shift to increased glucose utilization lowers myocardial oxygen demand. These effects are partially offset by a rise in intraventricular volume and pressure, raising the cardiac workload. In the ischemic setting, the net result favors a decrease of intracavitary tension and oxygen consumption by the heart at a given workload. When given before or during ischemia, beta-blocking agents have been shown to decrease postischemic contractile dysfunction, or "stunning," presumably by lowering myocardial oxygen demand and reducing the severity of ischemia.

Total coronary blood flow is decreased, and coronary vascular resistance is increased, by the action of beta-blockade (44). This may, in part, be an autoregulatory response to the decreased myocardial demand and oxygen consumption produced by beta-blocker therapy. Changes in regional intramyocardial blood flow may occur, as well, with shunting of flow to the subendocardium and ischemic areas (45). This shunting, in combination with an increased diastolic perfusion time, is of particular importance when the vasculature is already maximally dilated, as is the usual case in ischemic settings.

Clinical Trials with Beta-Blockers

Though beta-blockers are widely employed in the therapy of unstable angina, only a small number of prospective randomized trials have examined the benefits of beta-blockade in this syndrome.

Control of Ischemic Episodes

Extrapolation from trials designed to compare various antianginal regimens in small groups of patients suggests that beta-blockers reduce ischemic episodes in patients with unstable angina.

Andre-Fouet and others compared oral diltiazem use with propranolol (in dosages adjusted to decrease heart rate to less than sixty beats per minute) in the management of 70 patients with new onset, increasing exertional, or rest angina in the coronary care unit setting (46). No placebo control was used. The frequency of electrocardiographically determined ischemic events while taking test medications was compared to prehospitalization rates of ischemic events. Thirty-six patients were randomized to propranolol therapy. Although propranolol significantly reduced ischemic events, rest angina was not totally eliminated.

Parodi and others compared oral verapamil use with propranolol (300 mg/day) or placebo during serial 48-hour trial periods in a prospective, double-blind, double-crossover, controlled fashion in the management of 10 men with rest angina in a cardiac care unit (47). Episodes of electrocardiographically determined ST-shifts and instances of rest pain were compared in each patient with each therapy. At this dosage, propranolol was ineffective in limiting ischemic events or episodes of pain. In contrast, verapamil monotherapy significantly decreased diagnostic ischemic ST-segment shifts ($p < 0.01$).

In the Holland Interuniversity Nifedipine/Metoprolol Trial (HINT) (48), nifedipine, metoprolol (200 mg/day), and their combination were compared in a prospective, double-blinded, placebo-controlled fashion in the management of 537 patients admitted to coronary care units with the diagnosis of unstable angina. While not statistically significant, trends were noted toward reduced electrocardiographically determined ischemic events and reduced progression to myocardial infarction within 48 hours, with the use of metoprolol therapy compared to placebo therapy (odds ratio 0.76, 95% confidence intervals 0.49,1.16).

Prevention of Progression to Acute Myocardial Infarction

Published data suggest a slight reduction in progression to myocardial infarction in patients receiving beta-blockade as therapy for unstable angina.

Trials of Beta-Blockers as Monotherapy. A randomized, placebo-control, double-blind study of morbidity and mortality comparing heparin, atenolol (100 mg/day) and their combination was performed by Telford and Wilson (49). They initially enrolled 400 patients admitted to a coronary care unit with the diagnoses of preinfarction angina, subendocardial infarction, or acute coronary insufficiency (CPK rise less than twice control). It should be noted that 186 patients were later withdrawn, and analysis was performed on the results from the remaining 214 patients. Test medications were given at least 6 hours after the onset of chest pain. In this setting, atenolol had no effect in reducing progression to myocardial infarction within a one-week period in the 60 patients randomized to its use. Norris and coworkers treated 20 patients with "*threatened myocardial infarction*" (defined as typical clinical presentation for myocardial infarction but

Table 2 Evolution of Infarction in Patients with "Threatened Myocardial Infarction" Randomized to Either Atenolol or Placebo Treatment

	Atenolol			Controls		
Group	Eventual infarct	Threatened infarct	%	Eventual infarct	Threatened infarct	%
Suspicious ECG initially	31	51	61	45	60	75
Normal ECG initially	6	25	24	17	34	50
Total without "definite" infarct initially	37	76	49	62	94	66

Patients treated with atenolol appeared to have a reduction in progression to myocardial infarction.
Source: Ref. 54 with permission.

without diagnostic electrocardiograms for up to 4 hours after the onset of chest pain) with intravenous propranolol (0.1 mg/kg) followed by oral therapy (320 mg propranolol/day) begun within 4 hours of the onset of the suspected myocardial infarction (50). This randomized control trial showed a significant reduction in myocardial infarctions in those patients treated with propranolol compared to placebo therapy (55% with propranolol versus 96% in the control population, $p < 0.05$). Yusuf and others also showed a trend toward significant reduction in progression to myocardial infarction when atenolol was begun intravenously within 12 hours of the onset of chest pain (51). One hundred seventy patients with *threatened myocardial infarction* were randomized to therapy with atenolol (5 mg intravenously immediately followed by oral therapy) versus placebo, in a prospective, randomized fashion. A reduction in progression to myocardial infarction by one sixth (49% with atenolol versus 66% in the control group [Table 2] was noted ($p < 0.02$).

The effect of metoprolol on reduction of morbidity and mortality in patients with *threatened myocardial infarction* was analyzed in a prospective, randomized, double-blinded, placebo-controlled fashion in the Goteberg Metoprolol Trial (52). A total of 1395 patients with suspected acute myocardial infarction were randomized to receive metoprolol (15 mg intravenously followed by 200 mg/day orally) versus placebo. Of those patients with abnormal electrocardiograms, a trend toward a reduction in progression to myocardial infarction within 72 hours of onset of treatment was noted with metoprolol use. This benefit was seen only if therapy was instituted within 12 hours of the onset of pain (55% with

Table 3 Evolution of Myocardial Infarction in Patients with Threatened Myocardial Infarction Randomized to Either Metoprolol or Placebo Therapy

	Placebo (%)	Metoprolol (%)	Difference (%)	*p*
All patients	58.8	57.2	2	0.2
≤12 hr[a]	60.7	54.7	10	0.062
>12 hr	54.7	62.5	–14	0.123
≤12 hr and heart rate ≥ 70 beats/min	69.5	58.7	16	0.016

Note beneficial reduction in progression to myocardial infarction in those patients treated with metoprolol within 12 hr of onset of chest pain.
[a]Start of treatment after onset of symptoms
Source: Ref. 52 with permission.

metoprolol versus 61% in the control group, $p < 0.06$ [Table 3]). When surveillance was extended to 90 days postinstitution of therapy, this reduction in infarction rate in patients randomized to metoprolol therapy persisted. These results were corroborated in patients with normal electrocardiograms and threatened myocardial infarction by the conclusions of the metoprolol "MIAMI" trial (53), which also showed a reduction in progression to myocardial infarction with metoprolol use (26% with metoprolol versus 31% in the control population).

When the results of the above three randomized controlled studies of patients with *threatened myocardial infarction* are pooled, reduction of progression to myocardial infarction with beta-blocker therapy is demonstrated (28.4% with beta-blockade versus 32.4% with control, $p = 0.04$ [Table 4])(54). Such "meta-analyses" assume similarities of the patient populations and the effect of intervention. Potential dissimilarities can be detected by use of tests of "heterogeneity" (55). Despite a negative "heterogeneity test" (as was obtained in the above meta-analysis), unrecognized selection bias may still exist in meta-analysis of these trials given the varied types, timing, and doses of beta-blockers, as well as the variations in concomitant drug administration (56).

However, the conclusion remains that beta-blocking agents reduce progression of unstable angina to myocardial infarction by greater than 10%, and therefore, their use is recommended at the current time for such syndromes.

Trials of Beta Blockers in Multidrug Regimens. Two notable studies have analyzed the potential benefits of multidrug regimens that included beta-blockers and calcium channel blockers for the therapy of unstable angina.

Muller and others compared increasing dosages of beta-blocker therapy to nifedipine alone or combined therapy in the control of ischemic pain in patients

Table 4 Meta-analysis of Development of Myocardial Infarction in Patients with Threatened Myocardial Infarction Randomized to Beta-Blocker Therapy or Placebo

	Allocated beta-blocker	Allocated control	Odds ratio	95% confidence interval	*p*
Proven MI among those with initial "threatened" MI	312/1110(28.4%)	401/1236(32.4%)	0.83	0.69–0.98	0.04

Note a reduction in the evolution of myocardial infarction with use of beta blocker therapy.
Source: Ref. 55 with permission.

admitted to a coronary care unit with unstable angina (57). A subgroup analysis, in this randomized, double-blind study, of 67 patients receiving propranolol before randomization showed that the addition of nifedipine was more effective in controlling painful ischemia than increasing the dosage of beta-blocker therapy. However, nifedipine used as monotherapy, in patients *not* previously receiving beta-blockade, was no more effective than beta-blockade in the control of ischemic episodes.

Gottlieb and colleagues compared the combination of propranolol (up to 320 mg/day) and nifedipine (up to 120 mg/day) with nifedipine monotherapy in the treatment of 81 patients admitted to a coronary care unit with rest pain (58). In this randomized, double-blind, placebo-controlled study, patients were followed for 30 days. While the addition of propranolol to nifedipine significantly decreased the number and severity of painful and electrocardiographically determined ischemic episodes in the first 96 hours of therapy, no significant differences were noted in the subsequent requirement for revascularization, progression to myocardial infarction, or of cardiac death, during follow-up. This may be due to a true lack of medical effect, or it may be secondary to inadequate statistical power to show benefit, resulting from the small sample size of this trial.

Recommendations

In summary, beta-blockade in the therapy of unstable anginal syndromes appears to reduce the number of ischemic events and may decrease progression to myocardial infarction during hospitalization. However, due to small sample sizes, no single study can convincingly make such a claim. With pooling of data these results do reach statistical significance. It seems prudent, therefore, to begin beta-blockade therapy immediately after onset of unstable angina, unless contraindications exist such as bronchospasm, congestive heart failure, or heart block. Patients already taking a beta-blocker who exhibit inadequate beta-blockade (as determined by heart rate and blood pressure responses) should have the dose of their beta-blocker increased. One may choose to add a second class of anti-ischemic agent in those patients already receiving adequate beta-blocker therapy, or, as subgroup analyses indicate, one may add beta-blockade in those patients already taking a calcium antagonist of the dihydropyridine group, such as nifedipine. Any of a number of intravenous formulations of beta-blockers are available and can be used safely (Table 5). In those patients with relative contraindications to beta-blockade therapy, the ultrashort-acting cardioselective agent, esmolol, with a biologic half-life of 9.5 minutes, has been shown to be safe and effective when used in open label trials (59,60). Once clinical stability as been achieved, continuation of beta-blocker therapy should be dictated by other concerns, such as hypertension, arrhythmias, or persistent chronic stable exertional angina.

CALCIUM ANTAGONISTS

Despite Food and Drug Administration approval of the calcium antagonists only within the past 10 years, this class of pharmaceuticals has become one of the most widely prescribed in the treatment of cardiovascular disease.

Pharmacology and Pathophysiology

The organic calcium antagonists are a class of agents of varying chemical structures, including lipophilic dihydropyridine derivatives (nifedipine, niludipine, nimodipine, nisoldipine, nicardipine), papaverine-like compounds (verapamil, gallopamil, tiapamil), a member of the benzothiazine family (diltiazem), and a chemically distinct entity (lidoflazine). These agents were designed to either inhibit activation or alter the kinetics of activation and inactivation of the "slow" voltage-dependent calcium channel. Specific inorganic polyvalent cations also inhibit calcium entry into cells, but do so via mechanisms other than those of the organic antagonists (61).

Three types of calcium channels have been identified, termed "L," "T," and "N," based upon their kinetics of inactivation, voltage dependence, and sensitivity to organic and inorganic antagonists (62). Of the three subtypes, only the L and T channels are present in cardiac tissue. Organic calcium antagonists interact solely with the L channels, though the L and T channels are structurally similar. The L channels have been further subtyped based upon their distribution. Knowledge of the cardiac L channel has been inferred from recent advances in the understanding of the nature and composition of the L channel present in skeletal

Table 5 Intravenous Beta Adrenoceptor Blockade: Pharmacokinetics and Dosages

Agent	Elimination half life (hr)	Cardioselectivity	Lipid solubility	Acute intravenous dose
Propranolol	3–4	None	High	0.033 mg/kg q 5 min (up to 0.1 mg/kg) to desired effect
Atenolol	6–9	Moderate	Weak	5 mg dose (may repeat in 5–10 min)
Metoprolol	3–4	Moderate	Moderate	5 mg doses q 2 min (up to 15 mg) to desired effect
Esmolol	9 min	Moderate	Weak	500 μg/kg bolus × 1 minute then 50 μg/kg/minute for 4 minutes. Upward titration by steps of 50 μg/kg/min with each step preceeded by repeat 500 μg/kg bolus over 1 minute (max 200 μg/kg/min)

Patients who are candidates for administration of intravenous beta-blockers for unstable angina should meet the following criteria: Heart rate > 60 bpm, blood pressure > 100 mmHg, EKG PR interval < 0.24 sec, absence of rales > 10 cm, absence of bronchospasm, and absence of shock.

muscle, which has been better studied. The L channel is composed of several distinct subunits—a tightly bound alpha-1, beta, gamma moiety and a more loosely bound alpha-2, delta structure (63). All three subtypes of organic calcium channel antagonists bind to the alpha-1 subunit. While the binding site of the dihydropyridines is distinct, it is allosterically related to the phenylalkylamine and benzothiazepine binding sites.

These L channels regulate the intracellular movement of calcium ions across the cell membrane during the plateau phase of the action potential. This "calcium-triggered calcium release" stimulates an ATP- and cAMP-dependent cascade of events leading to myocardial or vascular smooth muscle contraction. The force of contraction of the heart, as well as the tone of vascular smooth muscle, can, therefore, be controlled by modulating the channels that control calcium ion influx with organic calcium antagonists. Of note, the activation of skeletal muscle, which is dependent upon intracellular, rather than transcellular, flux of calcium, is little affected by these agents. However, myocardial pacemaker cells (especially those within the sinoatrial and atrioventricular nodes), dependent on calcium channel currents for depolarization, can be affected to varying degrees by these agents.

Continuing debate exists regarding appropriate nomenclature for these agents (61). The phrase "calcium channel blocker" is felt to be misleading in that these agents alter the kinetics of activation and inactivation of these channels, rather than "blocking" them. The term "calcium-entry blocker" is nonspecific, given alternative means of calcium ion entry into the cells other than the "slow" channel, such as transport via the sodium-calcium exchanger or the potential for passive diffusion at various sites within the cell membrane, the name "calcium antagonist" was introduced in 1971 to describe the reversibility of the effects of these drugs by increasing the intracellular calcium concentration. This phrase is the least misleading of the commonly employed terminologies and, therefore, will be utilized throughout the remainder of this chapter.

Potential clinical benefits of modulation of the calcium channel in the therapy of unstable angina include a potent vasodilatory action, prevention of coronary artery spasm, an increase in collateral blood flow in ischemic regions, and a decrease in myocardial oxygen consumption secondary to reductions in myocardial contractility, heart rate, and blood pressure.

As a group, the calcium antagonists act to increase coronary blood flow in a dose-dependent fashion. Inhibition of vascular smooth muscle contraction produces dilation of both conductance and resistance vessels. The calcium blockers also inhibit both ergonovine-induced and sympathetically mediated coronary vasospasm and vasoconstriction. Verapamil, nifedipine, and diltiazem have all been shown to decrease postischemic contractile dysfunction, or "stunning."

Experimentally, all three subclasses of calcium antagonists decrease peripheral vascular resistance and will lower blood pressure and loading conditions of the left heart. This effect is most marked with nifedipine.

The calcium antagonists also have primary effects on myocardial hemodynamics. Experimentally, the rate of pressure development within the left ventricle, dP/dt, may be decreased by verapamil, increased by nifedipine (through stimulation of sympathetic reflexes), and is usually unchanged by diltiazem. Studies utilizing blood-perfused in vitro preparations of the sinoatrial or atrioventricular nodes, as well as direct injections into the A-V nodal artery, have revealed that each subclass of calcium antagonists affects the S-A and A-V nodes with varying degree and specificity (64). Clinically, diltiazem has a moderate effect on S-A nodal slowing, while verapamil has the greatest A-V nodel blocking ability. Nifedipine has no effect on A-V nodal conduction in clinically used doses. At "therapeutic" concentrations, nifedipine's baroreceptor-stimulated sympathetically induced increase in heart rate may play a more prominent role than its intrinsic effect of slowing of the conduction system. Diltiazem and verapamil may decrease heart rate.

Clinical Trials with Calcium Antagonists

Calcium antagonists are effective in the control of ischemic episodes in patients with unstable angina. Several prospective, randomized, control trials have been performed to evaluate their effects on morbidity and mortality. Most of these studies have utilized insufficient numbers of patients to exclude mild-to-moderate benefit. However, large beneficial effects of these agents are unlikely to be seen.

Nifedipine

Unstable Angina Trials. Previtali et al. evaluated the short-term control of ischemic events with nifedipine therapy versus placebo in 14 patients, each with greater than three episodes/day of rest angina (65). In their randomized, double-crossover, placebo-controlled trial, 48-hour periods were utilized to compare the effect of nifedipine with placebo. All patients had significant coronary artery disease, and seven of eight patients tested had ergonovine-induced vasospasm. In this small pilot study, nifedipine significantly reduced the number of all (painful and clinically silent) electrocardiographically detected episodes of ischemia (1 event/period with nifedipine treatment compared to 20 events/period with control therapy). Muller and colleagues revealed that the beneficial effect of nifedipine therapy in the control of painful ischemia was as effective as conventional therapy (66). Fifty-nine patients (not receiving prior beta-blockade) who were admitted to a coronary care unit with the diagnosis of unstable angina were randomized to receive either nifedipine monotherapy (80–120 mg/day) or conventional therapy consisting of propranolol (up to 240 mg/day) and isosorbide dinitrate (up to 80 mg/day) for a 14-day period. Both treatments were equally effective in reducing painful ischemia. A 14% incidence of progression to myocardial infarction in both subgroups was noted. A second subgroup analysis compared the initiation of nifedipine therapy with an increase in previously administered "conventional therapy" of beta-blockade and nitrates in 67 patients. Doses were only increased to 240 mg propranolol/day and 80 mg isosorbide dinitrate/day. A significant beneficial reduction in painful ischemic episodes with nifedipine was confirmed. However, the implied recommendation of the authors of this study to institute dihydropyridine therapy in those patients who present with unstable angina despite "maximal" beta-blockade must be interpreted cautiously given the doses and submaximal "beta-blocking" effects on heart rate and blood pressure achieved by the "conventional therapy" chosen in this protocol, as well as the now commonplace addition of platelet inhibitors as part of the patient's intensified antianginal regimen.

Gerstenblith and others conducted a randomized, double-blind, placebo-control trial evaluating the benefits of the addition of nifedipine to standard therapy (consisting of 160 mg propranolol/day and 40 mg isosorbide dinitrate/day) in 138 patients admitted to a coronary care unit with refractory pain (67). Painful episodes were reduced with nifedipine therapy compared with standard therapy. When "myocardial endpoints" (death, myocardial infarction, or coronary artery bypass) were viewed collectively, the investigators were able to show benefit with nifedipine therapy. However, when coronary bypass (for refractory pain) was excluded as an endpoint, there was no significant effect on progression to infarction or death in the 4 months of follow-up.

A lack of reduction in progression to myocardial infarction in patients with unstable angina who were treated with nifedipine monotherapy (60 mg/day) was confirmed by the HINT trial (48). In fact, nifedipine monotherapy *increased* progression to myocardial infarction (odds ratio of 1.51, 95% confidence intervals 0.87, 2.74). In the subgroup of patients previously receiving beta-blocking therapy (200 mg metoprolol/day), the addition of nifedipine significantly decreased the myocardial infarction rate within the next 48 hours (odds ratio of 0.86, 95% confidence intervals of 0.47, 0.97). The HINT Research Group hypothesized a protective role for nifedipine in those patients with unstable angina *despite prior beta-blocking therapy,* mediated, perhaps, by the antispasmodic actions of this agent.

The initiation of combined therapy with propranolol (up to 320 mg/day) and nifedipine (up to 120 mg/day) has been found to be of greater benefit in the control of ischemic pain, in a population of 81 patients with rest angina, than was nifedipine monotherapy (up to 120 mg/day) (58). No significant differences in revascularization requirement, progression to myocardial infarction, or death rate in the following 30 days was noted.

Threatened Myocardial Infarction Trials. The potential benefit of the addition of nifedipine (80 mg/day) to standard therapy in patients admitted to a coronary care unit with threatened myocardial infarction (typical ischemic pain of greater than 45 minutes duration accompanied by nondiagnostic electrocardiographic changes) was analyzed by the Nifedipine in Acute Myocardial Infarction Study

(NAMIS) (66). A randomized, double-blind, placebo-controlled study of 105 patients followed for a period of 2 weeks was conducted. Beta-blockers were continued only if patients were already receiving this medication. No benefit was shown in the reduction of progression to myocardial infarction or in mortality over the 6 months of follow-up in either the nifedipine- or propranol-treated groups, but a 75% rate of progression to myocardial infarction was seen in all subgroups tested. This trial (NAMIS) also evaluated the addition of nifedipine therapy to a subgroup of 66 patients with acute myocardial infarction. Somewhat surprisingly, when both subgroups of patients with threatened myocardial infarction and acute myocardial infarction were combined, 2-week mortality was *increased* with nifedipine therapy compared with placebo (7.9% with nifedipine versus 0% with placebo [Table 6]). This difference was no longer significant at 6 months of follow-up (10.1% with nifedipine compared to 8.5% with placebo).

The Norwegian Nifedipine Multicenter Trial (NNMT), a similar randomized, double-blind, controlled study, also *failed to show reduction in progression to myocardial infarction* in 227 patients with threatened myocardial infarction who were treated with nifedipine (50 mg/day for 48 hours followed by 40 mg/day for 6 weeks) compared with placebo control in addition to standard therapy (68). The rate of progression to infarction in these patients was 70%.

The beneficial results of the addition of nifedipine treatment to "standard" therapy on morbidity and mortality noted in the HINT unstable angina trial (48) contrasts with the negative data observed in the NAMIS and NNMT threatened myocardial infarction trials (66,68). In the HINT trial, subgroup analysis was designed to look at the effect of nifedipine therapy on those patients previously prescribed beta-blocking agents. During the first period of the trial, prior blocking therapy was maintained, without standardization of dose. During the later phase, all patients already receiving beta-blocking therapy were switched to a standard dose of 200 mg metoprolol/day. In the NAMIS trial, subgroup analysis of the effect of the addition of nifedipine to those patients previously taking beta-blocking agents was not performed. In fact, while prior beta-blockade therapy was maintained in these patients, the total number of patients, the type of beta-blocker, and the doses of medication were not specified. In the NNMT trial, nifedipine was added to other medical treatments prescribed according to "local practice." The number of patients taking beta-blocking agents and the doses of each of medications were not specified. Due to the differing designs of each of these trials, as well as the lack of comparable subgroup analyses, direct comparison of the results of these studies is limited.

Verapamil

Several randomized, placebo-controlled trials have evaluated the efficacy of verapamil in the reduction of ischemic events in patients with unstable angina.

Mehta et al. evaluated the addition of verapamil (320–480 mg/day) to topical nitrates (if started before randomization) in the control of ischemic events over a

Table 6 Mortality of Patients with Either Threatened or Acute Myocardial Infarction Randomized to Receive Nifedipine Therapy or Placebo

	2 weeks					6 months				
	Placebo		Nifedipine			Placebo		Nifedipine		
Patient group (*n*)	*n*	%	*n*	%	p-value	*n*	%	*n*	%	*p*-value
Randomized, eligible (171)	0/82	0	7/89	7.9	.018	7/82	8.5	9/89	10.1	NS
All randomized (181)	2/88	2.3	7/93	7.5	.19	10/88	11.4	10/93	10.8	NS

Note an increase in 2-week mortality (not present a 6 months follow-up) in the group treated with nifedipine.
Source: Ref. 56 with permission.

96-hour period in 15 patients admitted to a coronary care unit with rest angina (69). Nonresponders to placebo or verapamil were either switched to verapamil therapy or were placed on higher dosages of verapamil. Response was considered positive if symptoms were reduced at any point prior to the termination of the study. As might be expected with this type of trial, 92% of the tested patients decreased their symptoms with verapamil therapy, compared to 16% with placebo alone. Of the initial 65 patients screened for inclusion, only 15 patients met criteria for enrollment, due to a high spontaneous rate of reduction of episodes of rest pain prior to randomization. Parodi et al. reported on the beneficial effects of verapamil therapy in the treatment of rest angina (47,70). In two separate placebo-control, blinded, double-crossover trials, verapamil (400 and 480 mg/day) was shown to be effective in reducing the frequency of painful and electrocardiographically determined ischemic events by 80% compared with controls. These studies, however, were small, enrolling only 12 and 10 patients, respectively. In the latter trial propranolol monotherapy (300 mg/day) did not significantly decrease the frequency of rest pain. The beneficial results noted above with verapamil were confirmed in an identical setting by Capucci and others (71), who showed a significant reduction in painful rest epidodes in 18 patients with 480 mg/day of verapamil. In this trial, only a trend toward reduction of ischemic episodes was noted with propranolol monotherapy (240 mg/day) when compared with placebo.

There are no large-scale randomized control trials comparing the effects of multiple doses of verapamil therapy on the occurrence of ischemic events. While there is some recent evidence that verapamil may reduce a combined endpoint of reinfarcation and/or death in a highly selected subset of patients *postmyocardial infarction* (72), to date, there are no large-scale trials in the literature evaluating the effect of verapamil therapy on the reduction of myocardial infarction rate or death in patients with *unstable angina syndromes*.

Diltiazem

Two randomized, blinded studies have analyzed the benefits of diltiazem therapy in patients with unstable angina.

In an uncontrolled, randomized comparison of diltiazem and propranolol (dosages adjusted to decrease heart rate to less than 60 beats per minute), both agents significantly decreased episodes of ischemic pain in patients admitted with any form of unstable angina to a cardiac care unit (46). Theroux et al. evaluated the benefit of diltiazem therapy (360 mg/day) versus propranolol (up to 240 mg/day) or placebo in 100 consecutive patients admitted to a cardiac care unit with the diagnosis of unstable angina (73). Both agents significantly reduced painful ischemic episodes. In a 5-month follow-up, neither agent showed any reduction in the rate of readmissions for recurrent angina, progression to myocardial infarction, need for coronary artery bypass, or death when compared with controls.

Pepine et al. compared morbid and mortal endpoints at one year of therapy for patients enrolled in three similar trials using diltiazem, nifedipine, or verapamil as monotherapy in the treatment of rest unstable angina (74). In all three groups, there was no significant difference in hospitalizations for recurrent angina, progression to myocardial infarction, coronary artery bypass, or death at one year of follow-up. Unfortunately, no comparisons with the control or nonresponding populations were made.

Recommendations

In summary, all three subclasses of calcium antagonists effectively decrease the number of episodes of ischemic pain in small numbers of patients with various unstable anginal syndromes. However, as confirmed by a meta-analysis of six randomized control trials for unstable angina (enrolling collectively over 1100 patients) and of 17 randomized trials for threatened or suspected myocardial infarction (enrolling collectively over 10,000 patients), no reduction in progression to myocardial infarction or death was observed with the use of calcium antagonists (Table 7) (75). Therefore, at present, we recommend only the judicious addition of calcium antagonists to maximal "conventional therapy" of beta-blocking agents and organic nitrates for the control of ischemic episodes. Monotherapy with nifedipine should be avoided in patients with unstable angina and should be added with great caution to regimens employing nitroglycerin, given the risk of hypotension. Diltiazem and verapamil should be used cautiously in patients with congestive heart failure and in those already prescribed beta-blockers, because of the synergistic negative inotropic and chronotropic actions of these agents.

CONCLUSIONS

Natural history studies have claimed that patients with unstable angina who are treated "conservatively," without the routine use of beta-blockers and calcium antagonists, do as well as patients treated with "aggressive" medical regimens that include these agents (76–78). Problems in study design, including heterogeneity of both enrollment criteria and concomitant drug administration, as well as patient selection bias and small sample sizes, make the results of these single-center, nonrandomized trials of the natural history of unstable angina unconvincing.

Relief of Symptoms

The goals for treatment of patients with any of the heterogeneous unstable angina syndromes are many and include clinical stabilization with a reduction in the occurrence of ischemic episodes, and prevention of progression from unstable angina to myocardial infarction and death. In the short-term control of symp-

Table 7 Summary of Randomized Trials of Calcium Antagonists in Patients with Unstable Angina

			No. who developed infarct/ No. randomized		No. of deaths	
Trail	Treatment	Duration of treatment	Allocated to calcium blocker	Allocated to control	Allocated to calcium blocker	Allocated to control
Placebo as control:						
Gerstenblith *et al.*	Nifedipine	4 months	11/68	12/70	7/68	5/70
HINT	Nifedipine	48 hr	78/341	77/327	1/341	2/327
Hagemeijer *et al.*	Diltiazem	48 hr	NA	NA	0/30	0/30
Subtotal			89/409	89/397	8/439	7/427
Standard treatment as control:						
Muller *et al.*	Nifedipine	48 hr	13/68	10/65	4/68	0/65
Theroux *et al.*	Diltiazem	5·1 months	5/50	4/50	2/50	2/50
André-Fouet *et al.*	Diltiazem	48 hr	3/34	1/36	0/34	0/36
Subtotal			21/152	15/151	6/152	2/151
Total			110/561	104/548	14/591	9/578

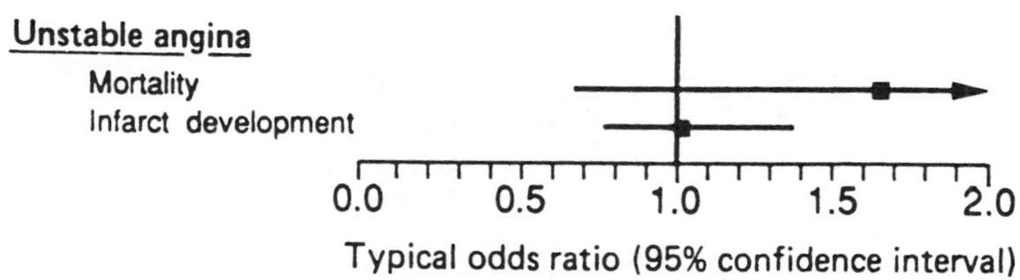

With meta-analysis, note a lack of a significant reduction in endpoints with calcium antagonist therapy for unstable angina.
NA = not available.
Source: Ref. 75 with permission.

toms, organic nitrates, beta-blocking agents, and calcium antagonists as monotherapy have all been shown to reduce the frequency of painful, as well as clinically silent, ischemic events. Analysis of the effects of these agents on reduction of other morbid and mortal events is more complex.

Reduction in Rate of Infarction and Ultimate Mortality

Pharmacotherapeutic interventions discussed in this chapter have all been shown to decrease symptoms, but evidence of a reduction in the proportion of patients who evolve an acute myocardial infarction or die is less convincing. The ability to detect only a small beneficial effect of medical therapy, as we might expect with these agents, requires trials enrolling large numbers of patients. For example, statistically significant documentation of a 10–20% reduction in a particular event rate requires enrollment of approximately 3000 patients in a study. Appropriate planning of sample size has been exemplified by the recent randomized control trials evaluating the effects of lytic therapy in the treatment of acute myocardial infarction. In contrast, the numbers of randomized control trials evaluating organic nitrates, beta-blockers, and calcium antagonists for the treatment of unstable angina syndromes are small, as are the number of patients enrolled in each trial. Some study designs have been flawed; enrollment criteria have not been uniform, "conventional therapy" has often been poorly defined, and "positive" results have been published in the form of subgroup analyses, different from the hypotheses intended to be studied by the original protocols.

Therapeutic Recommendations

We suspect that future studies with improved designs will further define the treatment benefits of organic nitrates, beta-blocking agents, calcium antagonists, and their combinations in the treatment of specific subclassifications of unstable angina. At this time certain conclusions can be drawn regarding medical therapy for unstable angina (Fig. 2). Patients with unstable angina should be maintained on antiplatelet and/or anticoagulant therapy—the merits of which are described elsewhere in this text. All patients should receive organic nitrates for relief of ischemic episodes. For patients not already taking beta-blockers who present with unstable angina, we recommend the institution of beta-blockade therapy to reduce the occurrence of ischemic episodes. Persons already on beta-blockers who exhibit inadequate beta-blockade (demonstrated by blood pressure and pulse responses) should have the dose of their beta-blocker increased. Beta-blockade in the setting of unstable angina may reduce progression to myocardial infarction and death. While aspirin therapy has also been shown to reduce progression to myocardial infarction and death in patients with unstable angina, any additive therapeutic benefit of beta-blockers in combination with aspirin therapy remains to be established.

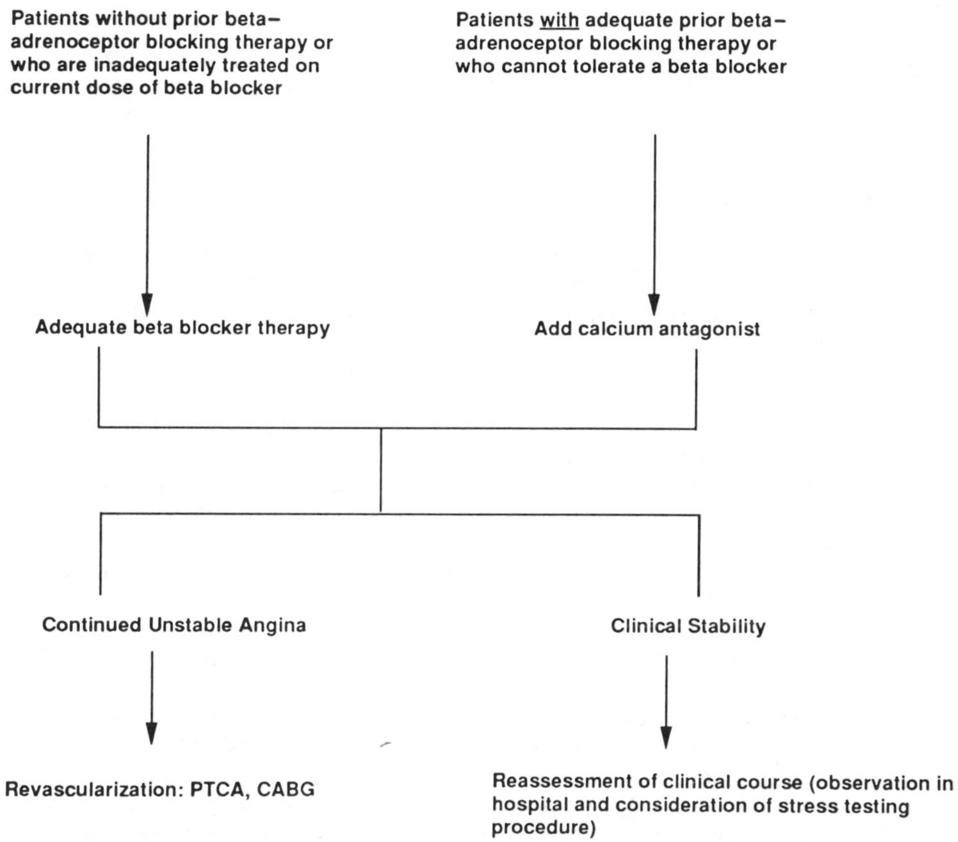

Figure 2 Recommendations for medical therapy of patients with unstable angina. Goals: (1) Clinical stabilization (reduction of number of ischemic events). (2) Reduction of proportion of patients evolving acute myocardial infarction. (3) Reduction in ischemic heart disease mortality. Treatment: All patients: nitrates, ASA and herparin (provided risks of bleeding are judged to be acceptably small), ? lytic therapy (remains investigational).

Of the calcium antagonists, nifedipine has been the best studied in the treatment of unstable angina. While verapamil and diltiazem can also be employed, one must use greater caution in patients on beta-blockers, due to the hazards of exaggerated negative chronotropic and inotropic effects. There appears to be no support for the institution of either nifedipine monotherapy or combination therapy with calcium antagonists and beta-blockers for patients with unstable angina who are not receiving beta-blockers at the time of presentation. In fact, evidence suggests that monotherapy with nifedipine should be avoided.

For those patients who become, or remain, unstable despite adequate beta-blockade, several analyses suggest that the addition of nifedipine therapy may reduce the number of ischemic episodes and possibly the progression to myocardial infarction and death.

REFERENCES

1. Braunwald E. Unstable angina: a classification. Circulation 1989; 80:410–14.
2. Fuster V, Stein B, Ambrose JA, Badimon L, Badimon JJ, Chesebro JH. Atherosclerotic plaque rupture and thrombosis: evolving concepts. Circulation 1990; 82:II-47–II-59.
3. Kloner RA, Przyklenk K, Patel B. Altered myocardial states: the stunned and hibernating myocardium. Am J Med 1986; 86:14.
4. Rahimtoola SH, The hibernating myocardium. Am Heart J 1989; 117:211–21.
5. Parker JO, Farrell B, Lahey KA, Moe G. Effect of intervals between doses on the development of tolerance to isosorbide dinitrate. N Engl J Med 1987; 316:1440–4.
6. Thadani V. Nitrate therapy for myocardial ischemic syndrome: current perspectives including tolerance. Curr Prob Cardiol 1988; 13:723–84.
7. Furchgott RF. Role of endothelium in response to vascular smooth muscle. Circ Res 1983; 53:557–73.
8. Wolin MS, Wood KS, Ignarro LJ. Guanylate cyclase from bovine lung: a kinetic analysis of the regulation of the purified enzyme by protoporphyrin IX, heme, and nitrosyl-heme. J Biol Chem 1982; 257:13312–20.
9. Rapoport RM, Murad F. Agonist-induced endothelium-dependent relaxation in rat thoracic aorta may be mediated through cGMP. Circ Res 1983; 52:352–7.
10. Ignarro LJ, Lippton H, Edwards JC, Baricos WH, Hyman AL, Kadowitz PJ, Gruetter CA. Mechanism of vascular smooth muscle relaxation by organic nitrates, nitrites, nitroprusside and nitric oxide: evidence for the involvement of S-nitrosothiols as active intermediates. J Pharmacol Exp Ther 1981; 218:739–49.
11. Rackley CE. Role of isosorbide dinitrate in patients with unstable angina pectoris. Am Heart J 1985; 110:269–72.
12. Araujo LI, Camici P, Spinks T, Jones T, Maseri A. Beneficial effect of nitrates on myocardial glucose utilization in unstable angina pectoris. Am J Cardiol 1987; 60:26H–30H.
13. Distante A, Maseri A, Severi S, Biagini A, Chierchia S. Management of vasospastic angina at rest with continuous infusion of isosorbide dinitrate. A double crossover study in a coronary care unit. Am J Cardiol 1979; 44:533–9.
14. Curfman GD, Heinsimer JA, Lozner EC, Fung HL. Intravenous nitroglycerin in the treatment of spontaneous angina pectoris: a prospective, randomized trial. Circulation 1983; 67:276–82.
15. Yusuf S, Collins R, MacMahon S, Peto R. Effect of intravenous nitrates on mortality in acute myocardial infarction: an overview of the randomized trials. Lancet 1988; ii:1088–92.
16. Come PC, Pitt B. Nitroglycerin-induced severe hypotension and bradycardia in patients with acute myocardial infarction. Circulation 1976; 54:624–8.

17. Beutler E. Methemoglobinemia and sulfhemoglobinemia. In: Beutler E, Williams WJ, Erslev AJ, Lichtman MA, eds. Hematology. New York: McGraw-Hill, 1990:743–6.
18. Shook TL, Kirshenbaum JM, Hundley RF, Shorey JM, Lamas GA. Ethanol intoxication complicating intravenous nitroglycerin therapy. Ann Intern Med 1984; 101:498–9.
19. Stewart DD. Remarkable tolerance to nitroglycerin. Philadelphia Polyclinic, 1888.
20. Dalal JJ, Yao L, Parker JO. Nitrate tolerance: influence of isosorbide dinitrate on the hemodynamic and antianginal effects of nitroglycerin. J Am Coll Cardiol 1983; 2:115–20.
21. Parker JO, Vankoughnett KA, Farrell B. Comparison of buccal nitroglycerin and oral isosorbide dinitrate for nitrate tolerance in stable angina pectoris. Am J Cardiol 1985; 56:724–8.
22. Keith RA, Burkman AM, Sokolowski TD, Fertel R. Vascular tolerance to nitroglycerine and cyclic GMP generation in rat aortic smooth muscle. J Pharmacol Exp Ther 1982; 221:535–1.
23. Kowaluk EA, Poliszczuk R, Fung HL. Tolerance to relaxation in rat aorta: compariton of an S-nitrosothiol with nitroglycerin. Eur J Pharmacol 1987; 144:379–83.
24. Needleman P, Johnson EM., Jr. Mechanism of tolerance development to organic nitrates. J Pharmacol Exp Ther 1973; 184:709–15.
25. Levy WS, Katz RJ, Buff L, Wasserman AG. Nitroglycerin tolerance modified by angiotensin converting enzyme inhibitors. Circulation 1989; 80:214.
26. Dupuis J, Lalonde G, Lemieux R, Rouleau JL. Tolerance to intravenous nitroglycerin in patients with congestive heart failure: role of neurohumoral activation and lack of prevention with n-acetylcysteine. J Am Coll Cardiol 1990; 16:923–31.
27. Rush ML, Lang WJ, Ran MJ. Studies on compensatory reflexes and tolerance to glyceryltrinitrate (GTN). Eur J Pharmacol 1971; 16:148–55.
28. Packer M, Kessler PD, Gottlieb SS. Does neurohormonal activation contribute to the development of nitrate tolerance in patients with chronic heart failure? Circulation 1988; 78:27.
29. Packer M. What causes tolerance to nitroglycerine—the 100 year old mystery continues. J Am Coll Cardiol 1990; 16:932–5.
30. Parker SD, Farrel B, Parker AC, Cohanim M, Parker JO. Neurohumoral responses and the hemodynamic adaptation to nitrates. Circulation 1990; 82:III-200.
31. Miller LF, Rumack BH. Clinical safety of high oral doses of acetylcysteine. Seminars in Oncology 1983; 10:76–85.
32. Munzel T, Holtz J, Mulsch A, Stewart DJ, Bassenje E. Nitrate tolerance in epicardial arteries or in the venous system is not reversed by n-acetylcysteine in vivo. Circulation 1989; 79:188–97.
33. Horowitz JD, Henry CA, Syrjanen ML, Louis WJ, Fish RD, Smith TW, Antman EM. Combined use of nitroglycerin and N-acetylcysteine in the management of unstable angina pectoris. Circulation 1988; 77:787–94.
34. Sussex BA, Campbell NR, Raju MK. Nitrate tolerance is modified by diuretic therapy. Circulation 1990; 82:III-200.
35. Yusuf S, Sleight P, Held P, McMahon S. Routine medical management of acute

myocardial infarction: lessons from overviews of recent randomized controlled trials. Circulation 1990; 82:II-117–II-134.

36. Gilman AG. G-protein and dual control of adenylate cyclase. Cell 1980; 36:577–9.
37. Thandrogen FT, Muntz KH, Buja LM, Willerson JT. Alterations in beta adrenergic receptors, adenylate cyclase and cyclic AMP concentration during acute myocardial ischemia and reperfusion. Circulation 1990; 82:30–7.
38. Ahlquist RP. A study of the adrenotropic receptors. Am J Physiol 1948; 153:586–600.
39. Strasser RH, Krimmer J, Marquetant R. Regulation of beta-adrenergic receptors: impaired desensitization in myocardial ischemia. J Cardiovasc Pharmacol 1988; 12:515–24.
40. Strasser RH, Dullaeus RB, Marquetant R. Dual sensitization of the beta-adrenergic system in early myocardial ischemia: independent regulation of beta receptors and adenylate cyclase. Circulation 1988; 78 (Suppl II):482.
41. Strasser RH, Marquetant R, Kubler W. Adrenergic receptors and sensitization of adenylyl cyclase in acute myocardial ischemia. Circulation 1990; 82:23–9.
42. Susanni EE, Manders WT, Knight DR, Vatner DE, Vatner SF, Homcy CJ. One hour of myocardial ischemia decreases the activity of the stimulatory guanine-nucleotide regulatory protein, Gs. Circ Res 1989; 65:1145–50.
43. Mueller HS, Ayres SM. Propranolol decreases sympathetic nervous activity reflected by plasma catecholamines during evolution of myocardial infarction in man. Clin Invest 1980; 65:338–46.
44. Parratt JR, Grayson J. Myocardial vascular reactivity after beta-adrenergic blockade. Lancet 1966; i:338–40.
45. Becker LC, Fortuin NJ, Pitt B. Effect of ischemia and antianginal drugs on the distribution of radioactive microspheres in the canine left ventricle. Circ Res 1971; 28:263–9.
46. Andre-Fouet X, Usdin JP, Gayet Ch, Wilner C. Comparison of short-term efficacy of diltiazem and propranolol in unstable angina at rest—a randomized trial in 70 patients. Eur Heart J 1983; 4:691–8.
47. Parodi O, Simonetti I, Michelassi C, Carpeggiani C, Biagini A, L'Abbate A, Maseri A. Comparison of verapamil and propranolol therapy for angina pectoris at rest: a randomized, multiple-crossover, controlled trial in the coronary care unit. Am J Cardiol 1986; 57:899–906.
48. Lubsen J, Tijssen JP. Efficacy of nifedepine and metoprolol in the early treatment of unstable angina in the coronary care unit: findings from the Holland Interuniversity Nifedipine/Metoprolol Trial (HINT). Am J Cardiol 1987; 60:18A–25A.
49. Telford AM, Wilson C. Trial of heparin versus atenolol in prevention of myocardial infarction in intermediate coronary syndrome. Lancet 1981; i:1225–9.
50. Norris RM, Clarke ED, Sammel NL, Smith WM. Protective effect of propranolol in threatened myocardial infarction. Lancet 1978; ii:907–9.
51. Yusuf S, Sleight P, Rossi P, Ramsdale D, Peto R, Furze L, Steery H, Pearson M, Motwani R, Parish S, Gray R, Bennett D, Bray C. Reduction in infarct size, arrhythmias and chest pain by early intravenous beta blockade in suspected acute myocardial infarction. Circulation 1983; 67:I-32–I-41.
52. Hjalmarson A, Herlitz J, Holmberg S, Ryden L, Swedberg K, Vedin A, Waagstein

F, Waldenstrom A, Waldenstrom J, Wedel H, Wilhelmsen L. The Goteborg Metroprolol Trial: effects on mortality and morbidity in acute myocardial infarction. Circulation 1983; 67:I-26–I-31.
53. The MIAMI Trial Research Group. Metoprolol in acute myocardial infarction (MIAMI): a randomized placebo-controlled international trial. Eur Heart J 1989; 6:199–226.
54. Yusuf S, Peto R, Lewis J, Collins R, Sleight P. Beta blockade during and after myocardial infarction: an overview of the randomized trials. Prog Cardiovasc Dis 1986; 27:335–71.
55. Yusuf S. The use of beta-blockers in the acute phase of myocardial infarction. In: Califf RM, Wagner GS, eds. Acute Coronary Care 1986. Boston: Martinus Nijhoff, 1985:73–88.
56. Lubsen J. Medical management of unstable angina: what have we learned from the randomized trials? Circulation 1990; 82:II-82–II-87.
57. Muller JE, Turi ZG, Pearle DL, Schneider JF, Serfas DH, Morrison J, Stone PH, Rude RE, Rosner B, Sobel BE, Tate C, Scheiner E, Roberts R, Hennekens CH, Braunwald E. Nifedipine and conventional therapy for unstable angina pectoris: a randomized, double-blind comparison. Circulation 1984; 69:728–39.
58. Gottlieb SO, Weisfeldt ML, Ouyang P, Achuff SC, Baughman KL, Traill TA, Brinker JA, Shapiro EP, Chandra NC, Mellits ED, Townsend SN, Gerstenblith G. Effect of the addition of propranolol to therapy with nifedipine for unstable angina pectoris: a randomized, double-blind, placebo-controlled trial. Circulation 1986; 73:331–337.
59. Kirshenbaum JM, Kloner RA, Antman EM, Braunwald E. Use of an ultra short-acting beta-blocker in patients with acute myocardial ischemia. Circulation 1985; 72:873–80.
60. Wallis DE, Pope C, Littman WJ, Scanlon PJ. Safety and efficacy of esmolol for unstable angina pectoris. Am J Cardiol 1988; 62:1033–7.
61. Nayler W. Calcium antagonists. New York: Harcourt Brace Jovanovich, 1988:82–8.
62. Nowycky MC, Fox AP, Tsien RW. Three types of neuronal calcium channels with different calcium agonist sensitivity. Nature 1989; 316:440–3.
63. Takahashi M, Seager MJ, Jones JF, Reber BF, Catterall W. Subunit structure of the dihydropyridine-sensitive calcium channels for skeletal muscle. PNAS 1987; 84:5478–82.
64. Ono H, Hashimoto K. In vitro tissue effects of calcium flux inhibition. In: Stone PH, Antman EM, eds. Calcium channel blocking agents in the treatment of cardiovascular disorders. Mount Kisco, NY: Futura, 1983:155–75.
65. Previtali M, Salerno JA, Tavazzi L, Ray M, Medici A, Chimienti M, Specchia G, Bobba P. Treatment of angina at rest with nifedipine: a short-term controlled study. Am J Cardiol 1980; 45:825–30.
66. Muller JE, Morrison J, Stone PH, Rude, RE, Rosner B, Roberts R, Perle DL, Turi ZG, Schneider JF, Serfas DH, Tate C, Scheiner E, Sobel BE, Hennekens CH, Braunwald E. Nifedipine therapy for patients with threatened and acute myocardial infarction: a randomized, double-blind, placebo-controlled comparison. Circulation 1984; 69:740–7.

67. Gerstenblith G, Ouyang P, Achuff SC, Bulkley BH, Becker LC, Mellits ED, Baughman KL, Weiss JL, Flaherty JT, Kallman CH, Llewellyn M, Weisfeldt ML, Nifedipine in unstable angina. A double-blind, randomized trial. N Engl J Med 1982; 306:885–9.
68. Sirnes PA, Overskeid K, Pedersen TR, Bathen J, Drivenes A, Froland GS, Kjekshus JK, Landmaark K, Rokseth R, Sirnes KE, Sundoy A, Torjussen BR, Westlund KM, Wik BA. Evolution of infarct size during the early use of nifedipine in patients with acute myocardial infarction: the Norwegian Nifedipine Multicenter Trial. Circulation 1984; 70:638–44.
69. Mehta J, Pepine CJ, Day M, Guerrero JR, Conti CR. Short-term efficacy of oral verapamil in rest angina. A double blind placebo controlled trial in CCU patients. Am J Med 1981; 71:977–82.
70. Parodi O, Simonetti I, L'Abbate A, Maseri A. Verapamil versus propranolol for angina at rest. Am J Cardiol 1982; 50:923–8.
71. Capucci A, Bracchetti D, Carini GC. Propranolol versus verapamil in patients with unstable angina. In: Zanchetti A, Krikler DM, eds. Calcium antagonism in cardiovascular therapy. Experience with verapamil. Amsterdam: Amsterdam Excerpta Medica, 1981:69–72.
72. The Danish Study Group on Verapamil in Myocardial Infarction. Effect of verapamil on mortality and major events after acute myocardial infarction (The Danish Verapamil Infarction Trial II-DAVIT II). Am J Cardiol 1990; 66:779–85.
73. Theroux P, Taeymans Y, Morissette D, Bosch X, Pelletier GB, Waters DD. A randomized study comparing propranolol and diltiazem in the treatment of unstable angina. J Am Coll Cardiol 1985; 5:717–22.
74. Pepine CJ, Feldman RL, Hill JA, Conti CR, Mehta J, Hill C, Scott E. Clinical outcome after treatment of rest angina with calcium blockers: comparative experience during the initial year of therapy with diltiazem, nifedipine, and verapamil. Am Heart J 1983; 106:1341–7.
75. Held PH, Yusuf S, Furberg CD. Calcium channel blockers in acute myocardial infarction and unstable angina: an overview. Br Med J 1989; 299:1187–92.
76. Mulcahy R, Daly L, Graham I, Hickey N, O'Donoghue S, Owens A, Rune P, Tobin G. Unstable angina: natural history and determinants of prognosis. Am J Cardiol 1981; 48:525–8.
77. Mulcahy R, Awadhi AHA, de Buitleor M, Tobin G, Johnson H, Contoy R. Natural history and prognosis of unstable angina. Am Heart J 1985; 109:753–8.
78. Mulcahy R, Conroy R, Katz R, Fitzpatrick M. Does intensive medical therapy influence the outcome in unstable angina? Clin Cardiol 1990; 13:687–9.

12

Percutaneous Transluminal Coronary Angioplasty for Unstable Angina

John A. Bittl and Thomas J. Ryan, Jr.

Brigham and Women's Hospital and Harvard Medical School
Boston, Massachusetts

INTRODUCTION

The approach to the patient with unstable angina has undergone major revision during the past 10 years. Previously, the treatment strategy was aimed at preventing propagation of the thrombus associated with the underlying unstable atheroma and reducing myocardial oxygen demand. It was common practice to stabilize the acute ischemic syndrome initially with intensive medical therapy and to reserve coronary artery bypass surgery for patients who continued to show evidence of ischemia (1,2). This approach changed after reports of successful use of coronary angioplasty for unstable angina appeared (3). Coronary angioplasty has been used in increasing numbers of patients with unstable angina as the skills of operators and balloon catheter design improved.

The foundation for an aggressive approach to the treatment of unstable angina comes from an improved understanding of the pathophysiology and natural history. It is now accepted from angiographic (4–6) and angioscopic (7,8) observations that plaque rupture and nonocclusive thrombus formation precipitate unstable angina and that thrombus is often present in patients with rest pain. Furthermore, adverse cardiac events (death, myocardial infarction, and need for urgent revascularization) are more common in patients with angiographic evidence of thrombus (6). Medical therapy has substantially diminished the risk of myocardial infarction in unstable angina by approximately 40% with aspirin, 44% with intravenous heparin, and 13% with beta-blockers (9). Unfortunately, it is impossible to compare the efficacy of medical and surgical therapy to coronary angioplasty for the treatment of unstable angina because of the heterogeneity of affected population, the continuing evolution of therapy for the syndrome, and the lack of completed randomized trials. Because of the perceived advantages of coronary angioplasty, a large proportion of patients presenting with unstable angina are now being treated with this intervention. For example, Leeman et al. (10) recently reported 104 consecutive patients with unstable angina admitted to two coronary care units and followed prospectively. Forty-one percent had coronary angioplasty, 46% were referred for coronary artery bypass surgery, and 13% had continued medical therapy. Thus, cardiac catheterization and coronary angioplasty, by providing an opportunity for prompt mechanical reperfusion of the ischemia-related artery, have become increasingly utilized in the current management of unstable angina.

The purpose of this chapter is to review the indications, techniques, and timing for cardiac catheterization and angioplasty in patients with unstable angina. We discuss success and complication rates, conduct of the procedure, approaches to the patient with intracoronary thrombus or hemodynamic instability and postprocedural management of anticoagulation.

DIAGNOSTIC CARDIAC CATHETERIZATION IN PREPARATION FOR ANGIOPLASTY IN PATIENTS WITH UNSTABLE ANGINA

Patient Selection

Patients who have failed medical therapy for unstable angina or who show evidence of widespread ischemia, such as fall in blood pressure or pulmonary congestion during ischemia, should undergo diagnostic cardiac catheterization with the ultimate goal of reperfusing the ischemia-related artery and preventing progression to acute myocardial infaction. Cardiac catheterization should also be considered for patients with mitral regurgitation that appears with episodes of angina, ST segment elevations during ischemia, or those progressing to acute myocardial infarction when thrombolytic therapy has failed or cannot be given (Table 1). Patients who experience prompt relief of pain, have normalization of electrocardiographic changes, and show no evidence of hemodynamic compromise with ischemia can be managed conservatively with cardiac catheterization and other interventions driven by clinical necessity.

Technical Aspects of the Diagnostic Procedure

Upon arrival in the cardiac catheterization laboratory, the patient should have vital signs measured quickly, electrocardiographic monitoring established, and the femoral area draped and prepared to allow easy placement of femoral arterial

Table 1 Indications for Emergency Cardiac Catheterization in Patients with Unstable Angina

Recurrence of ischemia on medical therapy
Evidence of widespread ischemia
Hypotension
Pulmonary edema
More than two leads with ST-segment depression
ST-segment elevation
Dynamic mitral regurgitation
Progression to acute myocardial infarction in which thrombolytic therapy has failed or cannot be given

and venous access. At the same time, attention must be given to the level of any ongoing discomfort and fear experienced by the patient. Pain refractory to intravenous nitroglycerin or beta-blockers can be treated with 2–4 mg morphine sulfate or 25–50 μg fentanyl intravenously. Appropriate informed consent and a reassuring explanation of the procedure often help the patient cope with the intimidating environment of the cardiac catheterization laboratory.

In the patient with hypotension accompanying ischemia refractory to inotropic agents and intravenous fluid administration, the contralateral femoral artery can be entered simultaneously for intra-aortic balloon support. No time should be wasted on insertion of prophylactic pacemakers or routine measurement of right heart pressures unless these procedures are clearly necessary. Thus, right heart catheterization should be performed only if such information may help in the acute managment of the patient by confirming low or high filling pressures. A temporary transvenous pacemaker is inserted for high-degree atrioventricular block that is hemodynamically compromising.

Coronary Arteriography

In the unstable patient, the primary objective of cardiac catheterization is to identify the artery responsible for ischemia and to determine its suitability for acute intervention, such as direct angioplasty or emergency bypass surgery. Full anticoagulation is not an absolute contraindication to cardiac catheterization in the unstable patient. A single-wall puncture needle may minimize bleeding complications in the patients at increased risk if the operator is skilled at such an approach. Otherwise, the routine technique for femoral artery puncture should be used. It is reasonable to place a 5 or 6Fr arterial sheath in the femoral artery for diagnostic coronary arteriography, espccially in patients who are at increased risk of bleeding because of anticoagulation or thrombolytic therapy. The 5 or 6Fr sheath can be replaced by an 7 or 8Fr sheath if coronary angioplasty is performed. The selection of contrast agent in this setting is the subject of controversy. Diatrizoate sodium may be less well tolerated than a lower osmolarity agent because of hemodynamic effects. The advantage of diatrizoate is that it is a better anticoagulant than the nonionic agents. Ioxaglate, a low-ionic agent that retains most of the anticoagulant properties of diatizoate sodium (11–13), is routinely used in our institution for angioplasty in the unstable patient with hemodynamic compromise.

Coronary arteriography of the suspected ischemia-related vessel, selected on the basis of electrocardiographic localization (14), is generally performed first. Then, while the contralateral coronary artery is being evaluated, the assistant prepares an appropriate angioplasty balloon. The left coronary artery is generally evaluated first in either the AP caudal view or LAO cranial view. The right coronary artery is initially evaluated with the nonangulated, or mildly cranially angulated, left anterior oblique view with subsequent views taken to maximize visualization of the offending stenosis or stenoses.

ANGIOPLASTY FOR UNSTABLE ANGINA

Analogous to the five different aproaches to coronary angioplasty in acute myocardial infarction (15), coronary angioplasty for unstable angina can be executed in three different ways (Table 2):

1. *Direct angioplasty* is performed emergently to dilate the culprit vessel without adjunctive use of thrombolytic agents. This is the most common approach for angioplasty of the ischemia-related artery.
2. *Immediate angioplasty with thrombolytic therapy* can be used for patients who have evidence of intracoronary thrombus without dissection.
3. *Deferred angioplasty* is performed 18 hours to 7 days after unstable angina in suitable candidates with ≥60% residual stenosis who cannot undergo angioplasty at the time of diagnostic catheterization because of logistic reasons (e.g., surgical backup) or because of high-risk features (e.g., intracoronary thrombus) that may improve with further medical therapy.

Table 2 Angioplasty Approaches for Unstable Angina

Direct angioplasty
Immediate angioplasty with thrombolytic therapy
Deferred angioplasty after prolonged heparin and aspirin

Direct Angioplasty for Unstable Angina

This is the most certain method for promptly restoring patency to the responsible artery in most patients with unstable angina. Reports from several centers suggest that the success rate is 80–93% with a mortality rate of 0–2%, emergency coronary artery bypass rate of 0–12%, and myocardial infarction rate of 0–13% (Table 3). In 60 patients who continued to experience unstable angina after maximal therapy with beta-blockers, calcium antagonists, and intravenous nitroglycerin, de Feyter and colleagues (16) successfully performed percutaneous transluminal coronary angioplasty in 56 patients (93%). There were no deaths, but four patients experienced abrupt closure, sustained myocardial infarction, and required emergency coronary artery bypass surgery. The investigators followed all patients for a least 6 months. Late cardiac death occurred in one patient, eight had recurrent angina, but none had myocardial infarction. Follow-up angiography was obtained in 46 patients, and only 13 (28%) had evidence of restenosis, which was defined by presence of >50% stenosis. Clinical evidence of restenosis, defined as emergence of angina or evidence of provocable ischemia on exercise testing with thallium, was found in 20% of the patients at 6 months. Therefore, it is clear that in unstable patients high initial success can be achieved by dilating the "culprit" lesion with low morbidity and mortality.

Table 3 Clinical Trials of PTCA for Unstable Angina

		Complications (%)			Restenosis		
n	Procedural success (%)	Death	MI	CABG	*n*/*n*	(%)	Ref.
60	93	0	7	7	13/46	(28)[a]	16
53	89	0	8	8	14/53	(26)[b]	21
43	88	—	9	12	—/—	(29)[b]	26
27	89	0	0	0	—/—	(17)[b]	27
16	87	0	13	0	4/14	(27)[a]	29
68	87	0	1.5	1.5	24/58	(41)[b]	25
200	90	0.5	8	9	51/158	(32)[a]	18
54	80	0	4	6	12/43	(28)[b]	30
90	93	1	0	0	14/49	(29)[a]	40
66	88	2	6	3	6/36	(17)[b]	24
126	—	—	—	—	56/126	(44)[a]	41

[a]Angiographic restenosis (>50% stenosis at coronary arteriography).

[b]Clinical restenosis (defined as either spontaneous angina or provocable ischemia on noninvasive testing).

Risk Factors

Risk factors for procedural complications and for restenosis have been examined by a number of investigators. The investigators for the 1985–1986 NHLBI Percutaneous Transluminal Coronary Angioplasty Registry found no significant difference in the incidence of periprocedural occlusion in patients with stable vs. unstable angina (5.8% vs. 7.6%, p = NS by χ^2) (17).

De Feyter and colleagues (18) have evaluated their experience with angioplasty for unstable angina. In 200 patients, they have reported an 89% success rate with at least one major complication occurring in 21 patients (10%): death in 1, myocardial infarction in 16, and urgent surgery in 18. The angiographic restenosis rate was 32% (51/158). The 2-year mortality rate was 3%. Multivariate analysis identified risk factors for *procedural complications:* ST-segment elevation, persistent negative T waves, and stenosis ≥65%. Risk factors for *restenosis* were presence of collateral vessels, ST-segment depression, multivessel disease, stenosis in the left anterior descending artery, and history of recent onset of symptoms. Ellis et al. defined other risk factors for poor outcome for angioplasty during acute myocardial infarction, which are also applicable to the patient with unstable angina (Table 4) (19).

The Timing of Angioplasty

The appropriate timing of angioplasty for patients with unstable angina has been retrospectively evaluated. Laskey et al. (20) found that the procedural success rate was higher for patients with unstable angina who were treated with heparin ≥24 hr before coronary angioplasty than for those patients who did not receive heparin (91% vs. 81% success rate, respectively; $p = 0.02$). Patients not receiving heparin were also more likely to experience abrupt closure (8% vs. 2%; $p < 0.01$). Other investigators have observed a trend toward improved outcome if angioplasty can be deferred for about 2 weeks after the onset of unstable angina (21).

Table 4 Risk Factors for Procedural Complications During Angioplasty Performed for Acute Ischemic Syndromes

Ejection fraction < 30%
Stenosis in arterial bend ≥ 45°
TIMI flow <Grade 2
Thrombus > 5 mm
Presence of other stenoses ≥ 50%
Patient age > 60 years
ST segment elevation
No prior heparin

Source: Modified from Refs. 18 and 19.

Much can be learned about the timing of angioplasty from the excellent clinical studies of thrombolytic therapy and angioplasty for myocardial infarction. It appears that the angiographic markers of the unstable lesion improve during the postinfarction period, suggesting that early remodeling the of the unstable plaque has taken place. Davies et al. (22) observed that globular filling defects, present initially at angiography in patients with acute myocardial infarction, had disappeared at a second angiographic study 2–10 days after streptokinase and heparin therapy. Topol et al. (23) observed that 14% of 98 patients, all of whom had significant stenoses during an emergency coronary arteriogram performed for acute myocardial infarction, had insignificant lesions one week later. This suggests that deferred angioplasty is preferable to emergency angioplasty for acute myocardial infarction. Since the pathologic processes leading to acute myocardial infarction and to the syndrome of unstable angina are probably similar, deferred angioplasty may also prove to be superior to emergency angioplasty in unstable angina. This issue is being examined in the ongoing National Heart, Lung, and Blood Trial—Thrombolysis in Myocardial Infarction III (TIMI III).

Angioplasty Procedure

The procedure is performed after emergency coronary arteriography has defined the anatomy of the ischemia-related artery. The 5 or 6Fr arterial sheath is then exchanged for an 8Fr sheath that can accommodate an angioplasty-guiding catheter, which is then advanced to the left main or right coronary artery. The patient should be treated with aspirin (325 mg orally), a frequently overlooked medication critical for successful outcome, and a total dose of heparin of 10,000–15,000 units intravenously. If blood pressure is >100 mmHg, intravenous nitroglycerin in a dose of 25 μg/min is begun. Even if the ischemia- or infarct-related artery is totally occluded, a floppy guidewire is generally able to penetrate a recent occlusion since it contains soft thrombus. For similar reasons, a balloon catheter selected to match the size of the artery is relatively easy to pass through the occlusion for one or two 2-minute inflations. The guidewire should be extended to permit unimpeded angiography with contrast medium in multiple views and easy access to the dilated site if acute closure occurs. If more than a small, focal dissection with impairment of flow is seen, the segment can be redilated with a standard angioplasty balloon for a longer duration if inflation is well tolerated. In some cases, repeat dilation with a Stack perfusion catheter (ACS) will be needed to repair dissections. After successful angioplasty, the patient is treated with 325 mg aspirin orally daily and heparin (700–1200 units/hr) to achieve a partial thromboplastin time of 60–80 sec, and intravenous nitroglyerin, as well as an oral calcium channel blocking agent to reduce the risk of vasospasm. The arterial and venous sheaths are left in place for 18–24 hr and removed after heparin has been discontinued for 3–4 hr. The heparin infusion can be restarted without a loading dose 3–4 hr after sheath removal if no hemmorrhagic complication is encountered.

Complex Angioplasty for Unstable Angina

Unstable Angina After Myocardial Infarction. Patients who develop unstable angina after myocardial infarction are at particularly high risk for poor outcome. De Feyter and colleagues (21) reported their experience in 53 patients who experienced unstable angina 48 hr to 30 days after acute myocardial infarction. The procedural success was 89% with a trend toward lower success rates when angioplasty was performed within 14 days after myocardial infarction compared to angioplasty performed after 14 days. Although no deaths were encountered, six patients had unsuccessful angioplasty attempts, four required emergency bypass surgery, and a total of four patients (8%) experienced myocardial infarction. Angina recurred in 14 patients for a clinical restenosis rate of 26%. More recently, Morrison (24) reported successful angioplasty procedures in 58/66 (88%) patients who experienced unstable angina within 30 days of documented myocardial infarction. One patient died, two patients required emergency bypass surgery, and four had myocardial infarction. The clinical restenosis rate was 6/36 (17%). The use of coronary angioplasty for the treatment of unstable angina after myocardial infarction was also evaluated by Safian et al. (25). These investigators performed angioplasty in a group of 69 patients with angina an average of 2.3 months after non–Q wave myocardial infarction. The procedural success rate was 87% (59/68), and one patient required emergency bypass surgery (1.5%). Long-term follow-up was available for 58/59 patients who had successful angioplasty. Recurrent angina developed in 41% (24/58). Therefore, coronary angioplasty can be used successfully in patients who develop unstable angina after myocardial infarction.

"Culprit Vessel Angioplasty." Many patients with unstable angina have multivessel disease. The approach of "culprit vessel" angioplasty may be appropriate for such patients in an attempt to reduce the risk of progression to myocardial infarction. De Feyter and colleagues (26) examined their experience with coronary angioplasty of the ischemia-related artery in 43 patients with multivessel disease and unstable angina. They reported an 88% success rate, 12% risk of emergency coronary artery bypass surgery, and 9% incidence of myocardial infarction. The success and complication rates for patients undergoing culprit vessel angioplasty were not different from a group of 111 patients with unstable angina who had angioplasty for single-vessel coronary artery disease. However, recurrence of angina and noninvasive evidence of provocable ischemia was greater in the multivessel disease group.

Wohlgelernter and colleagues (27) also have evaluated the approach of "culprit vessel" angioplasty for unstable angina in patients with multivessel coronary artery disease. In 27 patients, they achieved an 89% success rate without procedure-related complications. In an average of 16 months of follow-up for patients with initially successful angioplasty, the clinical recurrence rate was 17%.

Therefore, in patients with unstable angina and multivessel disease, coronary angioplasty of the offending vessel is highly successful. Since the major limitation is incomplete revascularization, symptoms may recur and ischemia may easily be provoked, requiring more complete revascularization with PTCA or bypass surgery.

Angioplasty for Unstable Angina with ST Elevation. Patients with unstable angina and ST segment elevations (transmural ischemia) may have a worse prognosis than those with ST depressions (28). Nevertheless, in a small series of patients with unstable angina and ST elevations, initial success rate of coronary angioplasty was 87%, and there were no deaths or urgent coronary bypass surgery, although two patients (13%) sustained a myocardial infarction. Angiographic restenosis was subsequently documented in 4/15 patients (27%) (29). Patients presenting with unstable angina and ST segment elevations may be excellent candidates for emergency angioplasty and thus avoid coronary artery bypass surgery.

The Elderly Patient. Coronary angioplasty can be performed for the elderly patient with unstable angina in whom the risk of surgery is increased. Holt and colleagues (30) reported their experience with coronary angioplasty in 54 patients >70 years old. Angioplasty was successful in 43 (80%), with emergency coronary artery bypass surgery required in 3 patients (6%) and Q wave myocardial infarction sustained by 2 patients (4%). The clinical restenosis rate was 12/43 (28%). Therefore, the elderly patient with unstable angina, who may be at increased risk bypass surgery, can be treated with coronary angioplasty.

Angioplasty of Bypass Grafts. The success of coronary angioplasty of lesions in bypass grafts contributing to the syndrome of unstable angina has been reported by Morrison (31). Angioplasty of a vein graft was attempted in 17 patients and was successful in 16; the remaining patient required a perfusion catheter and emergency bypass surgery and had uneventful recovery without myocardial infarction. Four patients had left internal mammary lesions: three were successfully dilated with balloon angioplasty, and the occluded native left anterior descending artery was successfully recanalized in the fourth patient. Although this preliminary report suggests favorable success rates for coronary angioplasty of bypass grafts in patients with unstable angina, certain recommendations need to be emphasized. The older (>3 yr) vein graft often contains large, friable lesions with thrombus and thus poses a greater risk of embolization (32). The presence of a large (>5 mm) filling defect should thus be considered a relative contraindication to the procedure. Furthermore, the risk of restenosis in older vein grafts is >80% (32). Dilatation of the internal mammary is required most often at the anastomotic site. Intubation of the ostium of the internal mammary artery is associated with dissection, which may require mechanical repair (33). Instrumentation of the body of the vessel can produce intense vasospasm refractory to intraarterial nitroglycerin but responsive to intraarterial verapamil or papaverine (33).

Immediate Angioplasty with Adjunctive Thrombolytic Therapy for Intracoronary Thrombus

Adjunctive Use of Thrombolytic Therapy

The use of adjunctive thrombolytic therapy associated with balloon angioplasty for unstable angina is currently being evaluated by several investigators. Surypranata et al. (34) used intracoronary streptokinase in 12 patients who experienced abrupt closure during balloon angioplasty for unstable angina. Intracoronary streptokinase alone was successful in restoring flow to the artery in three patients, and four patients had successful repeat balloon angioplasty with a larger balloon, four patients required emergency bypass surgery (with one death), and one patient received conservative therapy for a persistently occluded vessel and myocardial infarction. Thus, a total of 6/12 of the patients experienced myocardial infarction after abrupt closure despite treatment with intracoronary streptokinase.

More recently, Schieman et al. (35) reported their experience with intracoronary urokinase as adjunctive treatment for flow-limiting thrombus formation during PTCA in patients with acute ischemic syndromes. Intracoronary urokinase (mean dose 141,000 units over approximately 30 min; range 100,000–250,000 units) was used in 10 patients with unstable angina who developed impending vessel closure during angioplasty. Urokinase and repeat balloon angioplasty were successful in restoring flow and relieving ischemia in 9/10 patients. No patient experienced acute myocardial infarction, needed bypass surgery, or had clinical or antiographic evidence of reocclusion.

When to Use Adjunctive Thrombolytic Therapy

The safety and efficacy of angioplasty with adjunctive thrombolytic therapy has not been reported in large studies. Instead, the experience has been anecdotal. Certain subgroups of patients may benefit from the use of adjunctive thrombolysis (34,36), but the precise setting where this is useful is not clear.

It is reasonable to consider the use of intracoronary thrombolytic agents before angioplasty if >5 mm intraluminal filling defect is found, if there is no evidence of dissection, and if the clinical situation demands immediate revascularization. If direct angioplasty is performed without the use of adjunctive thrombolytic therapy and abrupt closure is encountered, thrombolytic therapy can be tried. Until further experience has been gained with adjunctive thrombolytic therapy during complicated PTCA, a significant dissection should be considered a contraindication to the use of thrombolytic agents because of the theoretical risk that they may precipitate mural hemorrhage and "paradoxically" contribute to vessel closure. We typically use urokinase 50,000 units intracoronary followed by 20,000 units per minute for a total of 250,000–500,000 units. Our anecdotal experience of about 50% success is similar to the report from Surypranata and colleagues (34).

Case Report: Intracoronary Urokinase to Remove Laminated Thrombus

A 71-year-old woman was readmitted to the coronary care unit with unstable angina one week after inferoposterior myocardial infarction. She presented to the hospital with 9 hours of severe chest pain and evidence of inferoposterior myocardial infarction. She was initially managed conservatively in hospital and had no complications until one week later when she developed angina associated with hypotension. Cardiac catherization showed evidence of inferior hypokinesis, occlusion of the mid-right coronary artery, and occlusion of the second marginal branch. The right coronary artery occlusion was easily penetrated with a guide wire, allowing dilatation with a 3.0-mm balloon, and a laminated thrombus was found (Fig. 1). This could not be dilated further until intracoronary urokinase was given (50,000 unit bolus followed by 20,000 units per minute for a total dose of 250,000 units). After urokinase, the artery had a 20% residual stenosis. Two days later, repeat coronary arteriography showed no change in the right coronary lesion (residual 20% stenosis without dissection or intraluminal filling defect). The second marginal branch was successfully dilated, leaving a residual 20% stenosis. One week later the patient underwent exercise testing: She exercised for 6'30'' on a Standard Bruce protocol, stopped because of fatigue at a peak heart rate of 118, and had no angina or electrocardiographic evidence of ischemia.

This case is an example of the inability of PTCA alone to dilate a stenosis comprised of laminated thrombus. The absence of dissection minimized the risk of mural hemorrhage, and adjunctive use of urokinase allowed the procedure to be completed successfully.

Deferred Angioplasty for Intracoronary Thrombus

In patients with unstable angina who are found to have an intraluminal filling defect with the appearance of thrombus, angioplasty can be deferred for 4–7 days while continued therapy with aspirin and intravenous heparin is used. This strategy has been reported by Douglas et al. (37). In 19 patients with large intracoronary thrombi and unstable angina or acute myocardial infarction, one week of heparin or aspirin therapy led to a decrease in the size of the intraluminal

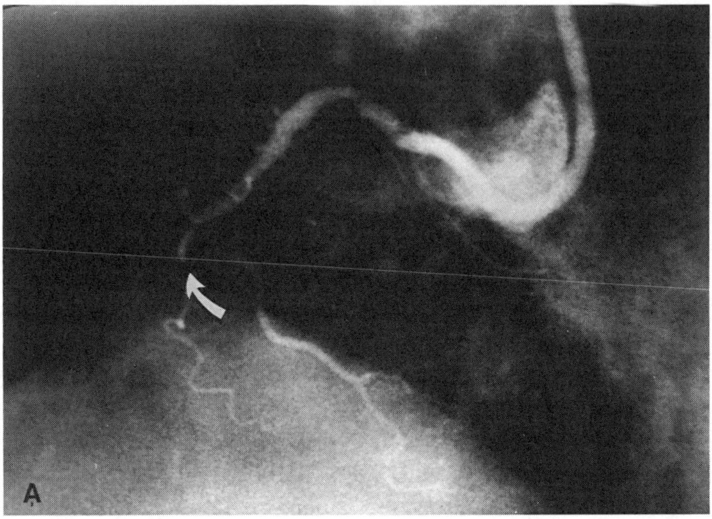

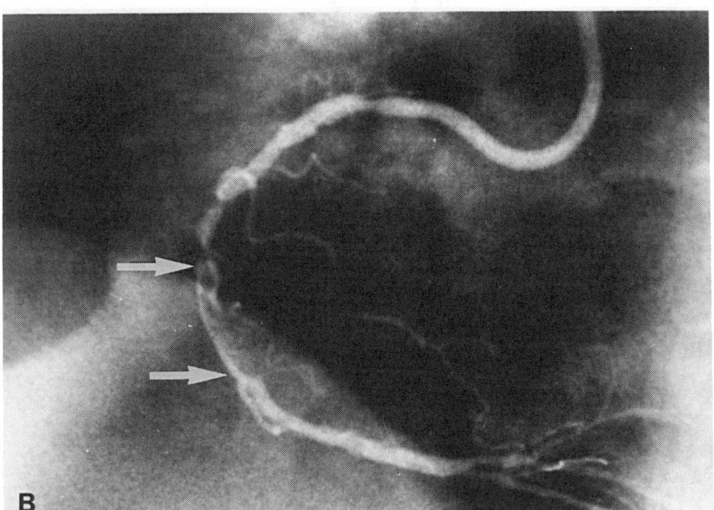

Figure 1 Urokinase therapy during immediate angioplasty for unstable angina. Total occlusion of the mid-portion of the right coronary artery (A, arrow) is dilated with 2.0-mm and 3.0-mm balloons, leaving significant residual stenosis and evidence of laminated thrombus (between arrows) without evidence of dissection (B). After a total of 250,000 units of intracoronary urokinase (UK) was given, the thrombus had almost completely disappeared (C). Follow-up angioplasty with a 3.0-mm balloon resulted in an irregular stenosis of 20% (D).

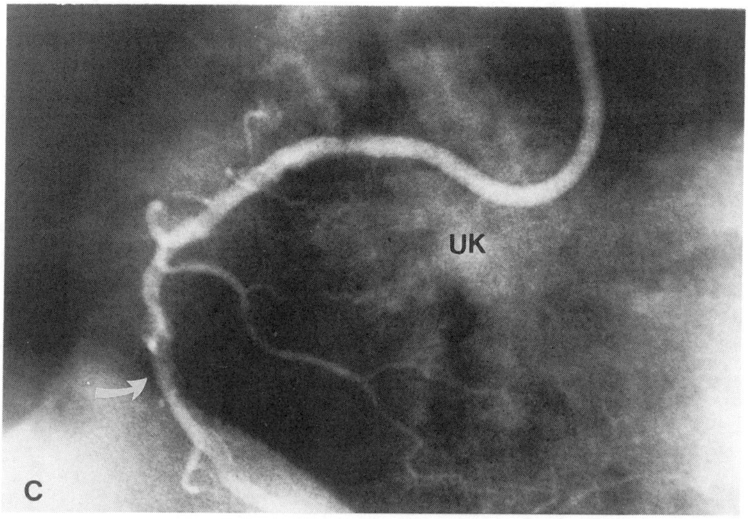
UK
C

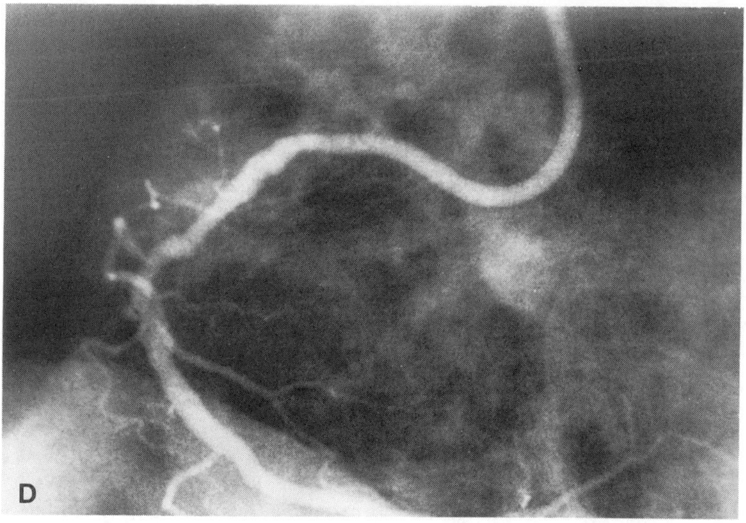
D

Table 5 Deferred Angioplasty for Unstable Angina in 13 Consecutive Patients with Intracoronary Filling Defects

	Number	%
Mean age (yr)	62±11	—
Sex: M/F	9/4	69/31
Age ≥ 70 years	4	31
No. of coronary arteries narrowed ≥50%		
1	10	77
2	3	23
3	0	0
Infarct-related artery		
Left anterior descending	6	46
Right coronary artery	4	31
Circumflex marginal	3	23
Success	13	100
Death, CABG, or Q wave MI	0	0
Reocclusion, non-Q wave MI, PTCA	1	8
Discharge without any complication	12	92

filling defect in 13 patients (68%). Coronary angioplasty was subsequently successful in all 15 patients in whom it was attempted.

We evaluated this strategy in 13 consecutive patients at the Brigham and Women's Hospital (Table 5). One patient had complete resolution of thrombus with a 40% residual stenosis and did not undergo angioplasty. In the remaining 12 patients, subsequent coronary angioplasty was successful in all 12. (One patient developed abrupt closure 24 hours after angioplasty, had successful repeat angiography and showed evidence of a small non–Q wave myocardial infarction by creatine kinase determinations. Fortunately, she had no evidence of regional wall motion abnormality on echocardiography or provocable ischemia on follow-up exercise testing.)

Thus, the delayed approach for angioplasty in the setting of an intraluminal defect appears to be a safe and effective strategy. It is unclear whether the adjunctive use of thrombolytic agents could shorten the hospitilization time required and permit equally successful results.

Effect of Angioplasty on Left Ventricular Function in Patients with Unstable Angina

The effect of coronary angioplasty on left ventricular function in patients with unstable angina was evaluated by de Feyter et al. (38). These investigators observed an increase in global ejection fraction from 0.55 to 0.60 ($p < 0.05$) in a group of patients with successful one-vessel angioplasty of the left anterior descending artery, and there was no evidence of restenosis or myocardial infarction. Significant improvements in regional, but not global, wall motion were also seen in patients who had angioplasty of the right and circumflex coronary arteries. Renkin et al. (39) extended these findings by reporting that patients with persistent negative T waves may show improvement in regional wall motion, measured as percent area shortening, after successful coronary angioplasty of the left anterior descending artery. Therefore, successful angioplasty can reverse ischemic dysfunction of myocardium.

Restenosis

Risk factors for restenosis after coronary angioplasty performed for unstable angina have been analyzed by Halon and colleagues (40). In 90 patients, procedural success was achieved in 84 (93%), while major complications occurred in only one patient (one death). Angiographic restenosis was found in 14 of 49 patients (29%). The lesion characteristics that predicted restenosis by multivariate analysis included the presence of luminal irregularities (complex lesion) and decreased flow (TIMI flow ≤ 2).

In a larger study reported recently, Frid et al. (41) from Duke University evaluated 396 patients undergoing first angioplasty. Angiographic follow-up was obtained in 86% of patients. The highest rates of restenosis were seen in 119 patients with unstable angina who responded to medical therapy (40% angiographic restenosis rate) and in 7 patients refractory to medical therapy (57% restenosis). In patients with stable anginal symptoms, the restenosis rate was only 21%.

Although aspirin has been shown not to reduce the rate of restenosis after PTCA (42), it is used after angioplasty for all patients who present with unstable angina. Calcium channel blockers are also frequently prescribed, but these agents have been shown to have no effect on restenosis after PTCA (43).

Selective Catheterization and Angioplasty

Do all patients with unstable angina require cardiac catheterization? Patients with new onset angina that is well tolerated may show marked improvement in symptom status after institution of medical therapy. If these patients have no evidence of high-risk features (Table 1) and have good exercise capacity, cardiac catheterization is not required. Instead, invasive procedures are reserved for those who continue to show evidence of either spontaneous or provocable ischemia.

While diagnostic cardiac catheterization is performed in many hospitals,

Table 6 Indications for Emergency Surgery in Unstable Angina

Patients with >3 contraindications to PTCA (see Table 4)
Failed PTCA
Intra-aortic balloon dependence not reversed by PTCA
Poorly tolerated reocclusion not amenable to PTCA or thrombolytic therapy

only about 12% of hospitals in the United States are equipped to perform coronary angioplasty.

Emergency Bypass Surgery (Table 6)

As many as 46% of patients with unstable angina are referred for coronary artery bypass surgery (10). The indications for surgical treatment of unstable angina are: contraindications to PTCA (Table 4), unsuccessful PTCA with ongoing ischemia, clinically significant reocclusion of the infarct-related artery not amenable to PTCA or treatment with thrombolytic agents, low output state dependent on intra-aortic balloon pump, and mitral valve replacement for mitral regurgitation.

CONCLUSIONS

Emergency cardiac catheterization and coronary angioplasty now play an important role in the management of patients who have unstable angina. Cardiac catheterization identifies the coronary anatomy for revascularization, defines the extent of myocardium at risk, and allows the unstable patient to receive appropriate revascularization therapy in a timely manner.

REFERENCES

1. Silverman KJ, Grossman W. Angina pectoris: natural history and strategies for evaluation and management. N Engl J Med 1984; 310:1712–7.
2. Plotnick GD. Approach to the management of unstable angina. Am Heart J 1979; 98:243–55.
3. Williams DO, Riley RS, Singh AK, Gewirtz H, Most AS. Evaluation of the role of coronary angioplasty in patients with unstable angina pectoris. Am Heart J 1981; 102:1–9.
4. Gotoh K, Minamino T, Katoh O, Hamano Y, Fukui S, Hori M, Kusuoka H, Mishima M, Inoue M, Kamada T. The role of intracoronary thrombus in unstable angina: angiographic assessment and thrombolytic therapy during ongoing anginal attacks. Circulation 1988; 77:526–34.
5. Ambrose JA, Winters SL, Stern A, Eng A, Teicholz LE, Gorlin R, Fuster V. Angiographic morphology and the pathogenesis of unstable angina pectoris. J Am Coll Cardiol 1985; 5:609–14.

6. Freeman MR, Williams AE, Chisholm RJ, Armstrong PW. Intracoronary thrombus and complex morphology in unstable angina. Relation of timing of angiography and in-hospital cardiac events. Circulation 1989; 80:17–23.
7. Sherman CT, Litvack F, Grundfest W, Lee M, Hickery A, Chaux A, Kass R, Blanche C, Matloff J, Morgenstern L, Ganz W, Swan HJC, Forrester J. Coronary angioscopy in patients with unstable angina pectoris. N Engl J Med 1986; 315:913–9.
8. Forrester JS, Litvack F, Grundfest W, Hickey A. A perspective of coronary disease seen through the arteries of living man. Circulation 1986; 75:505–12.
9. Yusef S, Wittes J, Friedman L. Overview of results of randomized clinical trials in heart disease. II. Unstable angina, heart failure, primary prevention with aspirin, and risk factor modification. JAMA 1988; 260:2259–63.
10. Leeman DE, McCabe CH, Faxon DP, Lorell BH, Kellett MA, McKay RG, Varricchione T, Baim DS. Use of percutaneous transluminal coronary angioplasty and bypass surgery despite improved medical therapy for unstable angina pectoris. Am J Cardiol 1988; 61:38G-44G.
11. Ing JJ, Smith DC, Bull BS. Differing mechanisms of clotting inhibition by ionic and nonionic contrast agents. Radiology 1989; 172:345–8.
12. Levi M, Pascucci C, Agnelli G, Sturk A, Hoek J, Wouter tCJ. Effect on thrombus growth and thrombolysis of two types of osmolar contrast media in rabbits. Invest Radiol 1990; 25:533–5.
13. Rasuli P, McLeish WA, Hammond DI. Anticoagulant effects of contrast materials: in vitro study of iohexol, ioxaglate, and diatrizoate. Am J Roentgenol 1989; 152:309–11.
14. Fuchs RM, Achuff SC, Grunwald L, Yin FCP, Griffith LSC. Electrocardiographic localization of coronary artery narrowings: studies during myocardial ischemia and infarction in patients with one-vessel disease. Circulation 1982; 66:1168–76.
15. Topol EJ. Coronary angioplasty for acute myocardial infarction. Ann Int Med 1988; 109:970–80.
16. de Feyter PJ, Serruys PW, van dBM, Balakumaran K, Mochtar B, Soward AL, Arnold AE, Hugenholtz PG. Emergency coronary angioplasty in refractory unstable angina. N Engl J Med 1985; 313:342–6.
17. Detre KM, Holmes DRJ, Holubkov R, Cowley MJ, Bourassa MG, Faxon DP, Dorros GR, Bentivoglio LG, Kent KM, Myler RK, Coinvestigators of the National H Lung, and Blood Institute's Percutaneous Transluminal Coronary Angioplasty Registry. Incidence and consequences of periprocedural occlusion: The 1985–1986 National Heart, Lung, and Blood Institute Percutaneous Transluminal Coronary Angioplasty Registry. Circulation 1990; 82:739–50.
18. de Feyter PJ, Suryapranata H, Serruys PW, Beatt K, van Domburg R, van der Brand M, Tijssen JJ, Azar AJ, Hugenholtz PG. Coronary angioplasty for unstable angina: immediate and late results in 200 consecutive patients with identification of risk factors for unfavorable early and late outcome. J Am Coll Cardiol 1988; 12:324–33.
19. Ellis SG, Topol EJ, Gallison L, Grines CL, Langburd AB, Bates ER, Walton JAJ, O'Neill WW. Predictors of success for coronary angioplasty performed for acute myocardial infarction. J Am Coll Cardiol 1988; 12:1407–15.

20. Laskey MA, Deutsch E, Barnathan E, Laskey WK. Influence of heparin therapy on percutaneous transluminal coronary angioplasty outcome in unstable angina pectoris. Am J Cardiol 1990; 65:1425–9.
21. de Feyter PJ, Serruys PW, Soward A, van der Brand M, Bos E, Hugenholtz PG. Coronary angioplasty for early postinfarction unstable angina. Circulation 1986; 74:1365–70.
22. Davies SW, Marchant B, Lyons JP, Timmis AD, Rothman MT, Layton CA, Balcon R. Coronary lesion morphology in acute myocardial infarction: demonstration of early remodeling after streptokinase treatment. J Am Coll Cardiol 1990; 16:1079–86.
23. Topol EJ, Califf RM, George BS, Kereiakes DJ, Abbottsmith CW, Candela RJ, Lee KL, Pitt B, Stack RS, O'Neill WW. A randomized trial of immediate versus delayed elective angioplasty after intravenous tissue plasminogen activator in acute myocardial infarction. N Engl J Med 1987; 317:581–8.
24. Morrison DA. Coronary angioplasty for medically refractory unstable angina within 30 days of acute myocardial infarction. Am Heart J 1990; 120:256–61.
25. Safian RD, Snyder LD, Synder BA, McKay RG, Lorell BH, Aroesty JM, Pasternak RC, Bradley AB, Monrad ES, Baim DS. Usefulness of percutaneous transluminal coronary angioplasty for unstable angina pectoris after non-Q-wave acute myocardial infarction. Am J Cardiol 1987; 59:263–6.
26. de Feyter PJ, Serruys PW, Arnold A, Simoons ML, Wijns W, Geuskens R, Soward A, van der Brand M, Hugenholtz PG. Coronary angioplasty of the unstable angina related vessel in patients with multivessel disease. Eur Heart J 1986; 7:460–7.
27. Wohlgelernter D, Cleman M, Highman HA, Zaret BL. Percutaneous transluminal coronary angioplasty of the "culprit lesion" for management of unstable angina pectoris in patients with multivessel coronary artery disease. Am J Cardiol 1986; 58:460–4.
28. Gerstenblith G, Ouyang P, Achuff SC, Bulkley BH, Becker LC, Mellits ED, Baughman KL, Weiss JL, Flaherty JT, Kallman CH, Llewellyn M, Weisfeldt ML. Nifedipine in unstable angina: a double-blind, randomized trial. N Engl J Med 1982; 306:885–9.
29. de Feyter PJ, Serruys PW, van der Brand M, Soward A. Coronary angioplasty for treatment of unstable angina with transient marked ST-segment elevation. Eur Heart J 1987; 8:569–74.
30. Holt GW, Sugrue DD, Bresnahan JF, Vlietstra RE, Bresnahan DR, Reeder GS, Holmes DRJ. Results of percutaneous transluminal coronary angioplasty for unstable angina pectoris in patients 70 years of age and older. Am J Cardiol 1988; 61:994–7.
31. Morrison DA. Coronary angioplasty for medically refractory unstable angina in patients with prior coronary bypass surgery. Cathet Cardiovasc Diagn 1990; 20:174–81.
32. Platko WP, Hollman J, Whitlow PL, Franco I. Percutaneous transluminal angioplasty of saphenous vein graft stenosis: long-term follow-up. J Am Coll Cardiol 1989; 14:1645–50.
33. Shimshak TM, Giorgi LV, Johnson WL, McConahay DR, Rutherford BD, Ligon R, Hartzler GO. Application of percutaneous transluminal coronary angioplasty to the internal mammary artery graft. J Am Coll Cardiol 1988; 12:1205–14.

34. Suryapranata H, de Feyter PJ, Serruys PW. Coronary angioplasty in patients with unstable angina pectoris: is there a role for thrombolysis? J Am Coll Cardiol 1988; 69A–77A.
35. Schieman G, Cohen BM, Kozina J, Erickson JS, Podolin RA, Peterson KL, Ross JJ, Buchbinder M. Intracoronary urokinase for intracoronary thrombus accumulation complicating percutaneous transluminal coronary angioplasty for acute ischemic syndromes. Circulation 1990; 82:2052–60.
36. Topol EJ, Nicklas JM, Kander NH, Walton JA, Ellis SG, Gorman L, Pitt B. Coronary revascularization after intravenous tissue plasminogen activator for unstable angina pectoris: results of a randomized, double-blind, placebo-controlled trial. Am J Cardiol 1988; 62:368–71.
37. Douglas JS, Lutz JF, Dlements SD, Robinson PH, Roubin GS, Lembo NJ, King SBI. Therapy of large intracoronary thrombi in candidates for percutaneous transluminal coronary angioplasty. J Am Coll Cardiol 1988; 11:238A (abstract).
38. de Feyter PJ, Suryapranata H, Serruys PW, Beatt K, van der Brand M, Hugenholtz PG. Effects of successful percutaneous transluminal coronary angiplasty on global and regional left ventricular function in unstable angina pectoris. Am J Cardiol 1987; 60:993–7.
39. Renkin J, Wijns W, Ladha Z, Col J. Reversal of segmental hypokinesis by coronary angioplasty in patients with unstable angina, persistent T wave inversion, and left anterior descending coronary artery stenosis. Additional evidence for myocardial stunning in humans. Circulation 1990; 82:913–21.
40. Halon DA, Merdler A, Shefer A, Flugelman MY, Lewis BS. Identifying patients at high risk for restenosis after percutaneous transluminal coronary angioplasty for unstable angina pectoris. Am J Cardiol 1989; 64:289–93.
41. Frid DJ, Fortin DF, Lam LC, Harlan WR, Navetta FI, Smith JE, Ramos R, Nelson C, Tcheng JE. Effect of unstable symptoms on restenosis. Circulation 1990; 82:III-427 (abstract).
42. Schwartz L, Bourassa MG, Lesperance J, et al. Aspirin and dipyridamole in the prevention of restenosis after percutaneous transluminal coronary angioplasty. N Engl J Med 1988; 318:1714–9.
43. Fanelli C, Aronoff R. Restenosis following coronary angioplasty. Am Heart J 1990; 119:357–67.

13

The Role of Surgery in the Management of Unstable Angina

Alfred F. Parisi

Brown University, The Miriam Hospital, and Roger Williams Medical Center
Providence, Rhode Island

INTRODUCTION AND PRACTICAL CONSIDERATIONS

Much of what we know about the results of surgery for coronary artery disease comes from randomized trials of medical versus surgical therapies (1–4). In these studies many criteria of therapeutic efficacy have been examined to evaluate the outcomes of these two approaches to patient management (Table 1). Survival is the most objective of these endpoints because of its ease of definition, binary nature, and the finality of mortality. As a consequence survival dominates much of the thinking with regard to the therapeutic benefits of either surgery or medicine. In some ways, particularly for the severely symptomatic patient, this has been unfortunate because it tends to subjugate other important potential benefits of a therapeutic intervention to being either purely secondary or inconsequential. Over the past 15 years the highest level of attention has been paid to which surgical subgroups (three-vessel disease versus lesser disease, normal versus abnormal left ventricular function, and combinations of the vessels diseased with left ventricular dysfunction) might have a *survival advantage*. This has tended to obscure several findings that became apparent from the earliest results of coronary surgery trials—first, that *superior angina relief* was achieved by revascularization, and second, that with the exception of left main disease, if outcomes after one year were considered without further reference to patient subgrouping, there was *no survival disadvantage* for surgical therapy.

Table 1 Endpoints of Trials Examining Medical and Surgical Therapy for Angina

Survival (mortality)
Change in angina
Subsequent nonfatal myocardial infarctions
Subsequent hospitalizations
Treadmill performance
Return to work
Overall quality of life
Crossover to alternative therapy

The above considerations are most pertinent to decision making in patients with unstable angina who are by definition severely symptomatic at the time of their clinical presentation. For these individuals the incremental value of outcomes of therapeutic alternatives must take account of symptomatic benefits, subsequent cardiac events, and quality of life issues if there is no survival disadvantage to surgical revascularization.

A second consideration regarding randomized unstable angina trials (5–11) is that surgery in these studies was in large part accomplished in the mid- to late 1970s and very early 1980s. Surgical techniques have improved significantly over the past decade, particularly with regard to myocardial preservation, improved methods of anesthesia, more widespread use of internal mammary grafts, and better post operative care. These advances have probably made the outcomes of published trials a "worst-case expectation" for surgical intervention. Medical treatment has also changed—it is based on a better pathophysiologic understanding of the mechanisms of unstable angina and introduction of new pharmaceuticals—particularly calcium channel blockers—which extend the medical therapeutic armamentarium. In addition, medical management with aspirin and dipyridamole has improved the patency expectations for saphenous vein grafts and thus has an important role in postoperative surgical management.

A final consideration relates to the "representativeness" of clinical trials relative to the individual under consideration. Trials that measure survival tend to eliminate as many irrelevant prognosis-limiting variables as possible. This idealized situation often does not pertain to the patient at hand. One very pertinent consideration is age—the number of patients over age 70 who have participated in randomized surgical trials is miniscule. Yet the proportion of patients operated today who are septugenarians and older is substantial. Many of these patients have unstable angina. Patients who have unstable angina in hospital after acute infarction are another important clinical subgroup. In the current era these patients frequently undergo revascularization interventions, in particular bypass surgery especially if they have triple-vessel disease and a large amount of myocardium at risk. Such patients differ substantially from the patients randomized in the large medical-surgical trials in the past decades. In that era a recent (<3 months old) myocardial infarction was an exclusion criterion vis-à-vis randomization.

How then is one to judge clinical trials of unstable angina and incorporate their results into a contemporary decision-determining data base? Should reports from smaller, single hospital studies temper this judgment? It is my contention that the most relevant data derives from *consensus*—findings mutually supported by comparable trials should be given the greatest weight. A comparison must be made between the patient-at-hand and patients who qualified for the trials—are they identical? If not, how far does the present patient deviate from ones previously randomized? The more significant this deviation, the less applicable the trial findings. Finally, there is no substitute for *common sense*. In a medical scenario where pharmaceuticals, angioplasty, and surgical revascularization all can play competing as well as complementary roles, the initial management strategy must always be weighed against available resources. What is the mortality/morbidity rate for interventional catheterization and surgical revascularization procedures in one's own (or referral) institution? Is it changing because of new technical advances? How suitable is the patient relative to the invasiveness of the procedure and its therapeutic goals? If intervention/revascularization is chosen, how suitable is the patient's coronary anatomy for the proposed procedure? While the existing body of information, to be reviewed and interpreted herein, will provide broad guidelines for clinical decision making, the needs of an individual patient and the state-of-the-art regarding available resources will always have to be factors in the choice of a final course of action.

OUTCOMES OF MAJOR PROSPECTIVE TRIALS

There have been two major multicenter trials of medical versus surgical therapy for patients with unstable angina. The first was the NHLBI-sponsored National Cooperative Study Group to compare surgical and medical therapy in which patients were randomized over the 4-year period from 1972 to 1976 (5–7). The second was the VA Cooperative Study of Medical Compared with Surgical Management of Unstable Angina in which randomizations occurred over the 6-year period between mid-1976 and mid-1982 (8–10).

NHLBI Trial

Requirements for Randomization

Candidates for this study needed to have "unstable angina pectoris of sufficient severity to warrant admission to an intensive care unit to rule out myocardial infarction." Both an age of 70 years, or greater, and a myocardial infarction within the preceding 3 months were exclusion criteria.

The protocol also required transient ECG changes during episodes of pain. ST segment elevation, ST segment depression, T-wave changes alone or in combination were considered qualifying so long as they reverted toward the control pattern after relief of pain and within 24 hours. Evolution of pathologic Q waves or a rise in serum enzyme studies within the first 24 hours compatible with acute myocardial infarction excluded the patient.

If the patient met the above criteria and had not failed a regimen of intensive medical therapy, informed consent was requested. Patients giving consent underwent left ventricular and coronary angiography within 72 hours of admission.

Angiographic criteria needed to proceed with randomization included a left ventricular ejection fraction greater than 30% and an end diastolic volume index of less than 125 ml/M^2. There had to be 70% luminal diameter narrowing of at least one major coronary vessel with distal vessel(s) suitable for surgery. Patients with left main coronary artery stenoses $>$ 50% were excluded. Patients needing additional concomitant cardiac surgery other than bypass (e.g., valve replacement, aneurymectomy) were excluded.

Randomization Procedure

A tentative surgical date was set prior to randomization. Patients assigned to surgery were to be operated within 8 days of admission. Patients assigned to medicine received propranolol and long-acting nitrates to control blood pressure and pulse; a systolic blood pressure of 110–120 and pulse rate near 60 beats/min were deemed adequate.

Characteristics of Patients Randomized

Of the patients screened, 288 were randomized—147 to medicine and 141 to surgery. Baseline clinical characteristics of the medical and surgical groups were, respectively, mean age, 53; proportion of men (82% vs. 86%); incidence of prior myocardial infarction (27% vs. 35%); history of diabetes (14% vs. 10%); hypertension (29% vs. 35%); smoking (73% vs. 75%); and hyperlipidemia (21% vs. 20%) and did not differ statistically.

Approximately 50% of the patients in each treatment group had new onset angina, while the remaining had a crescendo pattern. Overall, 90% of this population manifested rest pain in the hospital. The ECG changes in the medical and surgical groups were also comparable. ST depression was seen in approximately 60% of all patients and was twice as frequent as ST elevation (Table 2).

Hemodynamic and angiographic characteristics of the medical and surgical groups were also nearly identical—approximately one patient in four had a left ventricular ejection fraction $<$50% and/or left ventricular and diastolic pressure $\geq$13 mmHg. Multivessel disease was present in 76% of each treatment group (Table 3).

Results

Patients were followed over a mean observation period of 30 months. Endpoints reported included angina status, nonfatal myocardial infarction, later surgery for

Table 2 Angina Classification and ECG Changes in NHLBI Unstable Angina Trial

	M% (n = 147)	S% (n = 141)
Angina		
New onset	48	46
Crescendo	52	54
Rest	89	91
Effort	11	9
ECG Changes		
ST depression	58	63
ST elevation	29	26
T-wave inversion only	13	11

M = patients randomized to medicine.
S = patients randomized to surgery.
Source: Ref. 5.

Table 3 Hemodynamic and Angiographic Features of NHLBI Unstable Angina Trial

	M%	S%
Left ventricular ejection fraction		
30–49	23	23
50–59	22	24
60–69	19	19
70–85	21	22
Unknown	15	12
Left ventricular end diastolic pressure		
< 12	57	64
13–30	26	24
Unknown	17	12
Extent of coronary disease		
3VD	39	43
2VD	37	33
1VD	24	24

M = patients randomized to medicine.
S = patients randomized to surgery.
Source: Ref. 5.

angina in the medical group, work status, and mortality. Medical patients who had later surgery were considered in analyses of nonfatal infarctions, angina, or work status up to the time of surgery and thereafter were considered lost to follow-up.

Angina Status

The incidence of high grade (Class III or IV) *angina* was significantly lower in surgically treated patients during the first year of follow-up—irrespective of the number of coronary vessels involved (Fig. 1). During the first year multivessel disease patients treated surgically were nearly three times less likely to have high grade angina than their medically treated counterparts (14% vs. 40%, $p < 0.01$). Patients with single-vessel disease had an even greater reduction in the incidence of high grade angina (22% vs. 3%, $p < 0.05$) during the first year. This advantage persisted through the second follow-up year. The symptomatic advantage for surgically treated patients with multivessel disease was not maintained by the end of the second year, an outcome attributed to the high incidence of later surgery in the patients originally assigned to medical therapy. This certainly would explain the marked fall in high grade angina experienced by medical patients with double- and triple-vessel disease between year 1 and year 2 (Fig. 1).

Nonfatal myocardial infarctions (i.e., survival at least 30 days after infarc-

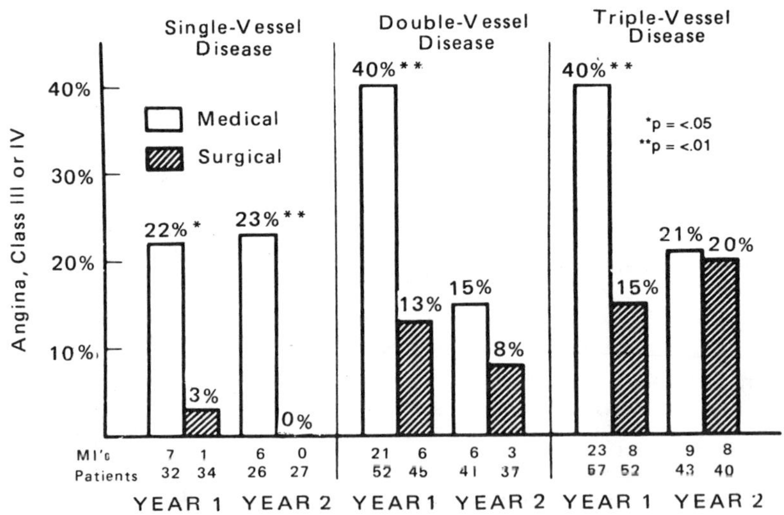

Figure 1 Worst degree of *angina* (class III or IV) at any follow-up during years 1 and 2 after randomization in the NHLBI Unstable Angina Trial. MI's = myocardial infarctions. (From Ref. 6 with permission of the *American Journal of Cardiology*.)

tion) were considered in two contexts—in-hospital and late. New pathologic Q waves were required for the diagnosis. The overall in-hospital myocardial infarction rate was 17% for all surgically treated patients and 8% for all medically treated patients ($p < 0.05$). Late infarctions (11% medical, 13% surgical) did not differ between the treatment groups.

Work status was not statistically significantly different with either surgical or medical therapy. In each group about half of those with triple-vessel disease and 70% with single- or double-vessel disease had returned to work during the first 2 years.

Of the 147 patients randomized to medicine, 53 (36%) had surgery during the mean 30 months of follow-up. Nearly half of these (19%) occurred within the first 12 months. The progression to surgery could not be predicted from the initial presentation or ECG changes. However, crossover to surgery was more likely depending on the number of coronary vessels involved—20% for single-vessel disease, 33% for double-vessel disease, and 49% for triple-vessel disease. For those medical patients who later underwent surgery, angina was reported as less in 78%, unchanged in 20%, and worse in 2%. Of note, a second operation for unacceptable angina was performed in five original surgically treated patients.

Survival

Overall survival was nearly identical in both treatment groups (Fig. 2). One-year survival was 93% for the medical group and 92% for the surgical group; at 2

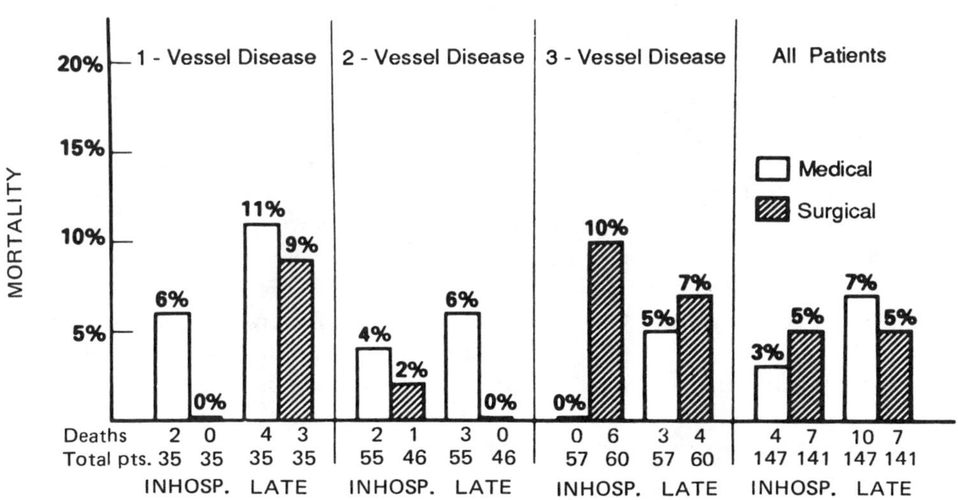

Figure 2 In-hospital (INHOSP.) and late mortality rates of medically and surgically treated patients (Pts) in the NHLBI Unstable Angina Trial. (From Ref. 6 with permission of the *American Journal of Cardiology*.)

years survival was 91% for and 90% for these respective groups. In-hospital mortality (3% medical, 5% surgical) was also comparable.

VA Trial of Unstable Angina

Requirements for Randomization

The VA study screened patients admitted to the hospital with chest pain. Unstable angina was distinguished by clinical criteria and stratified into subtypes 1 ("Progressive angina") and 2 ("Prolonged rest pain resistant to treatment"). Type 1 patients had a progression of previously stable angina which had at least doubled in the frequency of attacks or in its severity such that the average daily dose of nitroglycerin had doubled. Type 1 patients also included individuals who had new rest angina or new onset angina (less than 2 months in duration who were New York Heart Association Class III). Qualifying symptoms had to have been present within 10 days of entry for all Type 1 patients. Electrocardiographic changes consisting of ST segment depression of 1 mm or more or T-wave inversion were sought during in-hospital manifestations of chest pain. A positive exercise test was required if a patient did not have ST segment or T-wave changes during chest pain at rest. Type 2 patients had to have recurrent episodes of *prolonged* (>15 minutes) chest pain at rest which were considered resistant to or incompletely relieved by nitrates. As with Type 1 patients, at least one episode of pain was required within 10 days of entry. Moreover, electrocardiographic documentation of ischemia (ST elevation or depression, T-wave inversion) was required.

As in the NHLBI study, patients were excluded if they were 70 years of age or older or had ECG and/or enzymatic documentation of myocardial infarction during the screening process or within 3 months of the date of screening. The VA only randomized male patients and exluded any patient who had a previous operation for angina pectoris.

Patients who met clinical criteria were asked for informed consent for all the following: ventriculography, coronary arteriography, randomization and arteriography at one year as well as quarterly clinic visits during the first 2 years and semiannual visits thereafter. The angiographic criterion for eligibility was a proximal coronary lesion estimated to cause 75% lumen diameter reduction of a proximal coronary artery (i.e., ≥50% or more luminal narrowing in orthogonal views) with a distal vessel suitable for bypass grafting. Reasons for exclusion were left main stenosis, insufficient coronary disease, diffuse distal disease, and an ejection fraction less than 30%. A left ventricular aneurysm found at ventriculography was also disqualifying.

Randomization Procedure

Prior to randomization a "date of operation" was set by the local investigators. Patients were stratified by their clinical type of unstable angina (Type 1 vs. Type

2) *and* by their ventricular function—this led to randomization in four cells: Type 1, normal ventricular function; Type 1, abnormal ventricular function; Type 2, normal ventricular function; and Type 2, abnormal ventricular function. Ventricular function was defined as normal if the left ventricular ejection fraction was equal to or greater than 50% *and* if the left ventricular end-diastolic pressure was less than 16 mmHg. Therapy was considered to start on the preset "date of operation" for medical patients and on the actual date of operation for surgical patients.

Characteristics of Patients Randomized

Of 3159 patients screened, 468 were randomized—237 to medicine and 231 to surgery. There were 374 Type 1 patients and 94 Type 2 patients. The mean age of both the medically assigned patients and surgically assigned patients was 56 years. Additional baseline characteristics that were statistically indistinguishable for each group included history of myocardial infarction, diabetes, and entry-level blood pressure. These characteristics did not differ in accordance with the type of clinical presentation (Table 4).

Hemodynamic and angiographic characteristics of the medical and surgical groups were also statistically indistinguishable. More than one patient in four had abnormal left ventricular function, and multivessel disease was present in 81% of each treatment group (Table 5).

Results

The patients in the VA study were followed for a period of 5 years through clinic visits, and the survivors are still being followed annually through phone and mail contacts. The data presented herein, unless otherwise specified, are for a minimum of 60 months (mean 72 months) after date of assigned therapy or operation. All data reported are for treatment as originally assigned.

Freedom from Angina

The prevalence of patients who were *angina-free* was significantly higher in those patients assigned to surgery at 1, 3, and 5 years of follow-up (Table 6). The chances of being angina-free averaged nearly 3/10 for medically assigned patients but were 5/10 for surgically assigned patients. (These observations were supported by the lower use of long-acting nitrates at 1, 3, and 5 years and lower use of propranolol at 1 and 3 years). By 5 years 49% of the surgically assigned patients were NYHA Class 1 and 31% of medically assigned patients were Class 1 at 5 years ($p < 0.01$). It should be emphasized that these data are reported by treatment assigned and that these differences exist in the face of a continuous crossover of medically assigned patients to surgical therapy (see below).

Exercise-Induced Ischemia and Exercise Capacity

The VA data regarding angina and functional status were further substantiated by treadmill testing done on an annual basis from onset of treatment (Table 7). At 1

Table 4 Clinical Characteristics of Randomized Patients in VA Unstable Angina Trial

	All patients		Type 1		Type 2	
	M (n = 237)	S (n = 231)	M (n = 190)	S (n = 184)	M (n = 47)	S (n = 47)
Age (yr)	56.3 ± 6.9	55.7 ± 7.1	56.2 ± 6.9	56.0 ± 7.0	56.3 ± 7.1	54.8 ± 7.7
History of myocardial infarction	42.6	41.7	40.5	42.9	51.1	37.0
Diabetes	17.9	16.2	17.0	16.4	21.3	15.6
Systolic blood pressure	129 ± 18	133 ± 21	129 ± 17	133.1 ± 21.2	131.2 ± 20	130.3 ± 21.3
Diastolic blood pressure	79 ± 10	81 ± 11	79 ± 10	81.2 ± 11	80.1 ± 10.4	78.3 ± 13

Values are mean ± SD where applicable.
VA = Veterans Administration.
M = Patients randomized to medicine.
S = Patients randomized to surgery.
Source: Ref. 8.

Table 5 Angiographic Characteristics of Randomized Patients in VA Unstable Angina Trial

	All patients		Type 1[a]		Type 2[b]	
	M (n = 237)	S (n = 231)	M (n = 190)	S (n = 184)	M (n = 47)	S (n = 47)
Abnormal left ventricular function	28.7	28.6	30.0	27.2	23.4	34.0
Ejection fraction	63 ± 13	64 ± 14	63 ± 18	63 ± 14	63 ± 13	64 ± 13
Vessels diseased:						
One	18.6	18.8	17.5	18.6	23.4	19.6
Two	33.1	36.7	31.7	36.6	38.3	37.0
Three	48.3	44.5	50.8	44.8	38.3	43.5

M = Patients randomized to medicine.
W = Patients randomized to surgery.
Values are mean ± SD where applicable.
[a]"Progressive angina."
[b]"Prolonged rest pain."
Source: Ref. 8.

Table 6 Angina Status at 1, 3, and 5 Years After Randomization in VA Unstable Angina Trial

	M	S	
After 1 year	(n = 190)	(n = 171)	
% (n) angina free	31.7 (60)	57.3 (98)	*
% (n) not using propranolol	32.8 (62)	72.4 (123)	*
% (n) not using nitrates	33.7 (63)	71.9 (120)	*
NYHA Class 1 (%)	29.0	49.8	*
After 3 years	(n = 167)	(n = 162)	
% (n) angina free	29.7 (49)	48.1 (78)	*
% (n) not using propranolol	42.0 (71)	63.6 (103)	*
% (n) not using nitrates	37.2 (61)	63.0 (102)	*
NYHA Class 1 (%)	35.6	49.0	p = 0.10
After 5 years	(n = 158)	(n = 155)	
% (n) angina free	33.1 (52)	54.8 (85)	*
% (n) not using propranolol	51.0 (80)	51.5 (88)	p = 0.25
% (n) not using nitrates	45.5 (70)	61.8 (94)	*
NYHA Class 1 (%)	30.9 (47)	48.7 (73)	p = 0.01

n = number of patients.
M = Patients randomized to medicine.
S = Patients randomized to surgery.
*$p < 0.01$ between therapies.
Source: Ref. 11.

year 278 patients had been tested (147 medical; 131 surgical). *Surgically assigned* patients consistently had a *longer total exercise treadmill duration*—roughly on the order of 1 minute—than medically assigned patients on their annual tests through 5 years ($p < 0.01$, years 1–3; $p \leq 0.05$, years 4 and 5). Negative exercise tests, i.e., those not meeting the standardly accepted criterion of 1.0 mm ST depression during or after exercise, were significantly more common in the surgical group at 1 year (76% vs. 55%, $p < 0.01$). Thereafter, the surgically assigned patients continued to have a ≥70% incidence of negative tests, while the incidence of the negative tests in the medically assigned patients increased. It must be kept in mind that the crossover from medical to surgical treatment was 28% at 1 year, 34% at 2 years, and 43% by 5 years. These data are reported by original treatment assignment, and surgical crossover and more frequent use of calcium channel blockers by the mid-1980s are potential explanations for the increase in negative exercise test results in medically assigned patients. Selection bias for exercise testing may also play a role since the patients most likely to perform an exercise test are those who are more active and

Table 7 Outcomes of Exercise Testing in VA Study of Unstable Angina

	YEAR				
	1	2	3	4	5
Total Exercise Duration (sec)					
M	326	363	371	392	378
S	394	430	431	452	427
"Negative" ETT(%)					
M	55	66	66	65	66
S	76*	75	74	72	70
Angina Stopping Test					
M	28%		26%		23%
S	12%*		17%		12%*

M = Patients randomized to medicine.
S = Patients randomized to surgery.
$^*p < 0.01$
Source: Ref. 11.

experiencing less symptoms. These considerations notwithstanding, surgically assigned patients had consistently less angina as the principal reason to stop their exercise test. At 5 years nearly twice as many medically assigned patients stopped exercising because of angina (23% vs. 12%, $p < 0.01$).

Nonfatal Myocardial Infarctions

Nonfatal myocardial infarctions occurred 78 times over the first 5 years of follow-up, for an overall incidence of 17% (3.5%/year). A total of 42 of these occurred in the medically assigned patients and 36 in the surgically assigned patients (NS) (Table 8). When evaluated in terms of prerandomization stratification, there were no significant differences in this outcome whether the patient had "progressive angina" (Type 1) or "prolonged, refractory rest pain" (Type 2) or had normal or abnormal left ventricular function (Table 8).

Work Status

The medically and surgically assigned patients did not have a different experience with regard to *working status*. Three months after surgery nearly half the patients reported working full or part time (48% medical, 44% surgical). By 2 years this had decreased to 22% in the medical group and 30% in the surgical group. By 5 years these figures were 20% and 28%, respectively. It must be kept in mind that the mean age at entry into the study was 56 years in each group (Table 4, q.v.).

Table 8 5-Year Cumulative Incidence of Nonfatal Myocardial Infarction in VA Study of Unstable Angina

	M			S			
	n	Myocardial infarction	%	*n*	Myocardial infarction	%	*p*
All patients	237	42	17.7	231	36	15.6	0.54
Type 1	190	35	18.4	184	26	14.1	0.26
Normal LV function	133	27	20.3	134	21	15.7	0.32
Abnormal LV function	57	8	14.0	50	5	10.0	0.52
Type 2	47	7	14.9	47	10	21.3	0.42
Normal LV function	36	4	11.1	31	5	16.1	0.55
Abnormal LV function	11	3	27.3	16	5	31.3	0.82
LV function							
Normal	169	31	18.3	165	26	15.8	0.53
Abnormal	68	11	16.2	66	10	15.2	0.87

Five additional medical patients and three additional surgical patients had a myocardial infarction between data of randomization and start of therapy.
Type 1 = "Progressive angina."
Type 2 = "Prolonged rest pain."
Source: Ref. 10.

Table 9 Cumulative Percentage of Crossovers from Medically Assigned Treatment to Surgery in VA Study of Unstable Angina

Month	Number at Beginning of Interval	Crossovers During Interval	Lost or Withdrawn During Interval	Cumulative Occurrence (%) at End of Interval
0–6	237	50	7	22
7–12	180	14	3	28
13–18	163	15	1	33
19–24	149	2	1	34
25–30	146	4	4	36
31–36	138	2	4	37
37–42	132	5	6	40
43–48	121	1	3	40
49–54	117	4	1	42
55–60	112	1	2	43

Source: Ref. 10.

Surgical Crossover

As in the NHLBI study, the cumulative *crossover* rate from medicine to surgery was substantial. Most of the crossover occurred in the first 6 months—during this interval 50 patients originally assigned to medicine had surgery (Table 9). The cumulative crossover rate increased from 28% at the end of year 1 to 43% at the end of year 5.

Recurrent Hospitalizations

The VA also tracked recurrent hospitalizations in their patients. In the first 6 months after assigned therapy there were 74 new hospitalizations in the medical cohort and 54 in the surgical group. In the remaining 54 months of the first 5 years of follow-up there were 101 hospitalizations in the medical group and 103 in the surgical group. When hospitalizations are considered solely for cardiac reasons (primarily recurrent angina) there was an important difference between the two treatments, most of which appeared in the first 6 months (Fig. 3). This difference coincides with the pattern of crossover from medicine to surgery in the medically assigned patients.

Survival

Overall survival of the medically and surgically assigned cohorts did not differ (Fig. 4). Nine deaths occurred at or within 30 days of surgery (operative mortality 4.1%). As can be seen from Figure 4, these were the only surgical

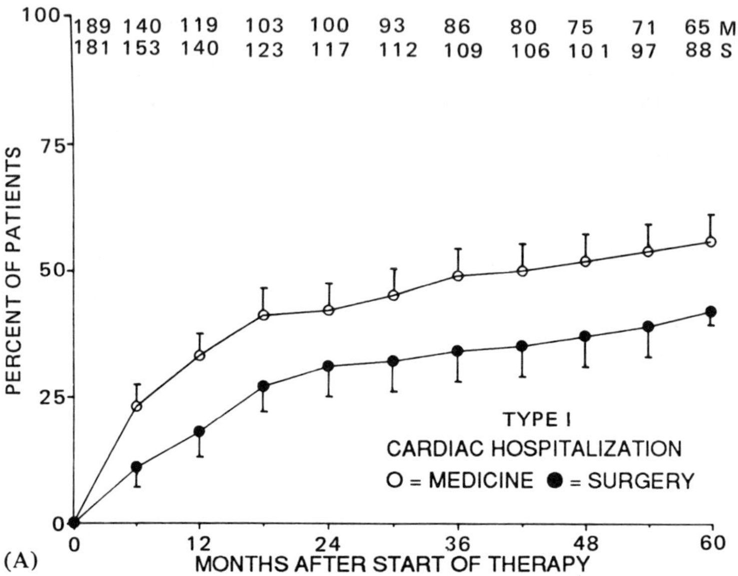

(A)

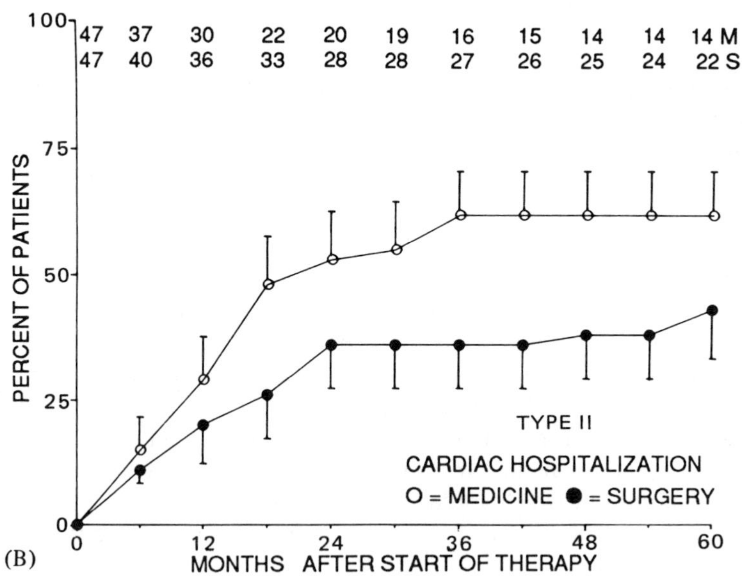

(B)

Figure 3 VA Trial of Unstable Angina Follow-up: (A) plot of cumulative rate of new hospitalizations for cardiac reasons for type 1 patient (with progressive angina); (B) plot of cumulative rate of new hospitalizations for cardiac reasons for type 2 patients (with prolonged rest pain). (From Ref. 10 with permission of the American Heart Association, Inc.)

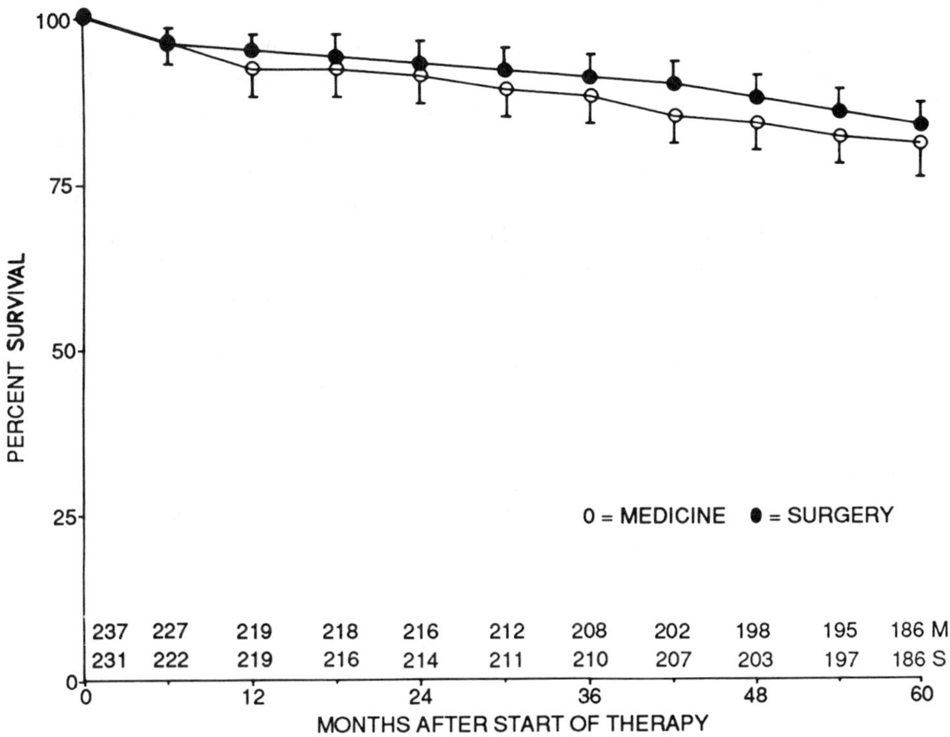

Figure 4 Survival in VA Trial of Unstable Angina: plot of overall survival of medical and surgical patients classified by treatment assigned. Vertical bars represent 1 SEM. Numbers of patients at risk in each time interval are listed above *x* axis. (From Ref. 10 with permission of the American Heart Association, Inc.)

deaths in the first 6 months after treatment assignment—by this time 10 medically assigned patients had succumbed. Survival did not differ statistically at 5 years using any of the prerandomization stratification criteria, i.e., Type 1 ("Progressive angina") vs. Type 2 ("Prolonged, refractory, rest pain") clinical presentation or normal vs. abnormal LV function.

Relationships Between Extent of Disease, Ventricular Function, and Survival

Because of the size of the study population and duration of follow-up, the VA study has been able to perform a number of analyses relating to long-term survival and angiographic measures of the severity of disease. The simplest and most striking of these evaluations relates to the number of diseased vessels determined on the baseline coronary angiogram (Fig. 5). Between 3 and 3½ years after treatment assignment, patients with three-vessel disease in the surgical group began to show a survival advantage that was not evident in patients with single- and double-vessel disease. This difference persisted to at least five years when the cumulative surgical mortality was 11% and the medical mortality was 29% ($p < 0.02$). If the combination of three-vessel disease and left ventricular dysfunction (as defined above) are used as patient characteristics, the cohorts under consideration became smaller ($n = 216$ for three-vessel disease; $n = 70$ for three-vessel disease and left ventricular dysfunction), but the survival advantage at 5 years for surgery increased. These latter subgroups had a 29% mortality when assigned to medical therapy and a 9% mortality when assigned to surgical therapy ($p < 0.05$).

Another evaluation which had an important relationship to 5-year survival

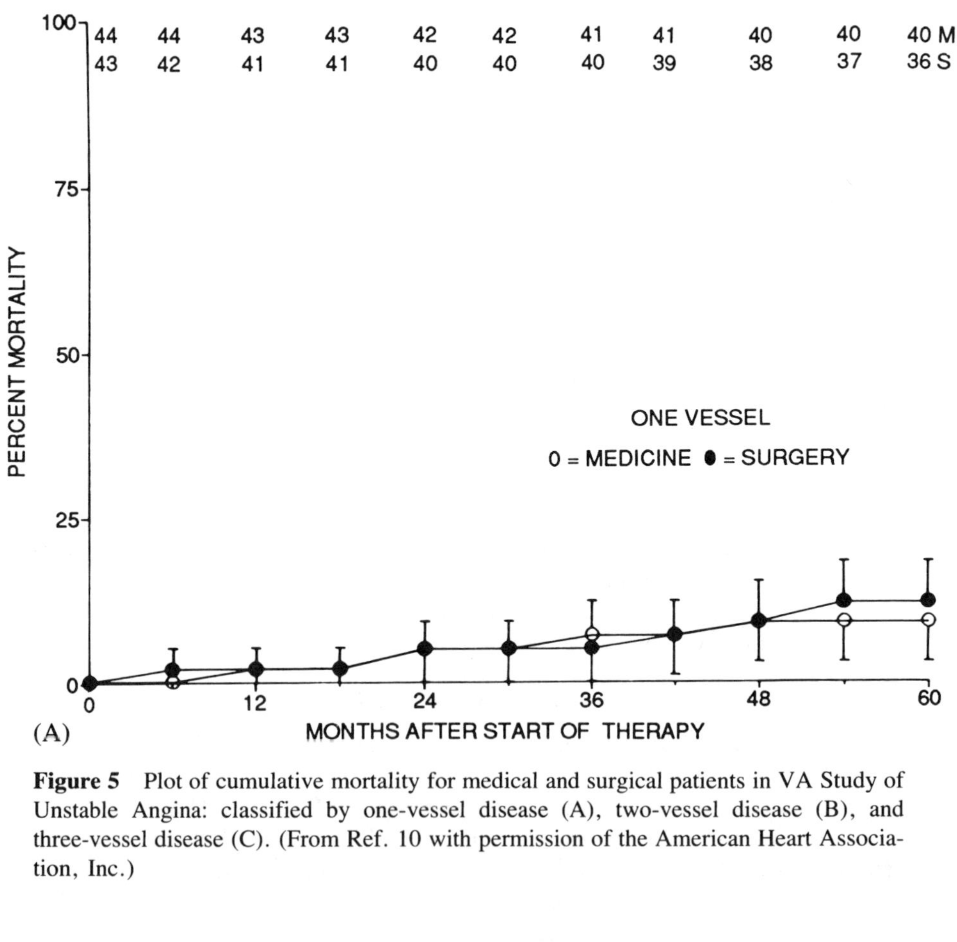

(A)

Figure 5 Plot of cumulative mortality for medical and surgical patients in VA Study of Unstable Angina: classified by one-vessel disease (A), two-vessel disease (B), and three-vessel disease (C). (From Ref. 10 with permission of the American Heart Association, Inc.)

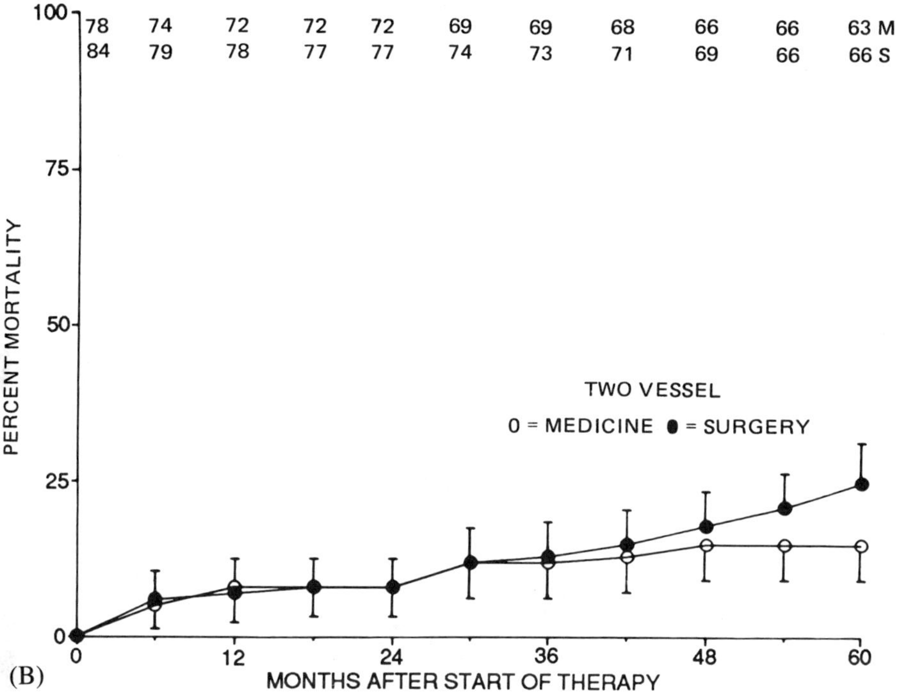

78 74 72 72 72 69 69 68 66 66 63 M
84 79 78 77 77 74 73 71 69 66 66 S
100
75
50
25
0
PERCENT MORTALITY
TWO VESSEL
0 = MEDICINE ● = SURGERY
0 12 24 36 48 60
MONTHS AFTER START OF THERAPY

(B)

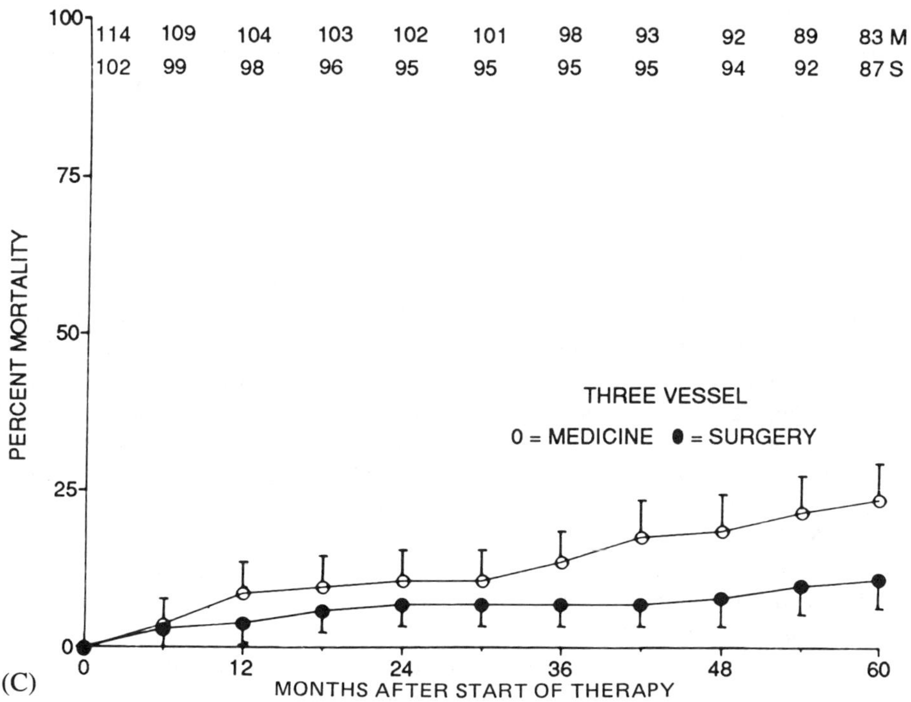

114 109 104 103 102 101 98 93 92 89 83 M
102 99 98 96 95 95 95 95 94 92 87 S
100
75
50
25
0
PERCENT MORTALITY
THREE VESSEL
0 = MEDICINE ● = SURGERY
0 12 24 36 48 60
MONTHS AFTER START OF THERAPY

(C)

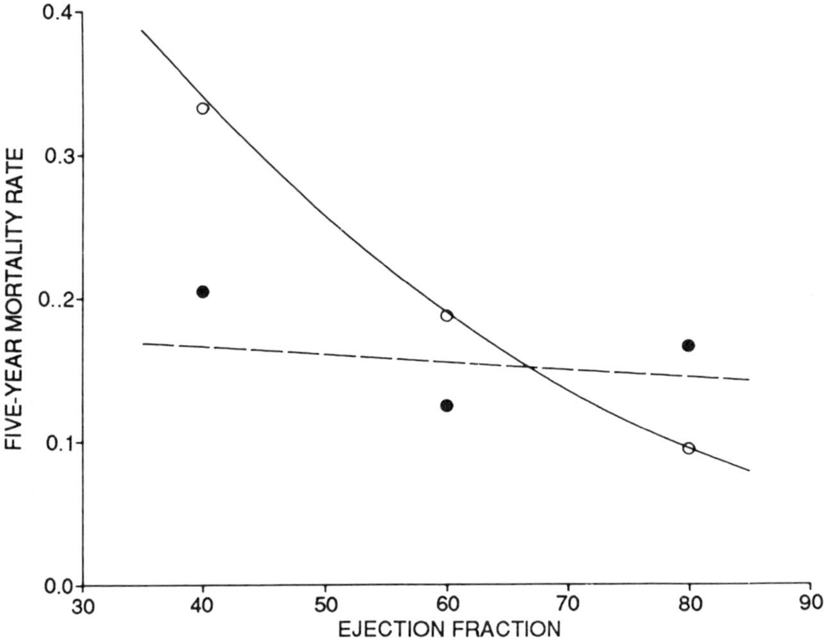

Figure 6 Plot of mortality for medical and surgical patients using ejection fraction as a continuous variable in the VA Study of Unstable Angina. Curves computed by logistic regression analysis based on 5-year mortality of medical and surgical patients by assigned treatment. For reference, points for mean observed percent mortality for medical patients (o) and surgical patients (●) are plotted for ejection fraction intervals 0.30–0.49, 0.50–0.69, and ≥0.70. (From Ref. 10 with permission of the American Heart Association, Inc.)

was left ventricular function as measured by ejection fraction. Probably because the majority of patients did not have prior myocardial infarctions the mean ejection fraction of all patients randomized was 63%, with only 18% of patients having an ejection fraction of less than 50%. If survival of the entire group of patients randomized was analyzed using *ejection fraction as a continuous variable,* important differences appeared in surgical and medical mortality (Fig. 6). The curves presented in Figure 6 are regression lines based on the survival of patients using their individual baseline ejection fractions. The mean observed percent mortality for ejection fraction ranges <50%, 50–70%, and >70% are shown for reference, but the regression curves are based on the overall data set for each assigned treatment.

Reduced ejection fraction had an important adverse influence on survival of medically assigned patients, and surgery improved the survival of patients with lower ejection fractions. This observation was substantiated by dividing the overall study population into terciles. Patients in the lowest ejection fraction tercile had a 5-year mortality of 27% when assigned to medical therapy but only a 14% mortality when assigned to surgical therapy ($p < 0.05$).

A Comparison of the VA and NHLBI Trials

It is useful in clinical trials of similar, or identical, problems to compare the study outcomes to ascertain the extent to which they are mutually supportive and to identify areas needing further clarification or investigation. Independent trials whose results concur make a considerably more compelling basis for establishing or changing behavior in clinical practice.

Before comparing outcomes, however, one must ask about the similarity of the protocols and of the patients randomized. Both studies enrolled patients with unstable angina. In each instance the chest pain syndrome was severe enough to warrant hospitalization. The VA study stratified its patients prior to randomization into those with an apparently less severe clinical presentation ("progressive angina", Type 1) versus those with a more severe clinical presentation (prolonged, refractory rest pain, Type 2). In addition, patients with normal and abnormal left ventricular function were differentiated. Similar patients would have been randomized in the NHLBI study. If randomization proceeds properly, the stratification process, or its absence, would not affect the overall outcome of either study. Prerandomization stratification is intended to eliminate subsequent bias in defining patient subgroups for later analyses. It also provides another line of assurance that randomization will be effective in certain segments of the prospective study population of high clinical interest. The protocols of these studies reveal that they were seeking nearly identical patients (Table 10). The VA study did not randomize women, but the basis for this was more pragmatic than scientific. Given this background it is not surprising that the outcomes of these two studies might have multiple similarities.

Baseline Characteristics

The baseline characteristics of the randomized patients in these studies were slightly different (Table 11). The VA patients were slightly older, with a more prevalent smoking history and diabetes. Consistent with this is a slightly greater prevalence of prior myocardial infarction and three-vessel disease. The NHLBI patients had a slightly greater prevalence of ejection fractions in the 30–49% range. None of these differences is very impressive. Furthermore, there is the agreement between survival outcomes at 1 and 2 years in the respective studies (Table 11). Each study showed that *overall* survival at 2 years was statistically indistinguishable between treatment groups. Most striking was the comparability of total overall survival in each study at 2 years—92% in the VA study and 91% in the NHLBI study.

Table 10 Comparison of the VA and NHLBI Trials of Unstable Angina

Protocol Requirements	NHLBI	VA
Clinical		
Symptoms requiring hospitalization	+	+
Most recent symptoms	[a]	<10 days
Age < 70	+	+
Male sex	0	+
No myocardial infarction < 3 mo	+	+
Acute myocardial infarction R/0	+	+
ECG changes during pain	+	+
Angiographic		
No left main disease	+	+
High grade coronary lesion	+	+
Ejection fraction ≥ 30%	+	+

[a]Recent enough to warrant coronary care unit admission.

Table 11 Clinical, Angiographic, and Survival Characteristics of Unstable Angina Patients in VA and NHLBI Trials

	VA		NHLBI	
	Medical	Surgical	Medical	Surgical
Age (yr)	56.3	55.7	52.7	53.0
Prior myocardial infarction	43%	42%	27%	35%
Smoking[a]	87%	93%	73%	75%
Diabetes	18%	16%	14%	10%
Mean blood pressure (S/D)	129/79	133/81	132/83	130/83
Vessel disease				
One	19%	19%	24%	24%
Two	33%	37%	37%	33%
Three	48%	44%	39%	43%
Ejection fraction 30–49%	19%	18%	23%	23%
Survival				
1 yr	92%	95%	93%	92%
2 yr	91%	93%	91%	90%

[a]At entry into the study in the medical group, 52.8% of the patients were current smokers, 34.6% had quit smoking, and 12.6% had never smoked; in the surgical group, 50% of the patients were current smokers, 42.5% had quit smoking, and 7.5% had never smoked.

S/D, systolic/diastolic; VA, Veterans Administration; NHLBI, National Heart, Lung, and Blood Institute.

Table 12 A Comparison of Late Clinical Outcomes in VA and NHLBI Trials of Unstable Angina

	NHLBI		VA	
	M	S	M	S
Nonfatal myocardial infarction	11%[a]	13%[a]	13.5%[b]	13.0%[b]
Crossover to surgery	31%[c]	—	34%[c]	—
Angina status				
3VD	21%[d]	20%[d]		
2VD	15%[d]	8%[d]	22.1%[e]	16.7%[e]
1VD	23%[d]	0%[d]		
Working status				
3VD	53%[f]	55%[f]	22%[g]	33%[g]
2VD	59%[f]	73%[f]		
1VD	73%[f]	67%[f]		

[a] These data are the incidence between initial hospitalization and 30 months.
[b] These data are the total cumulative incidence at 36 months.
[c] Crossover rate at 2 years.
[d] These data are angina Class III or IV at 24 months.
[e] Overall NYHA Class III or IV at 36 months.
[f] Work status at 24 months—baseline % working not defined.
[g] Work status at 24 months—38% medical and 46% surgical working at entry.

Nonfatal Myocardial Infarction

Comparison of data for nonfatal myocardial infarctions, angina, and working status are more difficult because of different methods of reporting between studies (Table 12). Nevertheless, based on observations from 2 to 3 years after randomization, there is a certain commonality of outcome. The incidence of late nonfatal myocardial infarction did not differ between medical and surgical assignment in either study and was nearly identical—12% in the NHLBI study and 13% in the VA study. Crossover rates to surgery in both studies were substantial and comparable at 24 months—31% in the NHLBI study and 34% in the VA study.

Severe Angina

In both studies the overall incidence of high grade angina (Class III–IV) was less than 25%, occurring less frequently in patients assigned to surgical therapy. However, the angina grade needs to be interpreted in the light of a high rate of crossover in the same time period. As indicated previously the NHLBI study showed a marked fall in high grade angina in medically assigned patients with multivessel disease between year 1 and year 2 after randomization (see Fig. 1). A similar pattern was observed in the VA study (Table 13). There is a noteworthy

Table 13 Occurrence of Angina NYHA Class III or IV in VA Study Follow-up

	M(%)	S(%)
1 yr	26	16
3 yr	22	19
5 yr	18	17

M = Patients randomized to medical therapy.
S = Patients randomized to surgical therapy.

decline in NYHA Class III or IV symptoms in medically assigned patients which was nearly equivalent to surgically assigned patients at 5 years. This outcome contrasts with the greater number of angina-free patients in those originally assigned to surgery (see Table 6) and like the NHLBI study implies that the more severely symptomatic medically assigned patients are those who later "cross over" to receive surgical treatment.

Work Status

Neither study showed that initial surgical assignment produced an advantage with regard to later work status. The VA population had fewer patients in its treatment groups working at 2 years than the NHLBI study, but less than 50% of the VA patients were working at baseline. Very likely many VA patients sought care at VA facilities because of its far greater accessibility to the unemployed. Since the average age of the VA patients was 56 at entry, it is also likely that those employed at baseline sought early retirement.

As far as one can ascertain from the 2- to 3-year follow-up of these independent trials, their results are concordant and represent a consensus for "state-of-the-art" medical and surgical therapy of unstable angina at the time of patient assignment to the respective treatment regimens.

OUTCOMES OF OTHER RANDOMIZED TRIALS

A few small randomized trials of medical versus surgical therapy based at individual medical centers were conducted in the 1970s. Although both surgical and medical treatment have advanced importantly over the intervening years, these studies are still of considerable historic interest. They not only indicated that randomized trials of medical versus surgical therapy were possible but also provided early insights into the short-term outcomes of these respective treatments.

In 1975 Selden and coworkers (12) reported the outcomes of 40 patients randomized during the preceding 3 years. By 4 months there were no deaths and two myocardial infarctions in 19 medically assigned patients and one death and three myocardial infarctions in 21 surgically treated patients. Of the 20 surgical survivors 19 were symptomatically Class 1–2 as compared to 7 of the 19 medical patients. In addition the surgical patients achieved a higher double product, higher workload, and experienced less angina during bicycle exercise testing. These observations were verified at subsequent catheterization. The revascularized patients had a higher angina threshold with atrial pacing and better myocardial extraction of lactate at their maximum-paced heart rates. At this time the surgical patients had a graft patency rate of 82%.

In 1978 Pugh et al. (13) reported on 27 randomized patients (14 medical, 13 surgical) at a mean follow-up of 18 months. There was one death in each group. Again surgically revascularized patients had superior symptom relief—7/12 survivors were pain-free and none had "severe" angina; by comparison 1/13 medical patients were pain free and 5/13 had severe angina.

In 1981 Brown et al. (14) presented 4-year follow-up data on the 83 patients randomized at Massachusetts General Hospital into the National Unstable Angina Pectoris Study. Late severe angina (NYHA Class III or IV) occurred in 28% of the medically treated patients and in 9% of the revascularized patients. In addition 23% of the medical patients underwent late elective CABG for relief of persistent angina.

Taken collectively these reports, two of which were forerunners of the national cooperative trials, showed that surgery offered superior symptom relief to patients with unstable angina and no survival disadvantage. Revascularization, as an urgent procedure, to promote survival in the ordinary patient with unstable angina did not seem indicated.

OUTCOMES OF NONRANDOMIZED AND SURGICAL SERIES

An overview of reports from surgical series over the past two decades is presented (Table 14). Patient selection criteria for various reported surgical series in the literature are not identical. This stems in part from the different feelings that physicians and surgeons have about what represents unstable angina. In addition, many of the surgical series have mixed patient populations with drug-*refractory* unstable angina patients reported along with patients who have drug-*responsive* unstable angina. Furthermore, some series also report patients who have had a myocardial infarction within the 30 days previous to surgery, i.e., postinfarction unstable angina. Such patients were excluded from the NIH and VA randomized trials of unstable angina.

Age

Many of these surgical series consist of patients who have been operated on with a mean age in the mid-50s. In the 1990s one would expect a mortality for surgical treatment of unstable angina of $< 5\%$. Of the studies reported after 1980, those

Table 14 Treatment of Unstable Angina: Nonrandomized Series

Authors	Year	Surgical Period	# Patients S/M	Age	# of Grafts	% Mortality S/M	% MI (peri-op)	Long-term F/U/Other Comments
Scanlon et al. (15)	1973	1970–72	48/82	30–70 (53)	1.2	12.5/27	25	None/
Wiles et al. (16)	1977	1974–75	124c/-	37–76 (55)	2.0	48%/-		None/
Golding et al. (17)	1978	1970–76	100c/-	36–72 (55)		4%		72/92 symptom free at 42 mo; postop graft patency—86% at 14 mo
Olinger et al. (18)	1978	1975–77	95c/-	34–76 (57) 38–74 (55)	2.5 2.6	1%	3	None/
Brawley et al. (19)	1980	1978–79	130/-	32–78 (57)	3.2	7.7%	8%	None/
Jones et al. (20)	1982	1974–80	78/	(57)	2.6	1.2%	3.8	
Hultgren et al. (21)	1984	1970–77	104/124	58M/55S	2.2	2%	13	7-yr survival—65%M; 85%S 5-yr angina free—62%S; 37%M

Rankin et al. (22)	1984	1981–82	100/-	33–79 (57)	3.6	4%—1 4%—2		Refractory unstable angina patients (100/531) 52 with postinfarct (group 2) 2-yr survival group 1 = 90%, group 2 = 88%
Rahimtoola (23)	1983	1970–82	1282/-	(57)		1.8%		5-yr survival—92% 10-yr survival—83%
Cobanoglu (24)	1984	1974–82	1163/-			1.7%		5-yr survival—92% 8-yr survival—89%
Naunheim (25)	1989	1985–87	129/-	36–86 (63)	3.3	6.2%	9	None
Huttunen (26)	1989	1983–87	100/-	30–66 (54)	4.6	1%	7	None

S/M = Patients receiving surgical or medical therapy respectively.
F/U = Follow-up.
c = Consecutive.

with mortalities of >5% had special extenuating circumstances applying to their patient groups. The most important of these is age. Brawley et al. (19) emphasizes the importance of age on surgical outcome in their 1980 paper. Of their 130 patients 12 were more than 70 years old. They experienced a surgical mortality of 33%. The only other surgical series reported since this time with a mortality in excess of 5% was that of Naunheim in 1989, where the mortality was 6%. The age profile in this series indicates that 29% of their patients were over 70 years of age, and this became a very important factor in survival. In this latter study there were eight operative deaths in 129 operated patients—the mean age was 63 in survivors and 71 in nonsurvivors. This study also reported that increased duration of cross-clamp time and cardiopulmonary bypass time were both significantly related to survival.

Perioperative Myocardial Infarction

Most of the surgical series indicate that perioperative myocardial infarction can be expected to occur in <10% of cases. Obviously the diligence with which perioperative myocardial infarction is sought will affect its reported incidence. Most series (and all those listed in Table 14) sought infarction by the postoperative appearance of new Q waves. More sensitive criteria of enzyme rises beyond the expected for uncomplicated surgery will lead to a higher incidence of possible infarction.

Only a few of these series have had concurrent medically treated patients as a reference group. In the series of Hultgren et al. (21) the angina-free rate was 62% at 5 years for surgically treated patients as compared to 37% for the medically treated patients. In addition, there was an 85% 7-year survival in their surgically treated patients compared to a 65% survival in the concurrently treated medical reference group. Similarly Rahimtoola et al. (23) in a very large series reported a 5-year survival in surgically treated patients of 92% and a 10-year survival of 83%.

Completeness of Revascularization

Overall assessment of surgical series during the past two decades indicates that a progressive emphasis has been placed on completeness of myocardial revascularization. The number of vessels bypassed per patient has increased substantially since the earliest reported series. This trend has been enhanced more recently by the culling of patients who have less than multivessel disease for initial treatment with angioplasty. Thus, in the present era older patients with complex, multivessel disease form a greater proportion of surgically treated patients who usually receive multiple coronary artery grafts.

The very early report of Scanlon et al. (15) appeared in the learning phases of patient selection and surgical technique. A number of these patients were probably inadequately revascularized as indicated by the average number of grafts of

1.2 per patient. Twelve of their patients had the long outmoded placement of internal mammary implants. The mortality of patients who had suffered recent myocardial infarctions was more than twice (22%) that of patients who did not have a recent myocardial infarction (10%).

Patient Selection

Wiles et al. (16) reported a consecutive series of 124 patients and demonstrated that surgical mortality in properly selected patients with unstable angina could be reduced to <5%. They emphasized risk factors associated with mortality and concluded that failure to respond to in-hospital maximum medical therapy, three-vessel disease, and hypertension were important factors in determining an immediate adverse outcome. However, as time has progressed subsequent studies have demonstrated that improved surgical skills and adjunctive measures have changed this perspective.

Golding et al. (17) also demonstrated that mortality in the early 1970s for patients who had emergency revascularization for unstable angina (selected as defined by the NIH National Cooperative Study Group) could be achieved at a rate of <5%. Of four operative deaths, three were demonstrated at post-mortem examination to have an unrecognized recent myocardial infarction. In this series the postoperative graft patency rate at 14 months was 86%, and long-term follow-up indicated that 72 of 92 survivors were free of symptoms at 42 months.

In 1978 Olinger et al. (18) had only one surgical death and a 3% incidence of perioperative infarction in a consecutive series of 95 patients (53 of whom had continuing angina despite propranolol therapy). What is not defined in this series is the larger population of patients with unstable angina who may not have been offered an operation. Therefore, comparison of these excellent results to other series with a worse surgical mortality is not possible. The report of Brawley et al. (19) gives a better perspective on preoperative surgical risk factors. One hundred and thirty of 471 patients undergoing the coronary bypass operation at the Johns Hopkins Medical Center had unstable angina. There was an 8% mortality in the patients with unstable angina compared to a 2% mortality in patients having surgery for chronic stable angina. Age greater than 70 years, poor left ventricular function, and distal coronary arteries unfavorable for grafting as well as the presence of left main disease all adversely influenced mortality. In 78 patients with unstable angina who had none of these risk factors the mortality was 1.3%. When elderly patients and patients with poor left ventricular function or poor distal vessels were excluded the operative mortality rate associated with coronary bypass in patients with unstable angina was 2% (2 of 101).

Jones et al. (20) selected a series of 78 patients who had prolonged (>20 minutes) chest pain with concurrent electrocardiographic changes as their group to compare with the National Cooperative Study Group patients of unstable angina. Myocardial infarction had been ruled out. This report also demonstrated that surgery can be performed in patients with unstable angina with a low mortality (1.2%) and low incidence of perioperative myocardial infarction (3.8%).

Hultgren et al.'s (21) study is of value since it reports a concurrent medically treated reference group. In the 7-year period between 1970 and 1977, 104 patients were treated surgically and 124 were treated medically. Their approach to the unstable angina patient required a 5-day hospital observation period for entry. Patients who died of an acute myocardial infarction or who had complications which would be a contraindication to surgical treatment during this period were excluded. A 5-day observation period will have the impact of lowering mortality both in medical as well as surgically treated patients. The reason why some patients were selected for surgery and others for medicine in this study is not defined. The implication is that it was a random process since the patients who had medicine or surgery had similar baseline clinical characteristics, electrocardiographic changes, lower performance, mean ejection fractions, extent of disease at cardiac catheterization. However, only 65% of the medical patients in this series had arteriography. At 5 years they experienced an identical mortality rate to those that did have arteriography (39% vs. 43%). This study demonstrated a superior degree of angina relief in the patients who had surgery and a better 5-year survival. There was, however, a high early incidence of perioperative infarction which in the 5-year period immediately preceding their report had been reduced to 3%.

The report of Rankin et al. (22) focused on *a subset of patients with unstable angina*. Of the 531 patients who were admitted with unstable angina to the Duke Coronary Care Unit in the one-year period from June 1981 to September 1982, 100 had *persistent angina* despite optimal medical therapy which included beta-blockade, nitrates, and nifedipine. This group of 100 patients was subdivided into those without evidence of myocardial infarction in the 30 days prior to catheterization (Group 1, $n = 48$) and those with evidence of myocardial infarction (Group 2, $n = 52$). These patients were all operated on irrespective of ventricular function, hemodynamic status, or coronary anatomy and received an average of 3.6 grafts per patient. Two hospital deaths occurred in each of the groups (4%). In follow-up there was a 90% survival in Group 1 and 88% in Group 2, and 81% of the surviving patients had NYHA Class 1 or 2 symptoms. Anticoagulation with heparin and intra-aortic balloon pumping placed percutaneously were employed liberally in the patients who had the most refractory syndromes. This study suggests that with appropriate patient selection and preoperative preparation, excellent results can be achieved with regard to surgical mortality in even persistently symptomatic patients who have had recent myocardial infarction. What is not clear from the report, however, is whether any patients were refused surgery during this same time period.

The largest surgical series in the literature comes from the University of Oregon, having been reported by Rahimtoola et al. in 1983 and again from a surgical perspective by Cobanoglu in 1984 (23, 24). The Oregon experience confirms that a surgical mortality of about 2% should be a usual expectation. In this series the 5-year survival exceeded 92% and the 10-year survival was 83%.

In 1989 Naunheim et al. (25) reported a series of patients with unstable angina again representing a *subset*. This included those patients who required intravenous nitroglycerin preoperatively in the hospital. Since there was no algorithm defining what steps would be required prior to the administration of intravenous nitroglycerin, it is not absolutely clear that all patients absolutely required this therapy. Patients were excluded if they had ongoing ischemia as a result of failed PTCA, postinfarction angina (within 30 days), and cardiogenic shock or hemodynamic instability. The overall mortality in this study was 6.2%. The age range in the report is among the widest in the literature. The mean age was 63 and the oldest patient was 86 years of age. These authors also emphasized aortic cross-clamp time and cardiopulmonary bypass time as critical factors that were related to operative death.

Another report by Huttunen (26) appeared in the Scandinavian literature in 1989. One hundred patients had *postinfarction unstable angina*. The patients all had refractory unstable angina despite maximum medication; all demonstrated ECG changes. Operation of 100 patients was gleaned from 111 patients with refractory unstable angina undergoing coronary arteriography during the reported study period. Of the 11 unoperated patients, 1 died before surgery, 6 had insignificant or no coronary artery stenoses, and 2 were judged to be inoperable, 1 had a successful PTCA, and 1 patient with a single-vessel disease in a marginal branch was managed medically. Thirty-five of the 100 patients had postinfarct angina. This paper also relates a very low surgical mortality (1%) again indicating that with careful patient selection and completeness of revascularization, excellent survival results can be achieved even when symptoms persist on a maximum medical regimen.

From the foregoing one may conclude that many medical centers have worked out algorithms for approaching patients with unstable angina. These approaches will vary from center to center. Nevertheless, important generalizations apply. For the most part an initial period of observation and intensive medical therapy is used. When necessary, percutaneous intra-aortic balloon counterpulsation is used to stabilize patients. Patients who have postinfarction angina are either not operated or are treated as a separate subgroup when considering both surgical mortality and other outcomes. The severity of the clinical syndrome particularly in the absence of myocardial infarction does *not* have an adverse impact on the long-term surgical mortality or long-term symptomatic outcome.

SURGERY FOR POSTINFARCTION UNSTABLE ANGINA

Several recent reports have culled out patients with postinfarction angina from the overall population who meet the definition of unstable angina. These patients differ from those entered into each of the major national randomized trials since postinfarction angina was an exclusion criterion.

Jones et al. (27) reported on 107 consecutive patients operated in 1983 and 1984 for postinfarction angina. These were subdivided into 38 who underwent CABG 7 days or less after infarction, 25 between 8 and 15 days, and 44 between 16 and 30 days (Groups 1, 2, and 3, respectively). Of the 9 inhospital deaths, 4 occurred in Group 1, 2 occurred in Group 2, and 3 in Group 3. They concluded that death was more likely to occur when coronary bypass was done within 7 days of acute myocardial infarction. The authors indicated that the mortality was acceptable given the clinical conditions of their patients. When shock developed after acute myocardial infarction there was an unacceptable outcome if CABG was done within 7 days even in patients who were stabilized.

Stuart et al. (28) conducted an analysis of risk factors associated with perioperative mortality in patients with unstable postinfarction angina. They focused on 225 patients who had urgent CABG between the years 1982 and 1986. The mean age was 62 years with a range of 35–87, and the operative mortality was 5.3%. Of the single independent predictors of perioperative mortality, the presence of transmural anterior infarction, need for preoperative intra-aortic balloon pumping, or the presence of preoperative congestive heart failure were all associated with adverse outcomes. The perioperative deaths (n = 12) occurred in the subset of patients with anterior myocardial infarction, intra-aortic balloon pumping, or both. Survival was 92% at 1 year, 91% at 2 years, 88% at 3 years and at 4 years, respectively. Ninety-six percent of the survivors had Class 1 or 2 angina only. They emphasized that while acceptable mortality could be achieved, surgery is done with increased risk in patients with preoperative transmural anterior infarction, intra-aortic balloon pumping, or both.

SUMMARY AND CONCLUSIONS

The patient's clinical status, extent of coronary disease, and left ventricular function are the key elements in the process of deciding whether or not to recommend surgery for unstable angina.

The clinical factors that influence immediate outcome favorably are age—particularly a young physiologic age—and absence of other important prognosis limiting systemic disease or organ dysfunction. Persistent or ongoing symptoms of unstable angina (whether or not in the postinfarction setting) are not contraindications to surgery and do not necessarily denote an adverse prognosis for surgically treated patients. Indeed, a revascularization procedure—provided it is technically feasible—is the means of choice for managing drug-resistant unstable angina syndrome.

For patients with drug-responsive unstable angina and adequate ventricular function (ejection fraction > 30%) surgery should be performed if the patient has a significant left main coronary artery stenosis. Revascularization surgery also offers a 5-year survival advantage when used as initial therapy in patients with three-vessel disease. The combination of three-vessel disease and left ventricular dysfunction is an even more compelling reason for operation. These statements are made with the understanding that the distal vessels are adequate for revascularization. If there is less than three-vessel disease, superior symptom relief is more likely following revascularization surgery.

Severe left ventricular dysfunction (ejection fraction < 30%) is not a contraindication to surgery, but the expectations for patients in this category are less well defined. Surgical mortality will most likely exceed 2% if there is a recent large (usually anterior) myocardial infarction and/or accompanying hemodynamic instability.

Surgery is at present the standard and preferred means of revasularizing patients with drug-resistant, refractory, or recurrent unstable angina. In addition, a survival advantage out to at least 5 years after surgical therapy accrues to those unstable angina patients who have angiographically proven three-vessel disease irrespective of their response to medical therapy. These data have been obtained using coronary bypass grafts; the present-day use of internal mammary artery grafts would likely increase these expectations. Until other means are proven to achieve the same ends in well-conducted trials, surgical revascularization will remain an important therapeutic consideration for every patient who presents with unstable angina.

ACKNOWLEDGMENT

The author expresses his gratitude to Elaine Palumbo for her excellent assistance and typing.

REFERENCES

1. Takaro T, Hultgren HN, Lipton MJ, Detre KM. The VA Cooperative Randomized Study of Surgery for Coronary Arterial Occlusive Disease. II. Subgroup with significant left main lesions—cardiovascular surgery 1975. Circulation 1976; 54 (suppl 3):107–17.
2. The Veterans Administration Coronary Artery Bypass Surgery Cooperative Study Group. Eleven-year survival in the Veterans Administration Randomized Trial of Coronary Bypass Surgery for Stable Angina. N Engl J Med 1985; 311:1333–9.

3. European Coronary Surgery Study Group. Prospective randomised study of coronary artery bypass surgery in stable angina pectoris. Lancet 1980; 2:491–5.
4. CASS Principal Investigators and Their Associates. Coronary Artery Surgery Study (CASS): A randomized trial of coronary artery bypass surgery. Survival data. Circulation 1983; 68:939–50.
5. Unstable angina pectoris: National Cooperative Study Group to Compare Medical and Surgical Therapy. I. Report of protocol and patient population. Am J Cardiol 1976; 37:896–902.
6. Unstable angina pectoris: National Cooperative Study Group to Compare Surgical and Medical Therapy. II. In-hospital experience and initial follow-up results in patients with one, two and three vessel disease. Am J Cardiol 1978; 42:839–48.
7. Unstable angina pectoris: National Cooperative Study Group to Compare Surgical and Medical Therapy. III. Results in patients with S-T segment elevation during pain. Am J Cardiol 1980; 45:819–24.
8. Luchi RJ, Scott SM, Deupree RH, Principal Investigators and Their Associates of Veterans Administration Cooperative Study No. 28. N Engl J Med 1987; 316:977–84.
9. Scott SM, Luchi RJ, Deupree RH, Veterans Administration Unstable Angina Cooperative Study Group. Veterans Administration Cooperative Study for Treatment of Patients with Unstable Angina. Results in patients with abnormal left ventricular function. Circulation 1988; 78(suppl I):113–21.
10. Parisi AF, Khuri S, Deupree RH, Sharma GVRK, Scott SM, Luchi RJ. Medical compared with surgical management of unstable angina. 5-year mortality and morbidity in the veterans administration study. Circulation 1989; 80:1176–89.
11. Booth DC, Deupree RH, Scott SM, Luchi RJ. Quality of life after bypass surgery for unstable angina. Five year follow-up results of a VA Cooperative Study. Circulation, 1991; 83.
12. Selden R, Neill WA, Ritzmann LW, Okies JE, Anderson RP. Medical versus surgical therapy for acute coronary insufficiency. A randomized study. N Engl J Med 1975; 293:1329–33.
13. Pugh B, Platt MR, Mills LJ, Crumbo D, Poliner LR, Curry GC, Blomqvist GC, Parkey RW, Buja LM, Willerson JT. Unstable angina pectoris: A randomized study of patients treated medically and surgically. Am J Cardiol 1978; 41:1291–8.
14. Brown CA, Hutter AM, DeSanctis RW, Gold HK, Leinbach RC, Roberts-Niles A, Austen WG, Buckley MJ. Prospective study of medical and urgent surgical therapy in randomizable patients with unstable angina pectoris: Results of in-hospital and chronic mortality and morbidity. Am Heart J 1981; 102:959–64.
15. Scanlon PJ, Nemickas R, Moran JF, Talano JV, Amirparviz F, Pifarre R. Accelerated angina pectoris. Clinical, hemodynamic, arteriographic and therapeutic experience in 85 patients. Circulation 1973; 47:19–26.
16. Wiles JC, Peduzzi PN, Hammond GL, Cohen LS, Langou RA. Preoperative predictors of operative mortality for coronary bypass grafting in patients with unstable angina pectoris. Am J Cardiol 1977; 39:939–43.
17. Golding LAR, Loop FD, Sheldon WC, Taylor PC, Groves LK, Cosgrove DM. Emergency revascularization for unstable angina. Circulation 1978; 58:1163–6.

18. Olinger GN, Bonchek LI, Keelan MH, Tresch DD, Siegel R, Bamrah V, Tristani FE. Unstable angina: the case for operation. Am J Cardiol 1978; 42:634–40.
19. Brawley RK, Merrill W, Gott VL, Donahoo JS, Watkins L Jr., Gardner TJ. Unstable angina pectoris. Factors influencing operative risk. Ann Surg 1980; 191:745–50.
20. Jones EL, Waites TF, Craver JM, Bone DK, Hatcher CR Jr, Thompkins T. Unstable angina pectoris: comparison with the National Cooperative Study. Ann Thorac Surg 1982; 34:427–34
21. Hultgren HN, Shettigar UR, Miller DC. Medical versus surgical treatment of unstable angina. Am J Cardiol 1982; 50:663–70.
22. Rankin JS, Newton JR Jr, Califf RM, Jones RH, Wechsler AS, Oldham HN Jr, Wolfe WG, Lowe JE. Clinical characteristics and current management of medically refractory unstable angina. Ann Surg 1984; 200:457–65.
23. Rahimtoola SH, Nunley D, Grunkemeier G, Tepley J, Lambert L, Starr A. Ten-year survival after coronary bypass surgery for unstable angina. N Engl J Med 1983; 308:676–81.
24. Cobanoglu A, Freimanis I, Grunkemeier G, Lambert L, Anderson V, Nunley D, Garcia C, Starr A. Enhanced late survival following coronary artery bypass graft operation for unstable versus chronic angina. Ann Thorac Surg 1984; 37:52–9.
25. Naunheim KS, Fiore AC, Arango DC, Pennington DG, Barner HB, McBride LR, Harris HH, Willman VL, Kaiser GC. Coronary artery bypass grafting for unstable angina pectoris: risk analysis. Ann Thorac Surg 1989; 47:569–74.
26. Huttunen K, Rehnberg S, Huttunen H, Soimakallio S, Suhonen M, Helin M. Clinical characteristics and coronary anatomy in refractory unstable angina pectoris leading to coronary artery bypass grafting. Scand J Thor Cardiovasc Surg 1989; 23:19–23.
27. Jones RN, Pifarre R, Sullivan HJ, Montoya A, Bakhos M, Grieco JG, Foy BK, Wyatt J. Early myocardial revascularization for postinfarction angina. Ann Thorac Surg 1987; 44:159–63.
28. Stuart RS, Baumgartner WA, Soule L, Borkon AM, Gardner TJ, Gott VL, Watkins L Jr, Reitz BA. Predictors of perioperative mortality in patients with unstable postinfarction angina. Circulation 1988, (suppl I):163–5.

14

Pros and Cons of Revascularization Versus a Conservative Approach

Joseph G. Murphy and Bernard J. Gersh

Mayo Clinic and Mayo Foundation
Rochester, Minnesota

INTRODUCTION

Unstable angina pectoris is not a uniform clinical entity, rather it encompasses several pathophysiologic syndromes considered intermediate between chronic stable angina and myocardial infarction. Implied in the term "unstable" is the concept of a recent change in the severity, character, or precipitating factors in a patient with previously stable angina or new-onset angina. The correct recognition and classification of unstable angina are important public health problems, because of both the frequency of its occurrence (750,000 hospitalizations annually in the United States) and the observation that up to 57% of patients with unstable angina undergo percutaneous transluminal coronary angioplasty (PTCA) or coronary artery bypass grafting (CABG) within a year of presentation (1–3). Among patients hospitalized with unstable angina, the condition may herald the onset of myocardial infarction in up to 10%.

There are no published randomized trials comparing PTCA with medical therapy in unstable angina, and there is a relative paucity of randomized trial data comparing CABG with medical therapy. Consequently, the decision to use coronary revascularization in unstable angina must to a considerable extent be extrapolated from studies in patients with chronic stable angina.

This chapter outlines our approach to revascularization versus conservative management of the patient with unstable angina based on the results of the three randomized trials of surgical revascularization versus medical management of unstable angina and on extrapolation from the randomized trials of operation in patients with chronic stable angina.

In this context, the major lessons from the randomized trials of CABG versus medical therapy in chronic stable angina emphasize that the "sicker" the patient—based on the severity of the angina or ischemia, the number of diseased epicardial vessels, and the extent of left ventricular dysfunction—*the greater the benefit of revascularization versus medical therapy*. Stratification of patients into categories of risk using these factors provides a logical basis to identify subgroups likely to benefit most from a conservative or a more aggressive strategy.

CLASSIFICATION OF UNSTABLE ANGINA

Braunwald (4) suggested a classification of unstable angina on which a logical basis for treatment and prognosis may be developed (Table 1). This chapter addresses the relative merits of conservative therapy versus revascularization utilizing this framework. This classification has two gradations of the severity of unstable angina (II, III), based on the presence and duration of rest pain, and a third category (I) for progressive angina without rest pain. There are two classes

Table 1 Classification of Unstable Angina

	A. Angina develops in presence of extracardiac condition that intensifies myocardial ischemia (secondary UA)	B. Angina develops in absence of extracardiac condition (primary UA)	C. Angina develops within 2 weeks after AMI (postinfarct UA)
I. New onset of severe angina or accelerated angina; no rest pain	IA	IB	IC
II. Angina at rest within past month but not within past 48 hours	IIA	IIB	IIC
III. Angina at rest within past 48 hours	IIIA	IIIB	IIIC

Abbreviations: AMI, acute myocardial infarction; UA, unstable angina.
Source: Ref. 4 by permission of the American Heart Association.

of unstable angina (A,B) based on the presence or absence of an extracardiac condition that intensifies myocardial ischemia. There is a third class (C) for angina after myocardial infarction. Thus, this classification has a total of nine subgroups. The severity gradings are as follows:

I: New onset of severe angina or accelerated angina but no rest pain
II: Angina at rest within the past month but not within the past 48 hours
III: Angina at rest within the past 48 hours

The clinical classes are the following:

A: Angina develops in the presence of extracardiac conditions that intensify myocardial ischemia
B: Angina develops in the absence of an extracardiac condition
C: Angina develops within 2 weeks after an acute myocardial infarction

Other classification schemes of unstable angina have also been suggested based on the presence or absence of electrocardiographic changes and the level of antianginal medication needed to suppress symptoms.

NATURAL HISTORY OF UNSTABLE ANGINA

The natural history of unstable angina pectoris in the current era is difficult to assess because of two factors: the diversity of pathophysiologic mechanisms responsible for the same clinical features in different patients and the fact that a therapeutic intervention of some type is used in nearly all cases. One, therefore, has to go back almost 20 years before the era of coronary revascularization for information on the "natural" history of unstable angina; this information demonstrates clearly that affected patients are at increased risk of myocardial infarction and sudden death. In 1973, Gazes et al. (5) reported on the mortality in 140 patients with unstable angina who were followed for 10 years before the advent of PTCA and CABG. The 1-, 5-, and 10-year mortality rates were 18%, 39%, and 52%, respectively. In 1985, Mulcahy et al. (6) reported the natural history of unstable angina managed conservatively without PTCA or CABG. The 1-year cardiac mortality was 8–10%, and the 1-year nonfatal infarction rate was 12–14%.

Three presentations at the 1990 American Heart Association Annual Scientific Sessions (1–3) emphasized the current high rate of myocardial infarction and revascularization during the first year after development of unstable angina. Karlsson and Wallentin (1) reported a mortality rate of 2.2%, myocardial infarction rate of 9.6%, and revascularization rate of 56.3% at 1 month follow-up in 135 patients with unstable angina treated with recombinant tissue plasminogen activator. Cohen et al. (2) reported a 3-month myocardial infarction rate of 5% and a revascularization rate of 53% in the nonaspirin arm of a retrospective study of the effect of prior regular aspirin usage in patients with rest angina. Pérez Villa et al. (3) reported a 1-year death rate of 7%, myocardial infarction rate of 32%, and a revascularization rate of 57% in the placebo arm of a randomized trial of thrombolytic agents in unstable angina.

Several generalizations can be made, however, regarding the natural history of currently managed unstable angina pectoris based on the Braunwald classification outlined above (Table 1). Patients with progressive angina without rest pain appear to have a relatively benign acute course and in general manifest a good response to pharmacologic intervention aimed at decreasing recurrent ischemia or preventing progression to myocardial infarction.

Patients with angina at rest in association with ST-segment or T-wave changes on a baseline electrocardiogram have a worse prognosis in that they have a high incidence of acute myocardial infarction and mortality and so require more aggressive therapeutic approach. A subset of these patients with ST changes in the anteroseptal leads, which have been correlated with significant stenosis of the left anterior descending coronary artery, appears to be a particularly high-risk group (Fig. 1) (7). Patients who are refractory to pharmacologic treatment also appear to have a more ominous prognosis, which dictates urgent, aggressive intervention.

Patients with early (within 30 days) postinfarction angina at rest with ST-segment or T-wave changes, or patients with angina pectoris induced by light exercise, appear to have a high incidence of recurrent myocardial infarction and

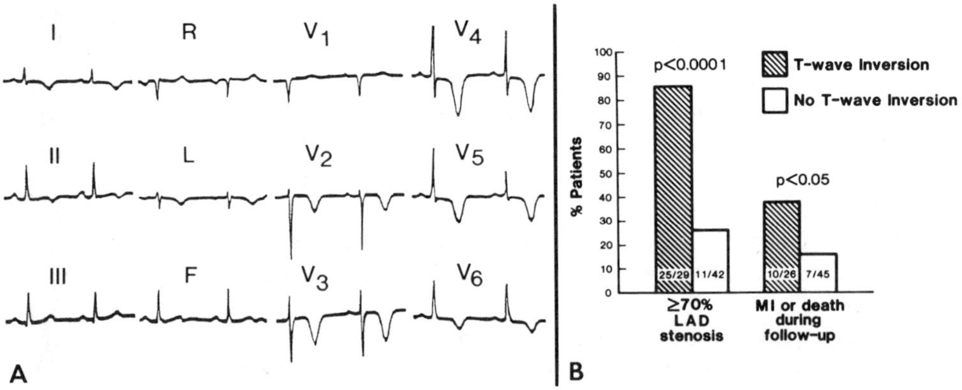

Figure 1 (A) Symmetrical anterior T-wave inversion with isoelectric ST segment is frequently associated with critical stenosis of left anterior descending coronary artery. (B) Prevalence of significant stenosis of left anterior descending coronary artery (LAD) and the incidence of cardiac events in patients with and without new T-wave inversion. MI, myocardial infarction. (From Ref. 7 by permission of Cahners Publishing Company, a Division of Reed Publishing USA.)

mortality and comprise a subgroup in which more aggressive strategies (such as CABG) are indicated. Postinfarction angina is associated with a high recurrence rate of second infarctions and a significant mortality. Schuster and Bulkley (8) differentiated between ischemia in the infarct zone and ischemia at a distance in association with postinfarction angina. They reported a mortality at 6 months of 44% when the ischemia was confined to the infarct zone and of 72% when ischemia was in a distant area of myocardium.

PRINCIPLES OF THERAPEUTIC STRATEGIES IN UNSTABLE ANGINA

Medical Therapy

The goals of acute management in unstable angina, be it conservative or invasive, are to prevent progression to myocardial infarction, to decrease symptoms, and to prevent sudden death. The initial management of unstable angina pectoris will be pharmacologic in nearly all cases.

Patients should be reassured, mildly sedated if necessary, and placed on bed rest with continuous electrocardiographic monitoring. Myocardial oxygen demand should be minimized by correction of factors that increase oxygen consumption (such as hypertension and tachycardia). Several large-scale randomized trials have confirmed the effectiveness of aspirin in unstable angina (9). Nitrates and β-adrenergic blockers have also been shown to be effective for relieving pain. The role of calcium channel blockers as monotherapy in unstable angina remains unproved, but enthusiasm for this approach appears to be waning. A subset of patients with unstable angina in which dynamic coronary obstruction due to coronary vasospasm is the principal cause of coronary obstruction can be expected to respond well to calcium channel blockers.

It is generally agreed that the initial steps to be taken in the patient with unstable angina are to correct precipitating factors and to stabilize the patient with pharmacologic means. After stabilization, the conservative approach would be to mobilize the patient gradually and to follow this step by an exercise study (either a treadmill or stationary cycle study with or without the addition of radionuclide ventriculography, thallium-201 scintigraphy, or exercise echocardiography) (Fig. 2). In patients who are unable to perform an exercise study, a dipyridamole thallium study or dobutamine echocardiography can be substituted. Holter monitoring to define episodes of silent ischemia also has been shown to have prognostic significance in patients with unstable angina (Fig. 3) (10). The rationale for the conservative approach is to use noninvasive studies to discriminate between patients who are at low and those who are at high risk for future cardiac events. Although noninvasive stress testing is an effective method for identification of high-risk subpopulations, it will lead to both false-positive

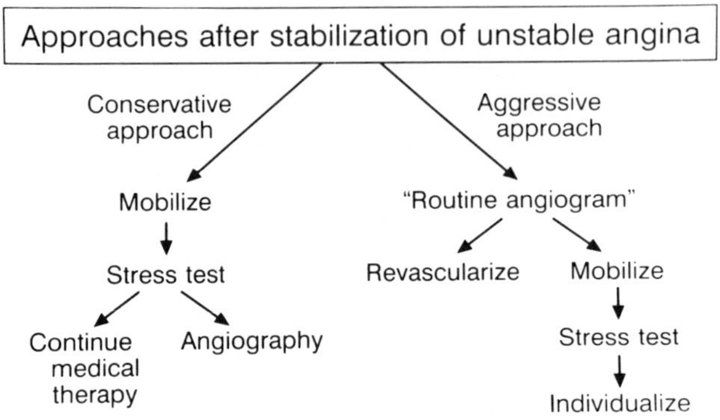

Figure 2 Approaches after stabilization of unstable angina.

and false-negative diagnoses in individual patients. The alternative approach of "routine" angiography after stabilization is discussed elsewhere in this chapter (Fig. 2).

Operation

The rationale for early surgical myocardial revascularization in patients with persistent or recurrent angina pectoris after acute myocardial infarction relates to the high rates of reinfarction and cardiac-related mortality and the need for

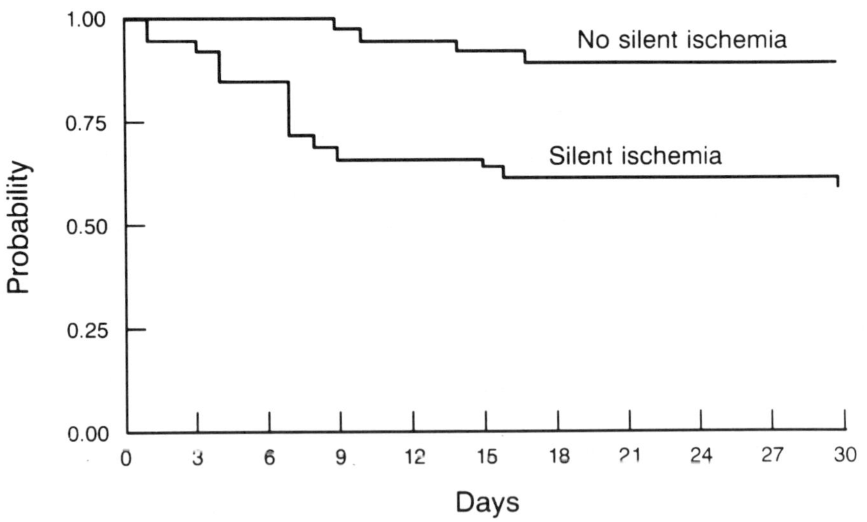

Figure 3 Prognosis of patients with unstable angina according to presence or absence of continuing silent ischemia. Probability of not experiencing myocardial infarction or revascularization for recurrent angina. (From Ref. 10 by permission of the journal.)

subsequent interventional therapy in patients who are managed initially with medical therapy. Most of the reported surgical data in unstable angina come from studies of patients with postinfarction angina (Braunwald category C). Extrapolation from these studies can, however, reasonably be made to patients with classification B unstable angina with the caveat that left ventricular dysfunction (an important determinant of therapeutic benefit with revascularization versus conservative therapy) will be more frequent among patients with previous infarction than among patients without prior infarction. Surgical revascularization is generally not warranted in patients with category A disease (unstable angina in the presence of extracardiac factors that precipitate myocardial ischemia).

Several studies have demonstrated that CABG early after myocardial infarction can be accomplished with low mortality. The variables that independently predict increased operative risk and postoperative morbidity, however, remain incompletely defined. Improvements in surgical technique and myocardial preservation have certainly decreased the operative mortality in postinfarction patients with unstable angina, which now is reported to be between 3.3% and 8.4% with a perioperative myocardial infarction rate of approximately 15% (Table 2).

The results obtained by acute operation and angioplasty cannot be compared directly because patients who undergo angioplasty are a select group with predominantly single-vessel disease and preserved left ventricular function, whereas patients selected for operation tend to have multivessel (frequently triple-vessel) disease, left main stem disease, and compromised left ventricular function, factors known to influence prognosis adversely.

Preoperative ventricular function is a strong predictor of surgical risk in postinfarction angina. In patients with depressed left ventricular function, delay-

Table 2 Operative Mortality with Coronary Artery Bypass Grafting in Postinfarction Unstable Angina

Study	Year	No. of patients	Mean EF (%)	Left main CAD (%)	Three-vessel disease (%)	Death (%)
Breyer et al.[11]	1985	75	54	20	76	8.0
Jones et al.[12]	1987	107	NA	NA	NA	8.4
Naunheim et al.[13]	1988	185	NA	NA	NA	6.5
Kouchoukos et al.[14]	1989	240	NA	13	70	3.3
Gardner et al.[15]	1989	300	47	NA	NA	5.0

Abbreviations: CAD, coronary artery disease; NA, not available (data were not given in reference).

ing operation for at least 6 weeks after infarction appears to result in a lower operative mortality (16).

Coronary Angioplasty

PTCA is an attractive alternative to surgical revascularization in unstable angina. Balloon angioplasty generally can be performed more quickly than CABG and frequently may be done as part of diagnostic angiography. However, the success rate is lower and the occurrence of procedural complications is higher than with elective coronary angioplasty (Table 3). Procedure-related mortality is reported to be between 0 and 2%. Complications resulting in an acute myocardial infarction occur in up to 8% of patients, and emergency CABG is required in approximately 5% (22). It is hoped that newer interventional technologies such as stents may reduce the need for emergency CABG in this setting.

The short-term prognosis appears excellent after an initial successful coronary angioplasty, with low late mortality and reinfarction rates. Recurrence of angina appears to be comparable to the rate in patients after elective PTCA for stable angina. Unstable angina is, however, an independent predictor of restenosis after PTCA.

De Feyter (23) reviewed the results of balloon angioplasty in 352 patients with postinfarction angina from six large centers (24–29). Success rates for PTCA varied between 76 and 91%. Major complications occurred in 3–12% of patients (death, 0–2%; myocardial infarction, 0–8%; emergency CABG, 1.5–12%). These rates are higher than those reported from other studies confined primarily to patients with stable angina.

Differences between patients with unstable angina and those with stable angina need to be emphasized because they might have a major bearing on the

Table 3 PTCA in Unstable Angina Pectoris

Study	No. of patients	Follow-up (months)	Success (%)	MVD[a] (%)	Death, early[b]/ late (%)
Faxon et al.[17]	442	18	61	—	0.9/2.6
Myler et al.[18]	807	37	84	10	0.2/3.0
Quigley et al.[19]	25	14	81	52	0.4/0.0
Plokker et al.[20]	469	19	88	28	1.5/2.5
Bentivoglio[21]	952	—	84	53	1.3-NA[c]
de Feyter et al.[22]	200	24	89.5	33	1.5/2.0

[a]MVD, multivessel disease.
[b]Early death, in-hospital death (that is, during hospitalization for PTCA).
[c]NA, not available (data were not given in reference).

results of the same procedure in the two syndromes. PTCA in unstable angina is associated with increased risks of major complications. Patients with angina at rest, patients with early postinfarction angina, and those refractory to treatment are at particular risk of procedural complications, whereas patients with progressive angina appear to be at a lower risk. The higher incidence of complications is understandable in light of the increasing knowledge of the pathophysiology of the "acute ischemic syndromes." Pathophysiologic features of these coronary syndromes include endothelial ulceration adjacent to an atherosclerotic plaque, subsequent platelet adhesion and aggregation, and alteration of prostaglandin metabolism of both vessel wall and platelet, leading to local vasoconstriction and spasm.

Regional left ventricular wall function is often impaired in unstable angina as a result of chronic ischemia (hibernating myocardium) or prolonged postischemic dysfunction (stunned myocardium), and additional dilations of the nonculprit lesion may jeopardize myocardium, which in the event of failure could result in serious, if not fatal, left ventricular dysfunction.

To expand the potential use of PTCA as an alternative to CABG in patients with unstable angina and multivessel disease, dilation of only the "culprit" lesion has been recommended as an initial approach to stabilize the patient's condition. This strategy is initially successful in most patients; however, it is associated, not unexpectedly, with a higher occurrence of angina pectoris after the procedure, which may necessitate later CABG or PTCA of other vessels at a late stage. This approach does not provide long-term treatment in all patients. One potential benefit of the culprit-lesion approach, however, is that subsequent interventions can be employed on a more "elective" basis and at a lower risk. Nonetheless, among patients with multivessel disease it is frequently not possible to identify the "culprit lesion," which exposes the patient to the risk of an inappropriate dilation at the time of greatest risk.

Although successful multilesion and multivessel dilations in a single-vessel angioplasty procedure are accepted practice in patients with *stable* angina, there is less experience with multiple dilations in unstable angina.

COMPARATIVE STUDIES OF SURGICAL REVASCULARIZATION VERSUS MEDICAL THERAPY

Chronic Stable Angina

As a framework for evaluating the role of CABG versus medical therapy in patients with unstable angina, it is relevant to review what has been learned from the randomized trials, which were confined primarily to patients with chronic *stable* angina. The numerous registry and data base studies of patient subsets other than those in the randomized trials, including some at "higher risk," also provide a useful frame of reference.

Despite differences among the three major randomized trials of CABG versus medical therapy, they do provide a consensus in that operation improves survival over medical therapy in patients with left main coronary artery disease, in patients with *mild to moderate* angina in association with triple-vessel disease and left ventricular dysfunction, and probably in patients with double-vessel disease in association with significant stenosis of the left anterior descending coronary artery. Moreover, CABG was superior to medical therapy for the relief of symptoms (at least over the short-term) in virtually all of the subgroups.

The registry and data base studies also have provided persuasive, although not definitive, evidence for the superiority of CABG over medical therapy in other subsets of patients. In patients with *severe* angina or ischemia and triple-vessel disease, the benefit of CABG was noted in patients with *and* without left ventricular dysfuction, but in patients with double-vessel disease, survival benefit was evident only in patients with left ventricular dysfunnction. In patients with left main "equivalent" coronary artery disease, survival was better in surgically treated than in medically treated patients.

It is reasonable to extrapolate these data to patients with unstable angina, particularly if they are used in conjunction with the information emanating from the three randomized trials confined specifically to patients with unstable angina, defined by angina at rest. Moreover, no further randomized trials of operation versus medical therapy are in progress nor are any under consideration.

It should be emphasized further that the results of coronary revascularization with CABG cannot be extrapolated directly to PTCA; the optimal method of myocardial revascularization is the focus of several ongoing randomized trials of the 1990s.

Unstable Angina

Randomized Trials

There have been three large trials of medical versus surgical treatment of unstable angina (Table 4). In 1976, Bertolasi et al. (9) reported the first large-scale trial of conservative versus surgical therapy for unstable angina. This study, done in Argentina, had a mean follow-up of 32 months and reported a clear beneficial effect of operation on the late survival and late nonfatal myocardial infarction rates. The weaknesses of this study were that it probably included many patients with non–Q-wave myocardial infarctions, the crossover rate was not reported, and patients with left main coronary artery disease were included.

In 1978, the National Cooperative Study Group—National Institutes of Health (31) reported a 30-month average follow-up of 288 randomized patients; symptom relief was superior in the surgical group, but no overall late survival differences were found between the medical and surgical groups. This study differed from the study by Bertolasi et al. (9) because patients with left main

Table 4 Randomized Trials of Medical Versus Surgical Treatment

	Trial		
	VA Cooperative study[30]	NCSG–NIH[31]	Bertolasi et al.[9]
No. of patients	468	288	113
Mean follow-up (months)	24	30	32
Medical to surgical crossover (%)	34	36	—
EF < 50%, no. of pts.	29	23	—
Three-vessel disease, no. of pts.	46	41	39
Medical treatment, no. of pts.	237	147	51
Early death	5 (2.1%)	4 (3%)	6 (12%)
All death	22 (9.3%)	14 (10%)	13 (25%)
Early MI	—	12 (8%)	7 (14%)
All MI	29 (12.2%)	28 (19%)	11 (22%)
Surgical treatment, no. of pts.	231	141	62
Early death	9 (3.9%)	7 (5%)	6 (10%)
All death	18 (7.8%)	14 (10%)	6 (10%)
Early MI	23 (10%)	24 (17%)	8 (13%)
All MI	27 (11.7%)	42 (30%)	8 (13%)

Abbreviations: EF, ejection fraction; MI, myocardial infarction; NCSG–NIH, National Cooperative Study Group–National Institutes of Health; VA, Veterans Administration.

coronary artery disease and patients with an ejection fraction of less than 30% were excluded. The nonfatal myocardial infarction rate was higher overall in the surgically treated group, but this difference principally was due to early perioperative infarctions and tended to equalize over time. The medical to surgical crossover rate was 36%.

The Veterans Administration (30) initiated a prospective, stratified, and randomized study of medical versus surgical treatment of unstable angina in 1976. This study enrolled 468 patients during a 6-year period. Patients were stratified by clinical presentation and by left ventricular function. At 5 years of follow-up, there were significant differences in survival for patients with three-vessel disease: 75% for medically treated patients and 89% for surgically treated patients ($p < 0.02$). The cumulative 5-year rate of repeat hospitalizations for cardiac reasons was less in the surgical group. Analysis of medical and surgical groups with ejection fraction as a continuous variable showed that mortality in the medical group depended on ejection fraction ($p = 0.004$), whereas mortality in the surgical group did not ($p = 0.76$). An impaired ejection fraction

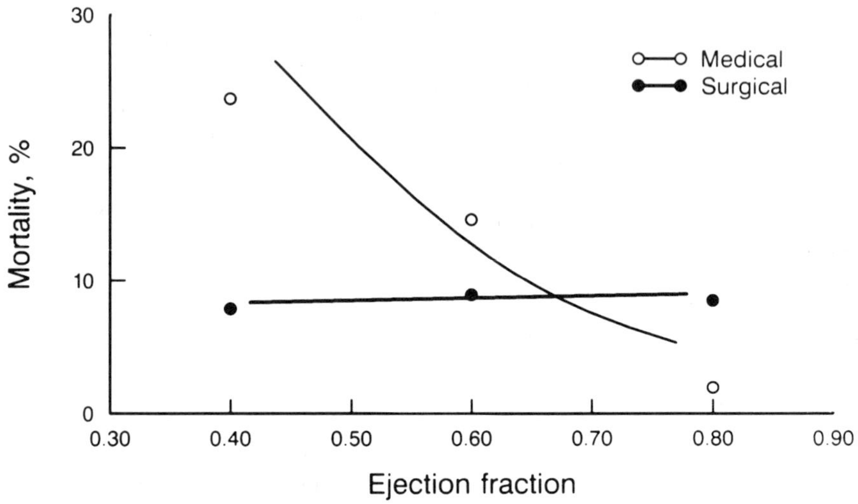

Figure 4 Effect of ejection fraction on late survival in patients treated with surgical revascularization or managed medically in the Veterans Administration Unstable Angina Trial. (From Ref. 34 by permission of the American Heart Association.)

had an adverse impact on the survival of medically treated patients but not on surgically treated patients, and mortality in the surgical group was improved compared with the medical group in the subgroup with the lowest ejection fraction (Fig. 4). This finding is in keeping with the results of trials of medical versus surgical therapy in chronic *stable* angina, in which the greater benefit with surgical therapy accrued to patients with poorer left ventricular function.

Nonadherence to assigned therapy ("crossovers") is a significant problem in medical-surgical trials of unstable angina. Many patients originally assigned to conservative treatment had CABG during follow-up. The National Heart, Lung, and Blood Institute study had a cumulative crossover rate of 31% by 24 months. In the Veterans Administration study, the crossover rate was 34% at 24 months and 43% at 60 months. Evaluation of outcomes by treatment initially assigned ("intention to treat") has long been advocated as the standard of assessment for all clinical trials, and this form of analysis preserves randomization, averts investigator bias in selecting patients for crossover, and makes no assumptions of outcomes had crossover failed to occur. The "intention to treat" principle evaluates an initial therapeutic strategy and not a specific therapy. Crossover reflects a failure of the initial strategy with subsequent adoption of the alternative therapy.

On balance, an intellectual argument can be made on the basis of randomized trials to treat patients with unstable angina medically and to intervene with coronary revascularization only in the face of refractory symptoms. Nonetheless, one must accept that unstable angina implies *severe ischemia*. In the face of added left ventricular dysfunction, the Veterans Administration trial suggests a policy of CABG as primary therapy (Fig. 4). In the absence of left ventricular dysfunction, one has to extrapolate from other data, which imply that *severe* ischemia is a bad prognostic feature, and the case for routine angiography with subsequent individualization of therapy is strong and logical—particularly because the trials have all documented the superiority of CABG over medical therapy for relief of symptoms. Moreover, the relatively high crossover rate during the first 2 years emphasizes that many patients come to CABG in any event. Added to this fact are further data that identify particular high-risk subsets (for example, patients with anterior T-wave inversion, a group not specifically addressed by the trials).

In summary, the randomized trials of unstable angina are helpful. Therapeutic decisions need to recognize the specific subsets that were included in the trials, and the results cannot be extrapolated to groups of patients who were excluded from these large studies.

Data Base Studies

Rahimtoola et al. (32) assessed the late results of CABG performed for unstable angina in 1282 patients between 1970 and 1982. The overall operative mortality was 1.8%. The actuarial 5- and 10-year survival rates were 92% and 83%, respectively. Preoperative left ventricular function was not a statistically significant determinant of late survival at 10 years. The finding that an abnormal preoperative left ventricular function does not adversely affect late survival was unexpected and contrasts with previous data base reports of CABG in patients with chronic stable angina. The authors suggested that the explanation for this effect may lie in the fact that left ventricular dysfunction in association with unstable angina may result from ischemia rather than permanent myocardial damage (Fig. 5).

The reoperation rates at 5 and 10 years postoperatively were 6% and 17%, respectively. No significant difference in late survival was observed among the three different clinical patterns of unstable angina: angina at rest, postinfarction angina, or progressive angina of recent origin. This study provides strong evidence that CABG is an effective long-term therapy for unstable angina with excellent late survival at least to 10 years postoperatively.

THE CASE FOR ROUTINE CORONARY ANGIOGRAPHY IN UNSTABLE ANGINA

Crucial to any management strategy, including revascularization, is the issue of routine coronary angiography in patients with unstable angina as opposed to the use of angiography only in the face of persistent ischemia (a finding implying

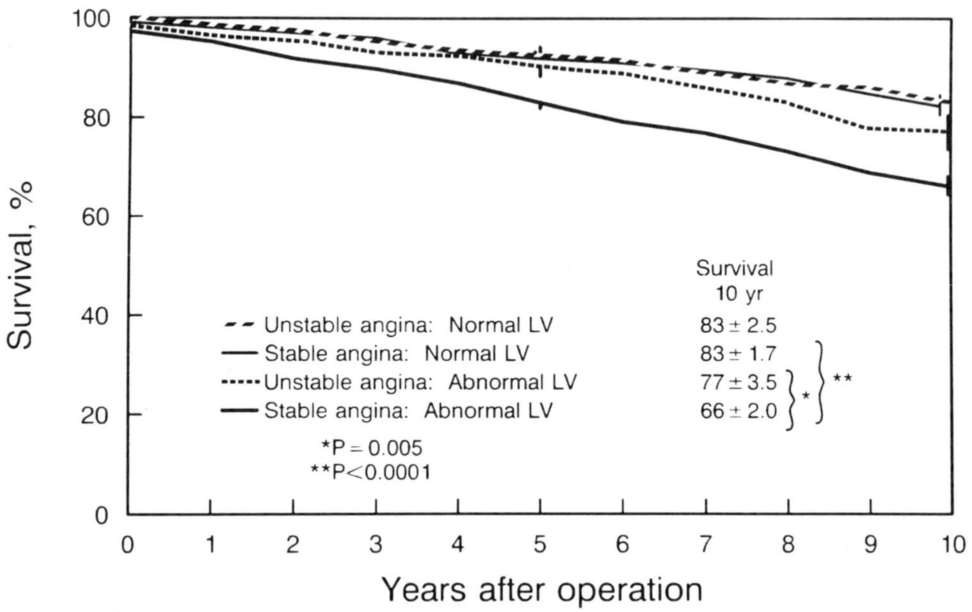

Figure 5 The 10-year survival after coronary artery bypass grafting in patients with and without left ventricular dysfunction (LV) in unstable and stable angina pectoris. (From Ref. 35 by permission of CV Mosby Company.)

failed medical therapy). If the latter approach is used, coronary angiography should be performed early in the event of recurrent rest pain with medical therapy or in the event of an initial favorable response followed by ischemia on mobilization or stress testing.

The alternative approach is to perform routine coronary angiography on all patients after initial stabilization of symptoms. The advantage of this strategy is that one can identify (early in the clinical course) a subset of patients in whom a subsequent therapeutic strategy is clearly evident, whether this be CABG, PTCA, medical therapy, or reassurance. If this approach is used, the following results can be expected (Fig. 6).

1. Approximately 10–15% of patients will have normal results or minimal coronary artery disease. It is well established that these patients have an excellent prognosis, although they may continue to have symptoms that may respond to nitrates or calcium channel blockers (syndrome X ?).
2. Coronary artery spasm as provoked by ergonovine challenge in association with normal results or minimal coronary disease can be expected to occur in

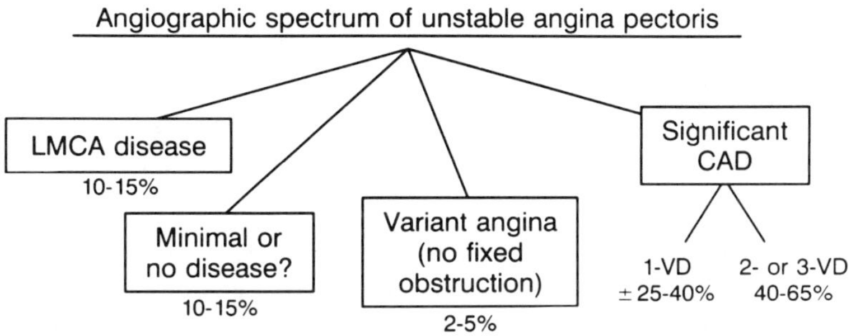

Figure 6 Angiographic spectrum in unstable angina pectoris. CAD, coronary artery disease; LMCA, left main coronary artery; VD, vessel disease.

approximately 2–5% of patients. The correct identification of this patient subgroup is important because of the significant beneficial effect of calcium channel blockade.

3. Approximately 10–15% of patients will have left main coronary artery disease. In general, all these patients will require CABG. Few would argue against the value of CABG in patients with significant left main coronary artery disease with or without symptoms (33). The Veterans Administration cooperative trial clearly demonstrated the beneficial effect of CABG in left main coronary artery disease in patients with chronic stable angina. It can reasonably be extrapolated from this study that the same or a greater benefit should be derived from operation in patients with unstable angina and left main coronary artery disease. Although conservative management with subsequent exercise testing also would be expected to identify these patients correctly by the early development of markers of myocardial ischemia (chest pain, electrocardiographic wall motion, or myocardial perfusion changes), it must be emphasized that stress testing in this group of patients is associated with a significantly higher mortality than among normal persons.
4. Among the remaining patients with single-vessel or multivessel disease, subsequent decisions can be made on the basis of coronary anatomy, left ventricular function, age, and life-style. In many patients, knowledge of the severity of coronary angiographic anatomy would allow subsequent stratification of individualized patient risk and referral for appropriate therapy. Single-vessel critical coronary stenosis will be identified by routine angiography in approximately 25–40% of cases. In general, the preferred treatment options in this case are medical management or balloon angioplasty. Extrapolation from studies of single-vessel disease in chronic stable angina indicates that both strategies are effective and that late mortality is very low. Proximal left anterior descending coronary artery disease is

considered to be associated with a worse prognosis than other forms of single-vessel disease. Exercise testing is particularly helpful in single-vessel disease to identify the extent to myocardial ischemia and the subsequent therapeutic approach.

5. Multivessel coronary disease will be identified by angiography in 40–65%of patients.

The treatment strategy in patients with multivessel disease needs to be individualized. Extrapolation from studies in patients with chronic stable angina indicates that long-term prognosis is related to the number of vessels with critical stenoses, the extent of myocardial ischemia, and ventricular function. In patients with depressed left ventricular function, myocardial revascularization is indicated. In patients with triple-vessel disease, *particularly* in association with left ventricular dysfunction, operation can be offered with the strong expectation of prolonged survival. The approach to patients with double-vessel disease depends on the extent of left ventricular dysfuction, if any, the response to medical treatment, and the existence of "anatomically compelling" coronary disease. In many of these cases, knowledge of the coronary anotomy and exclusion of left main coronary disease provide one with the confidence to proceed with mobilization and stress testing.

In the light of the data presented above, it is clear that among patients with multivessel disease, left ventricular dysfunction, and severe ischemia, coronary revascularization is generally indicated. This observation supports the case for "routine" coronary angiography in (a) all patients with unstable angina with evidence of left ventricular dysfunction, (b) patients with persistent ischemia or angina despite aggressive medical therapy, and (c) patients with adverse prognostic features, such as recent myocardial infarction and persistent T-wave inversion in the precordial leads.

Prior studies have established the appropriateness of coronary revascularization in selected patient subsets; it is hoped that the preferred method will be determined in the 1990s. Several large multicenter studies (BARI, EAST, ACME, GABI, RITA) are currently in progress comparing PTCA with CABG in patients with single-vessel and multivessel disease and stable and unstable angina.

SPECIFIC RECOMMENDATIONS IN SUBSETS OF UNSTABLE ANGINA

Many patients in the categories outlined below who undergo "routine" angiography will be referred for revascularization on the basis of compelling anatomy. The discussion therefore refers to the remainder, in whom the decision to perform coronary angiography is based on the clinical findings.

Extracardiac Factors in Unstable Angina (Braunwald Category A)

Identification of extracardiac factors in patients with unstable angina is important because severe fixed coronary obstruction rather than plaque fissuring and intracoronary thrombus formation is frequently present. Unstable angina in this setting can be viewed as a change in the previously stable supply/demand ratio of myocardial oxygenation to myocardial work. Examples of precipitating clinical events include hypertension, blood loss, hypotension, tachyarrhythmias, and bradyarrhythmias. In general, the treatment of these conditions is to reverse the precipitating cause. Patients should be placed at bed rest and lightly sedated, and a vigorous antianginal medical program should be undertaken while the precipitating clinical events are reversed. Most patients will be controlled by conservative measures without invasive procedures. A complicating factor may occur when an initial extracardiac event precipitates a second intracardiac event that further worsens the myocardial ischemia. An example of this process is a tachyarrhythmia leading to hypotension followed by the development of an intracoronary thrombus secondary to increased platelet aggregation due to reduced low coronary blood flow altering rheologic properties in the vessel.

If the patient fails to respond to reversal of the initial extracardiac precipitating event and maximal antianginal medication, then coronary angiography is indicated to define the pathophysiology of the unstable angina syndrome further. If the patient does respond, it is important to perform a noninvasive exercise study *after* mobilization to reassess the "modified" oxygen supply/demand milieu after correction of the extracardiac precipitant.

Progressive Angina Without Rest Pain (Braunwald Category IB)

Patients with progressive angina without rest pain generally have a better short-term prognosis than patients with rest pain. They can initially be managed pharmacologically. The decision to proceed with angiography in these patients is guided by the occurrence of left ventricular dysfunction on noninvasive testing. If left ventricular dysfunction is present, angiography is usually indicated, with the purpose to perform coronary revascularization if multivessel disease is identified. Persistence of symptoms after initial medical treatment warrants angiography.

Chest Pain at Rest (Braunwald Categories IIB and IIIB)

Patients with chest pain at rest accompanied by significant ST-T changes on electrocardiography have an increased risk of mortality and morbidity. Although in most of these patients the clinical symptoms can be stabilized with pharmacologic treatment, including nitrates, β-adrenergic blockers, calcium antagonists, and heparin, further treatment of the underlying coronary lesion with either PTCA or CABG is indicated in most patients. A persuasive argument for routine angiography can be made in most patients *even* if they are stabilized. If PTCA is to be used, there may well be a difference between the outcome in categories IIB and IIIB. This difference may be related to the higher occurrence of intracoronary thrombus in category IIIB.

Angina After Myocardial Infarction

The late prognosis of myocardial infarction is determined primarily by the extent of residual ischemia, left ventricular dysfunction, and arrhythmias. Of these, residual ischemia is the most amenable to correction. Recurrent angina or ischemia on stress testing after myocardial infarction, particularly in association with left ventricular dysfunction, identifies a group at risk in whom a strong case can be made for revascularization.

The incidence of angina early after myocardial infarction during the hospitalization period is between 18% and 57% and varies with the patient population. Early postinfarction angina is considered to have poor short- and long-term prognoses. In particular, non–Q-wave infarction has been shown to be associated with a higher incidence of recurrent infarction than those with Q-wave infarction. There is no consensus regarding patient selection and the timing of surgical revascularization for patients with severe angina early after acute myocardial infarction. Recent reports have suggested that myocardial revascularization within the first 30 days after infarction can be accomplished with an acceptable operative mortality in selected patients, although overall mortality and morbidity rates remain higher than those reported for elective operation, particularly in those with left ventricular dysfunction. Accordingly, current strategy for the management of patients with early postinfarction angina is aimed at delaying operation until it can be performed with the least inherent risks. However, in patients with severe recurrent angina, the clinical situation may demand early intervention.

CONCLUSION

Most would agree that the initial approach for the patient with unstable angina involves a period of attempted stabilization with attention to extracardiac precipitating factors.

The second step includes routine angiography or an alternative approach based on mobilization, followed by stress testing with angiography for patients with recurrent ischemia at any stage in the clinical course or after mobilization.

The performance of angiography provides a further opportunity to individualize therapy based on an integration of the angiographic anatomy with the measurment of left ventricular function, the severity of ischemia, and other factors (such as age, life-style, and concomitant medical conditions). In many patients, the information obtained from the randomized trials of unstable angina and other studies of stable angina enables one to make a rational decision for or against coronary revascularization on the basis of coronary anatomy alone, but this must be modified by other clinical outcomes.

The preferred method of coronary revascularization remains an issue of major debate, which will continue throughout the 1990s. The incidence of procedure-related complications after PTCA in patients with rest angina is increased, and in the early postinfarction period both CABG and PTCA are associated with high risk. Ongoing randomized trials will likely clarify the issues in the next few years.

Nonetheless, it must be argued that unstable angina is a clinical syndrome that includes many patients at high risk for future cardiac events. The umbrella of this diagnosis embraces many patients at particularly high risk on the basis of severe ischemia, multivessel disease, and left ventricular dysfunction. The role of coronary revascularization in the management of *most* patients with unstable angina is not in dispute; the preferred method and additional indications for revascularization (for example, patients with reversible stunned myocardium) will be a focus of investigation throughout the 1990s.

REFERENCES

1. Karlsson J-E, Wallentin L. Thrombolysis with r - TPA during instability in coronary artery disease (TRIC) (abstract). Circulation 1990; 82 (Suppl 3):84.
2. Cohen M, Greenberg S, Hawkins L, Fuster V. Clinical and angiographic characteristics and outcome of patients with rest angina occurring in the setting of regular aspirin use (abstract). Circulation 1990; 82 (Suppl 3):84.
3. Pérez Villa F, Betriu A, Sanz G, Mont L, Roig E, Azqueta M, Navarro-López F. Does thrombolysis improve outcome in unstable angina? A 1-year follow-up study (abstract). Circulation 1990; 82 (Suppl 3):85.
4. Braunwald E. Unstable angina: a classification. Circulation 1989; 80:410–4.
5. Gazes PC, Mobley EM Jr, Faris HM Jr, Duncan RC, Humphries GB. Preinfarctional (unstable) angina—a perspective study—ten year follow-up. Circulation 1973; 48:331–7.
6. Mulcahy R, Awadhi AHA, de Buitleor M, Tobin G, Johnson H, Contoy R. Natural history and prognosis of unstable angina. Am Heart J 1985; 109:753–8.
7. Haines DE, Raabe DS, Gundel WD, Wackers FJT. Anatomic and prognostic significance of new T-wave inversion in unstable angina. Am J Cardiol 1983; 52:14–8.
8. Schuster EH, Bulkley BH. Early post-infarction angina: ischemia at a distance and ischemia in the infarct zone. N Engl J Med 1981; 305:1101–5.
9. Bertolasi CA, Tronge JE, Riccitelli MA, Villamayor RM, Zuffardi E. Natural history of unstable angina with medical or surgical therapy. Chest 1976; 70:596–605.

10. Gottlieb SO, Weisfeldt ML, Ouyanp P, Mellits ED, Gerstenblith G. Silent ischemia as a marker for early unfavorable outcomes in patients with unstable angina. N Engl J Med 1986; 314:1214–9.
11. Breyer RH, Engelman RM, Rousou JA, Lemeshow S. Postinfarction angina: an expanding subset of patients undergoing coronary artery bypass. J Thorac Cardiovasc Surg 1985; 90:532–40.
12. Jones RN, Pifarré R, Sullivan HJ, Montoya A, Bakhos M, Grieco JG, Foy BK, Wyatt J. Early myocardial revascularization for postinfarction angina. Ann Thorac Surg 1987; 44:159–63.
13. Naunheim KS, Kesler KA, Kanter KR, Fiore AC, McBride LR, Pennington G, Barner HB, Kaiser GC, Willman VL. Coronary artery bypass for recent infarction: predictors of mortality. Circulation 1988; 78 (Suppl 1):122–8.
14 Kouchoukos NT, Murphy S, Philpott T, Pelate C, Marshall WG Jr. Coronary artery bypass grafting for postinfarction angina pectoris. Circultion 1989; 79 (Suppl 1):68–72.
15. Gardner TJ, Stuart RS, Greene PS, Baumgartner WA. The risk of coronary bypass surgery for patients with postinfarction angina. Circulation 1989; 79 (Suppl 1):79–80.
16. Hochberg MS, Parsonnet V, Gielchinsky I, Hussain SM, Fisch DA, Norman JC. Timing of coronary revascularization after acute myocardial infarction: early and late results in patients revascularized within seven weeks. J Thorac Cardiovasc Surg 1984; 88:914–21.
17. Faxon DP, Detre KM, McCabe CH, Fisher L, Holmes DR, Cowley MJ, Bourassa MG, Van Raden M, Ryan TJ. Role of percutaneous transluminal coronary angioplasty in the treatment of unstable angina: report from the National Heart, Lung, and Blood Institute Percutaneous Transluminal Coronary Angioplasty and Coronary Artery Surgery Study Registries. Am J Cardiol 1983; 53:131C–5C.
18. Myler RK, Shaw RE, Stertzer SH, Bashour TT, Ryan C, Hecht HS, Cumberland DC. Unstable angina and coronary angioplasty. Circulation 1990; 82 (Suppl 2):88–95.
19. Quigley PJ, Erwin J, Maurer BJ, Walsh MJ, Gearty GF. Percutaneous transluminal coronary angioplasty in unstable angina: comparison with stable angina. Br Heart J 1986; 55:227–30.
20. Plokker HWT, Ernst SMPG, Bal ET, van den Berg ECJM, Mast GEG, van der Feltz TA, Ascoop CAPL. Percutaneous transluminal coronary angioplasty in patients with unstable angina pectoris refractory to medical therapy: long-term clinical and angiographic results. Cathet Cardiovasc Diagn 1988; 14:15–8.
21 Bentivoglio LG, Holubkov R, Cowley MJ, Holmes DR Jr, Kelsey SF, Myler RK, Sopko G, Detre K. Outcome of PTCA in stable and unstable angina pectoris. NHLBI PTCA Registry 1985–86.
22. de Feyter PJ, Suryapranata H, Serruys PW, Beatt K, van Domburg R, van den Brand M, Tijssen JJ, Azar AJ, Hugenholtz PG. Coronary angioplasty for unstable angina: immediate and late results in 200 consecutive patients with identification of risk factors for unfavorable early and late outcome. J Am Coll Cardiol 1988; 12:324–33.

23. de Feyter PJ. Coronary angioplasty for unstable angina (editorial). Am Heart J 1989; 118:860–8.
24. de Feyter PJ, Serruys PW, Soward A, van den Brand M, Bos E, Hugenholtz PG. Coronary angioplasty for early postinfarction unstable angina. Circulation 1986; 74:1365–70.
25. Suryapranata H, Beatt K, de Feyter PJ, Verrostte J, van den Brand M, Zijlstra F, Serruys PW. Percutaneous transluminal coronary angioplasty for angina pectoris after a non-Q-wave acute myocardial infarction. Am J Cardiol 1988; 61:240–3.
26. Safian RD, Snyder LD, Snyder BA, McKay RG, Lorell BH, Aroesty JM, Pasternak RC, Bradley AB, Monrad ES, Baim DS. Usefulness of percutaneous transluminal coronary angioplasty for unstable angina pectoris after non-Q-wave acute myocardial infarction. Am J Cardiol 1987; 59:263–6.
27. Gottlieb SO, Walford GD, Ouyang P, Gerstenblith G, Brin KP, Mellits ED, Riegel MB, Brinker JA. Initial and late result of coronary angioplasty for early postinfarction unstable angina. Cathet Cardiovasc Diagn 1987; 13:93–9.
28. Hopkins J, Savage M, Zalewski A, Dervan JP, Goldberg S. Recurrent ischemia in the zone of prior myocardial infarction: results of coronary angioplasty of the infarct-related artery. Am Heart J 1988; 115:14–9.
29. Holt GW, Gersh BJ, Homes DR Jr, Vlietstra RE, Reeder GS, Bresnahan JF, Smith HC. The results of percutaneous transluminal coronary angioplasty (PTCA) in post infarction angina pectoris (abstract). J Am Coll Cardiol 1986; 7:62A.
30. Luchi RJ, Scott SM, Deupree RH, the Principal Investigators and Their Associates of Veterans Administration Cooperative Study No. 28. Comparison of medical and surgical treatment for unstable angina pectoris: results of a Veterans Administration cooperative study. N Engl J Med 1987; 316:977–84.
31. National Cooperative Study Group. Unstable angina pectoris: national cooperative study group to compare surgical and medical therapy. II. In-hospital experience and initial follow-up results in patients with one, two and three vessel disease. Am J Cardiol 1978; 42:839–48.
32. Rahimtoola SH, Nunley D, Grunkemeier G, Tepley J, Lambert L, Starr A. Ten-year survival after coronary bypass surgery for unstable angina. N Engl J Med 1983; 308:676–81.
33. Takaro T, Pifarre R, Fish R. Left main coronary artery disease. Prog Cardiovasc Dis 1985; 28:229–34.
34. Scott SM, Luchi RI, Deupree RH, and the Veterans Administration Unstable Angina Cooperative Study Group. Veterans Administration Cooperative Study for treatment of patients with unstable angina: results in patients with abnormal left ventricular function. Circulation 1988; 78 (Suppl 1):113–21.
35. Rahimtoola SH. The hibernating myocardium [editorial]. Am Heart J 1989; 117:211–21.

15

Natural History and Prognosis of Unstable Angina

John F. Keaney, Jr.

Brigham and Women's Hospital and Harvard Medical School
Boston, Massachusetts

INTRODUCTION

Ischemic heart disease comprises a broad spectrum of clinical syndromes. Acute myocardial infarction is the most dramatic in presentation and may be associated with hemodynamic compromise; in marked contrast is the entity of chronic stable angina pectoris with episodes of pain occurring in response to clearly measured and reproducible degrees of exertion. Intermediate between these two well-defined clinical problems is the entity of unstable angina pectoris. The term unstable angina has been used to denote angina of recent onset, angina occurring at rest, and/or chest pain that was once stable in character and now occurs with increasing frequency in the setting of progressively less activity. The diversity of clinical syndromes presenting as unstable angina can be exemplified by the synonyms used in its description, including impending myocardial infarction, preinfarction angina, intermediate coronary syndrome, coronary failure, acute coronary insufficiency, atypical angina, spasmodic angina, and impending infarction.

In 1951 the term "intermediate coronary syndrome" was independently described by Graybiel (1) in the United States and Vakil (2) in India. The intermediate coronary syndrome of Graybiel and Vakil has since evolved into the present-day definition of unstable angina. They described a syndrome of viselike chest pain, intermediate in intensity between angina and myocardial infarction, which occurred episodically—lasting from 15 minutes to several hours with equivocal or poor responses of the chest pain to nitrates or bed rest. They also indicated a lack of specific clinical or electrocardiographic evidence of acute myocardial infarction.

At the time Graybiel and Vakil offered their exhaustive description of what is now known as unstable angina, there were few therapeutic interventions available, and therefore comprehensive and complete descriptions concerning the natural history of unstable angina are found in this era. Any present-day discussion concerning the natural history of unstable angina must take into account interventions and therapies that have altered the "natural" history of unstable angina. Patients with the diagnosis of unstable angina may have been exposed to different intensities of medical therapy, percutaneous angioplasty, and surgical revascularization. At one extreme is the patient with a first episode of angina occurring at a relatively young age, on no medications, and without any significant previous cardiovascular history. At the other extreme is the elderly patient on multiple antianginal medications with a history of previous coronary artery bypass grafting who then develops unstable angina. It is clear that the natural history of unstable angina, as it relates to each of these patients, will be different.

Early reports published in the 1950s and 1960s concerning the prognosis of patients with unstable angina relied heavily on a relatively small number of clinical and historical variables. The presence of persistent electrocardiographic changes, failure to respond to nitrates, and the response to bed rest were all considered important prognostic indicators (2–4). However, as technology has become more advanced, and the pathophysiology of unstable angina becomes clearer, a number of other historical, clinical, and diagnostic variables have been used to discriminate between patients at high or low risk for evolving myocardial infarction or death.

In the following section, the natural history of unstable angina will be discussed, with special attention directed towards the changing natural history of this syndrome in the setting of developing changes in medical practice. In addition, we will review the evidence linking multiple clinical, historical, and diagnostic variables to the prognosis of the patient with unstable angina.

NATURAL HISTORY

In 1955 Levy described a series of 158 patients followed over a period of 6 years from 1948 to 1953 (3). The patients were drawn from his own consultative practice. The patients were required to demonstrate either a sudden change in a previously stable anginal pattern characterized by angina occurring more frequently or induced more easily than previously, or a sudden recurrence of anginal pain after a symptom-free interval. Patients who presented with their first manifestation of coronary artery disease, evidence of myocardial infarction, and those with suspected myocardial infarction were excluded from the study. Levy was able to obtain follow-up data on approximately 90% of his patients, 126 of whom were male, 32 of which were female. On the basis of arbitrary clinical characteristics, the patients were divided into separate groups, which later carried different prognoses. The first group of patients Levy described was characterized by angina which resolved promptly with bed rest. Approximately 18% of all patients fell into this category, and they did relatively well with no evidence of myocardial infarction or recurrent unstable angina. In 40% of the patients, evidence of a non–Q-wave myocardial infarction developed. Twenty-three percent of the patients developed signs and symptoms of a classic Q-wave myocardial infarction with a mortality of approximately 16%. Three percent of the patients continued to have unstable angina but without any evidence of myocardial infarction, and a time course of 10 weeks was required before the anginal pattern returned to normal. Levy also reported an approximately 16% incidence of sudden death and an overall mortality of 32%. The only medications used in this study included nitroglycerin and digoxin.

In 1961 Vakil (2) described a series of 251 patients drawn from his own practice with the diagnosis of intermediate coronary syndrome. Entry into the series required fulfillment of four rather rigid criteria, including (a) chest pain longer than 15 minutes; (b) absence of myocardial infarction; (c) availability of at least two electrocardiograms providing objective evidence of ischemia; and (d) follow-up within 3 months. In this series, Vakil reported 93 cases of myocardial infarction within 3 months of enrollment for an incidence of 37%. In addition, 40% of the 251 patients developed evidence of recurrent unstable angina after recovering from the acute attack. Surprisingly, only two of the 251 patients died during the course of the study, resulting in a mortality of less than 1%.

In 1973, Gazes et al. followed 140 patients for the 10-year period between 1961 and 1971 (4). Patients were selected on the basis of recent anginal chest pain occurring at rest and followed longitudinally for the development of myocardial infarction or death. The authors retrospectively developed a profile of patients at high risk for subsequent events based on the presence of frequent in-hospital angina, prior stable angina, and ischemic electrocardiographic changes during episodes of chest pain. When compared with the entire study group, the high-risk subgroup had a greater incidence of myocardial infarction (35% vs. 21%) and markedly increased mortality from myocardial infarction (63% vs. 41%). Cumulative survival for the entire study group at 1, 5, and 10 years was 82%, 61%, and 48%, respectively, while the corresponding rates in the high-risk subgroup fell to 57%, 27%, and 19%, respectively. Therefore, these early studies in a heterogeneous population of patients with unstable angina suggested that the likelihood of developing a myocardial infarction varied greatly (0–37%), as did the associated mortality (0–63%).

PROGNOSIS

Due to the heterogeneous nature of patient populations with unstable angina, the subsequent incidence of nonfatal myocardial infarction and death has been difficult to obtain (Table 1). When the earlier series of patients with unstable angina are compared to the more recent randomized trials, it is obvious that the

Table 1 Myocardial Infarction and Mortality in Patients with Unstable Angina

Study	Therapy	n	Date	Mortality/MI (%)						
				1 month	4 month	1 yr	2 yr	4 yr	5 yr	10 yr
Vakil (2)		251	1951						1/39	
Levy (3)		158	1951				33/63			
Gazes (4)	Med	140	1973			18/–			39/–	42/–
National Co-op (5)	CABG	141	1978	5/17*			7/11			
	Med	147		3/8			5/13			
Harris (12)	Med	461	1980						29/–	
Telford (6)	Heparin	100	1981	0/3**[a]						
	Placebo	114		2/16						
Gerstenblith (7)	Nifed	91	1982		–/8.8					
Lewis (8)	ASA	625	1983		1.6/3.4					
	Placebo	641			3.3/6.9					
Rahimtoola (13)	CABG	1282	1983						8/–	17/–
Cairns (9)	ASA	276	1985				3/4			
	Placebo	139					11.7/5**			
Mulcahy (14)	Nitrate	100	1985	4/9		12/14				
Gottlieb (15)	Med	70	1986	10/0						
VA Co-op (10)	CABG	231	1988					6.1/13.6*		
	Med	237						17.6/14.7		
Theroux (11)	Heparin	118	1988	–/1.7***[b]						
	ASA	121		–/3*						
	Hep + ASA	122		–/1.6***						
	Placebo	118		–/11.9						
Stuart (47)	CABG	225	1988	8/–		12/–				

*$p \le 0.05$; **$p \le 0.01$; ***$p \le 0.005$.

[a]7-day endpoint.

[b]6-day endpoint.

Med = medical therapy; H = heparin.

incidence of nonfatal myocardial infarction and death has decreased. In 1955 Levy reported a 5-year incidence of nonfatal myocardial infarction and death of 63% and 33%, respectively (3), contrasted with the Veterans Administration Cooperative Trial, published in 1988, which revealed a 4-year incidence of nonfatal myocardial infarction of 14.7% and a 4-year cumulative mortality of 17.5% (10).

More recent studies of unstable angina in general have a shorter period of follow-up. The advent of safe and effective procedures such as percutaneous transluminal coronary angioplasty and coronary artery bypass surgery has led to stabilization and early mechanical intervention in patients with unstable angina. It is necessary, therefore, to examine the available evidence concerning the prognosis of unstable angina in the context of the time period in which the studies were conducted.

Coronary Artery Bypass Surgery

In the late 1960s, the technology required for coronary angiography became widely available. Published series in patients with chronic stable angina estimated the incidence of one-, two-, and three-vessel coronary artery disease at approximately 45%, 25%, and 20%, respectively (16). In patients with unstable angina, the degree of coronary artery disease was judged to be more severe and more heavily weighted toward three-vessel coronary disease (13). In this same time period, coronary bypass surgery and myocardial protection had progressed to the point where surgery could be performed on "unstable patients." With these technological developments in mind, the National Heart, Lung, and Blood Institute conducted a multicenter prospective, randomized study comparing intensive medical therapy and urgent coronary bypass surgery. Two hundred and eighty-eight patients were randomized to either medical or surgical therapy. The difference in mortality between the medical and surgical groups was not statistically significant (3% and 5%, respectively). Initially, the rate of myocardial infarction was found to be significantly higher in the surgical group (11% vs. 8%), although in the last 2 years of the study, possibly because of advances in surgical technique, the rate of myocardial infarction between the medical and surgical groups became equal (5). A subsequent subgroup analysis examining the 202 patients with single-vessel left anterior descending coronary artery disease revealed a 23% incidence of myocardial infarction in the surgical group compared to 9% in the medical group (17). In the first year after therapy, 42% of the medically treated patients experienced New York Heart Association Class III or IV angina, as compared with only 13% of those patients treated surgically (17). Therefore, in patients with unstable angina, coronary artery surgery did not diminish early mortality but was associated with greater relief of angina than medical therapy during the first year of follow-up.

These findings were subsequently supported by Selden et al., who randomized 40 patients with unstable angina to medical or surgical therapy. Obviously, too few patients were studied to provide information about mortality, but surgically treated patients were found to have a better functional class, better anginal threshold in response to pacing, and greater myocardial lactate extraction (18). It seemed, therefore, that coronary bypass surgery held some advantage in the relief of symptoms and ischemia when compared to medical therapy alone.

In 1976 Bertolasi et al. compared medical versus surgical therapy in 113 patients, which suggested that revascularization conferred some protection against both death and nonfatal myocardial infarction (19). Patients treated medically experienced a 46% mortality and 38% rate of myocardial infarction compared with rates of 11% and 14%, respectively, in the surgically treated group over a 32-month follow-up period. It should be noted that in this study there was no strict randomization and the surgically treated group had better left ventricular function.

In 1983 Rahimtoola et al. (13) reported a series of 1282 patients with unstable angina treated with revascularization surgery (Fig. 1). The patients had a cumulative operative mortality of 1.8%. This represented the composite of an operative mortality between 1970 and 1973 of 2.5%, which then fell between 1974 and 1982 to 1.7%. The cumulative 5- and 10-year survival rates were 92% and 83%, respectively (Fig. 1). Approximately 61% of the patient population were symptom-free at 10 years, and 25% were considered minimally symptomatic. The rate of reoperation was 17% at 10 years. An association between abnormal left ventricular function and diminished survival was not demonstrated.

These observations contrasted sharply with those of DeServi et al. (20). In this study, 217 medically treated patients with unstable angina were followed for 3 years. There were 41 deaths representing a 3-year mortality of 21%. Subsequent analysis using the Cox proportional hazard model revealed three independent predictors of a poor outcome, which were, in order of significance, left ventricular end-diastolic pressure, left main coronary artery disease, and the number of diseased coronary arteries.

The influence of left ventricular function on mortality in patients with unstable angina was subsequently examined in the Veteran's Administration Cooperative Study (10). In the 6-year period between 1976 and 1982, 486 patients were enrolled and underwent cardiac catheterization at entry and at one year. One hundred and thirty-four patients had abnormal left ventricular function as defined by an ejection fraction less than 0.50 or a left ventricular end diastolic pressure greater than 16 mmHg. The 3-year mortality in the group treated surgically was 6.1% in comparison to a mortality of 17.6% in the medically treated group. This represented a 65% reduction in mortality that reached statistical significance. In subsequent subgroup analysis, surgery conferred a survival advantage in patients with an ejection fraction less than 0.49, while their counterparts with normal left ventricular function demonstrated no significant difference with medical or surgical therapy (Fig. 2). In addition, the rate of rehospital-

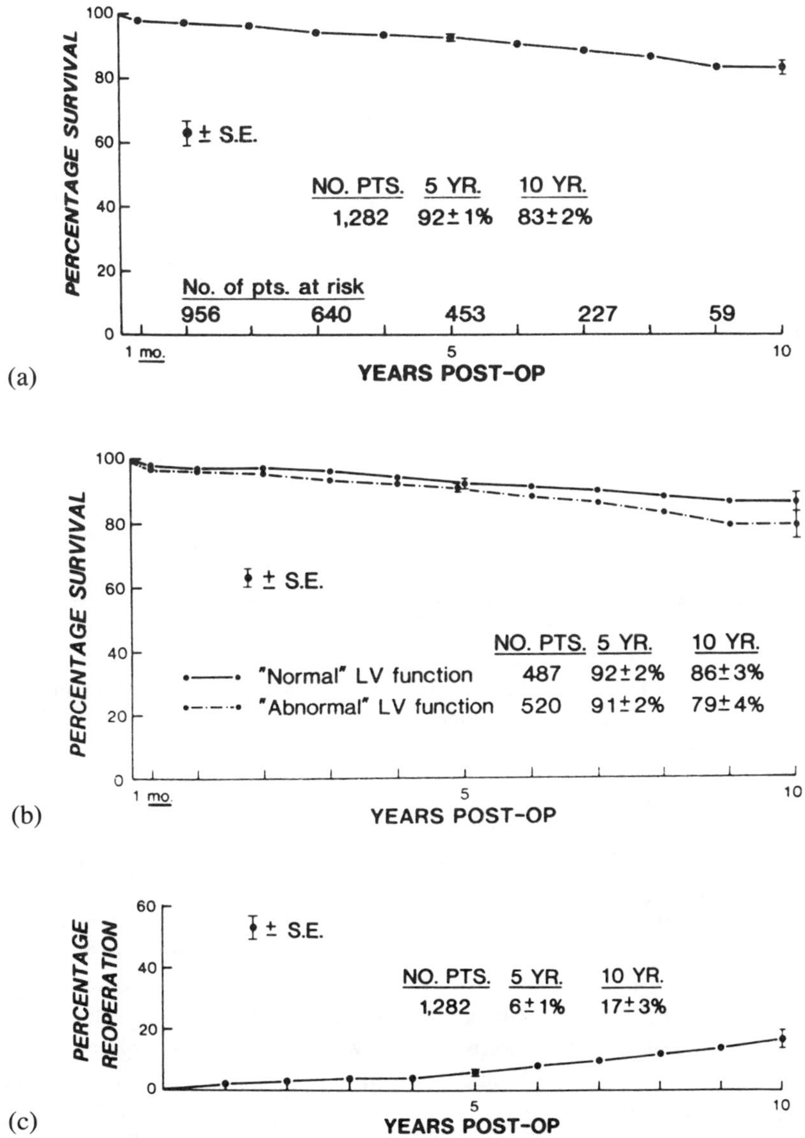

Figure 1 Cumulative survival and reoperation in 1282 patients with unstable angina treated with coronary bypass surgery. (a) Actuarial survival over 10 years for patients undergoing coronary bypass surgery for unstable angina. (b) Survival after bypass surgery as predicted based on left ventricular function (normal = LVEDP ≤15 mmHg *and* normal LV angiogram; abnormal = either LVEDP ≥15 mmHg *or* abnormal LV angiogram). (c) Cumulative rate of reoperation in patients treated surgically for unstable angina. (Adapted from Ref. 13 with permission.)

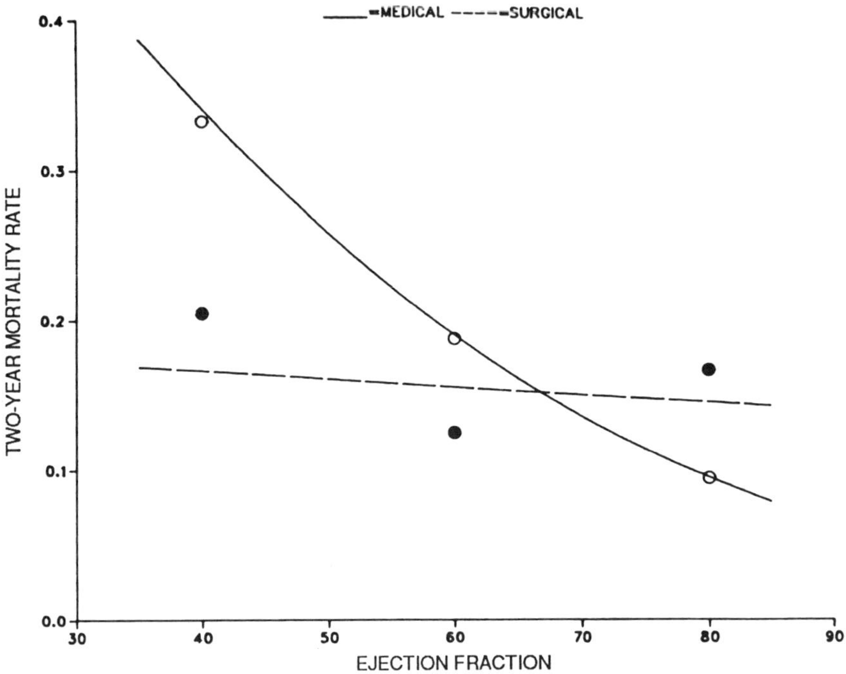

Figure 2 Mortality following surgical and medical treatment of unstable angina as a function of left ventricular ejection fraction. Impaired left ventricular ejection fraction is associated with a poor prognosis in medically treated patients suggesting that surgery should be recommended for patients with unstable angina and reduced ejection fraction because it improves survival. (From Ref. 21, with permission.)

ization for cardiac events was significantly less in the surgically treated patients. The rate of myocardial infarction in the two groups was similar, but perioperative infarctions comprised approximately two thirds of all infarctions in the surgical patients.

Data concerning the long-term survival of patients with unstable angina in response to surgical versus medical therapy have been difficult to determine. This is largely due to the rate of crossover between medical and surgical therapy in large-scale studies, e.g., 34% at 2 years in the VA Cooperative Study. If the operative mortality exceeds 2% for patients with unstable angina, the benefits of surgery for those with diminished left ventricular function are doubtful. On balance, patients with unstable angina and diminished left ventricular function will have improved survival with surgical therapy (10,19,21) compared to standard medical therapy.

Electrocardiographic Characteristics

Different electrocardiographic patterns associated with unstable angina (Table 2) have been observed. In the National Cooperative Study (22), 27% of the 288

Table 2 ECG Patterns in Unstable Angina with Associated In-hospital (≤1 Month), Early (<6 Months), and Late (>6Months) Mortality

Study	rx	*n*	ECG	Mortality (%)			MI (%)		
				Hosp	Early	Late	Hosp	Early	Late
National Co-op (22)	CABG	37	ST ↑ + CP	5.4	—	—	14	—	—
1980	Med	42		4.8	—	—	12	—	—
de Zwaan et al. (23)	Med	16	V_2V_3 TWI	18.7**	—	—	75	—	—
1982	CABG	10		0	—	—	10	—	—
Scarlovsky et al. (25)	Med	19	ST ↑ + CP	5.3**	—	—	100	—	—
1986	Med	13	ST ↓ + CP	77	—	—	100	—	—
de Zwaan et al. (24)	CABG	124	V_2V_3 TWI	2.5	1.7	0.8	5	5.2	8
1989	Med	54		2.5	3.5	14.8*	5	3.5	27*

*$p \leq 0.05$; **$p \leq 0.01$.
Hosp = ≤1 month; Early = ≤6 months; Late = ≥6 months; TWI = T-wave inversion; CP = chest pain.

patients experienced chest pain at rest with transient ST-segment elevation on the electrocardiogram. These patients were also characterized by a fixed, obstructive coronary lesion of ≥70% in one or more coronary arteries. These patients had a myocardial infarction rate of 12% and 14% with medical and surgical therapy, respectively, and the mortality rate was not significantly different. In patients with transient ST-segment depression or T-wave inversion on the electrocardiogram, no significant differences in myocardial infarction rate or mortality were found between treatment groups. These findings led the authors to speculate that patients presenting with unstable angina and ST elevation should be treated in the same manner as those presenting with different electrocardiographic patterns.

In 1982 de Zwaan et al. described a series of 145 consecutive patients admitted to the coronary care unit with the diagnosis of unstable angina (23). They reported an ECG pattern of precordial T-wave inversions which identified a subgroup of patients at high risk for subsequent myocardial infarction and death (Fig. 3). This electrocardiographic pattern was found in 18% of their patient population, and, over the course of several weeks, 10 out of 26 patients ultimately underwent coronary bypass surgery with no in-hospital deaths and a 10% incidence of in-hospital myocardial infarction. In 12 of 16 patients (75%) treated medically, an extensive anterior myocardial infarction developed, which was associated with an in-hospital mortality of approximately 19%.

The prognostic importance of anterior T-wave inversions in the setting of unstable angina was subsequently confirmed by the same authors in 1989 (24). Between 1980 and 1985, 204 patients with unstable angina and a typical pattern of anterior T-wave inversions were examined. This group represented approximately 14% of all patients hospitalized with the diagnosis of unstable angina in a single institution. Patients were followed for approximately 4.2 years, and all patients underwent coronary angiography. All patients demonstrated abnormalities in the left anterior descending coronary artery ranging from stenoses of 50% to total occlusions. Left ventricular angiography revealed wall motion abnormalities related to the left anterior descending coronary artery in 76% of patients. It would seem, then, that patients presenting with unstable angina and anterior T-wave inversions have a high likelihood of left anterior descending coronary artery disease and subsequent myocardial infarction. In this series, the presentation of unstable angina with anterior T-wave inversions carried a high rate of nonfatal MI (27%) and death (14.8%) when treated medically.

Patients who exhibit ST changes during chest pain, particularly ST-segment depression, appear to have an adverse prognosis in at least two studies. In the study of Gazes et al. (4), patients who presented with both chest pain and ischemic ST-segment depression had a 12-month mortality of 43% and a 10-year mortality of 81%. In addition, this group had an extremely high rate of myocardial infarction (34%) at only 12 weeks. These findings were substantiated in a much smaller study by Scarlovsky et al. (25), where patients presenting with unstable angina, ST-segment depression, and developing signs of myocardial infarction experienced a mortality of 77%.

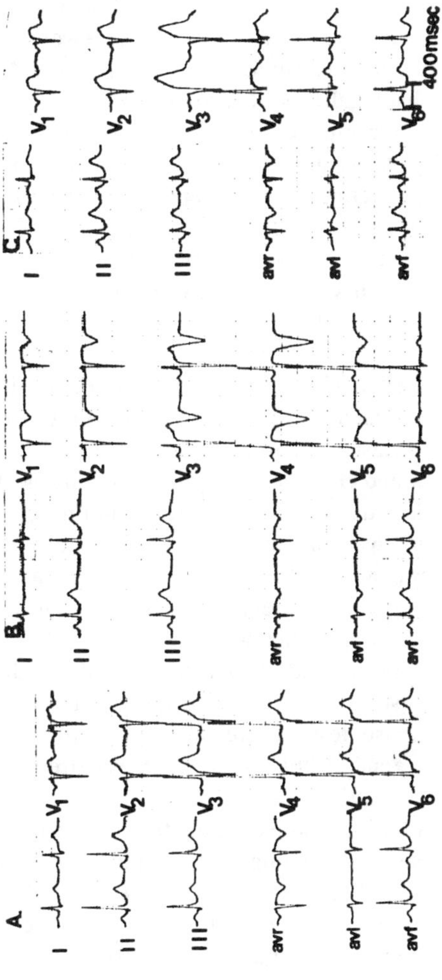

Figure 3 ECG pattern associated with LAD stenosis. Tracings obtained from a patient admitted with unstable angina. (A) ECG recorded on admission. (B) ECG obtained 23 hours after admission. Nine days after admission, the patient suffered intractable chest pain unresponsive to nitroglycerin, and ECG is shown in (C). The patient eventually succumbed to pump failure; post-mortem revealed proximal occlusion of the LAD. (Adapted from Ref. 24 with permission.)

Exercise Testing

In addition to the resting electrocardiogram, early exercise testing can provide important prognostic information after patients with unstable angina have been stabilized. Butman et al. (26) studied the value of early exercise testing in 78 such patients. Forty-six percent of the patients developed a positive exercise tolerance test as manifested by angina and/or ST-segment depression associated with exercise. In patients with a positive exercise test, 92% were found to have multivessel coronary artery disease on angiography, while only 43% of those patients with a negative test had multivessel disease. In the final analysis, the sensitivity of exercise testing for multivessel disease was 65% with an 89% specificity, allowing a 92% positive predictive value. In this series, exercise testing was also important in detecting those patients at risk for an unfavorable outcome. Using a definition of "unfavorable outcome" as NYHA Class III or IV angina, unstable angina, coronary artery surgery, myocardial infarction, or death, the authors found that patients with a positive exercise test after unstable angina were 2½ times more likely (83% vs. 33%) to experience an unfavorable outcome.

Swahn et al. (27) performed a similar study in 276 men with suspected unstable angina who were first treated for 2–7 days in the coronary care unit and then subjected to an exercise test. Major endpoints included cardiac death, Q-wave myocardial infarction, and coronary artery bypass grafting. It was found that the presence of ST-segment depression, symptom-limiting chest pain, and the magnitude of cardiac work were all independent predictors of subsequent coronary events (Table 3). For example, the occurrence of myocardial infarction or cardiac death was 10.6% in those patients with ST-segment depression or chest pain compared to 2.8% in patients without these findings. Likewise, coronary bypass surgery was performed in one third of those demonstrating ST-segment depression or chest pain on exercise testing, but in only 2% of patients with a negative exercise test. There were no complications of the exercise testing per se, and, in general, this procedure was extremely safe in this patient population.

Severi et al. (28) took the additional step of using the combination of a resting electrocardiogram and exercise stress testing as a prognostic tool in a study of 374 patients with unstable angina. Patients enrolled in the study were required to have a history of angina at rest with evidence of transient ST-T changes on the electrocardiogram during episodes of angina. Patients were then grouped in a two-by-two design according to normal or abnormal ECG and negative or positive exercise stress tests. Using baseline electrocardiographic criteria alone, survival at 8 years in those patients with a normal electrocardiogram was 98%, while those patients with an abnormal electrocardiogram had a cumulative 8-year survival of 79%. This trend was duplicated when using the exercise test as a discriminating factor. For any given electrocardiographic category, the prognosis

Table 3 The Prognostic Importance of Exercise Test Variables in Predicting Coronary Bypass Surgery, Myocardial Infarction, and Death

	Simple correlation		Multiple regression		
Exercise test criteria	*r*	*p*	*B*	*t*	*p*
ST depression					
ST max	0.490	<0.001	0.11	7.13	<0.001
No. of leads	0.471	<0.001			
Pain-limiting exercise	0.400	<0.001	0.19	3.70	<0.001
Intensity	0.346	<0.001			
Cardiac work					
△ Systolic BP from rest to exercise	–0.219	<0.001			
Maximum heart rate	–0.301	<0.001			
Maximum rate pressure product	–0.287	<0.001	-0.27×10^{-5}	–2.54	<0.05
Peak work load	–0.288	<0.001			

The presence of ST-segment depression, symptom-limited chest pain, and the peak rate-pressure product are all independent predictors of subsequent cardiac events.
Source: Ref. 27 with permission.

was worse in the setting of a positive exercise tolerance test. These findings were supported when the endpoint of coronary bypass surgery was used. Patients with abnormal electrocardiograms and positive exercise tests were more likely to require coronary artery surgery than those with normal stress tests and normal electrocardiograms.

The findings contained in these three studies are not surprising. Patients with normal electrocardiograms have, on balance, better left ventricular function (28), lower incidence of previous myocardial infarction (10), and are less likely to have multivessel coronary artery disease and generally exhibit a greater degree of myocardial flow reserve (26).

Silent Ischemia

Over the last 10 years, the availability of continuous electrocardiographic monitoring has provided significant insights into the correlation between angina as a symptom and myocardial ischemia as an electrocardiographic abnormality. Patients with unstable angina are now known to have a significant degree of silent myocardial ischemia (Fig. 4) (29). It is estimated that up to 50% of patients admitted to the coronary care unit with a clinical diagnosis of unstable angina may have some degree of silent ischemia as well (15). In addition, patients with unstable angina may experience silent episodes of ischemia that could comprise

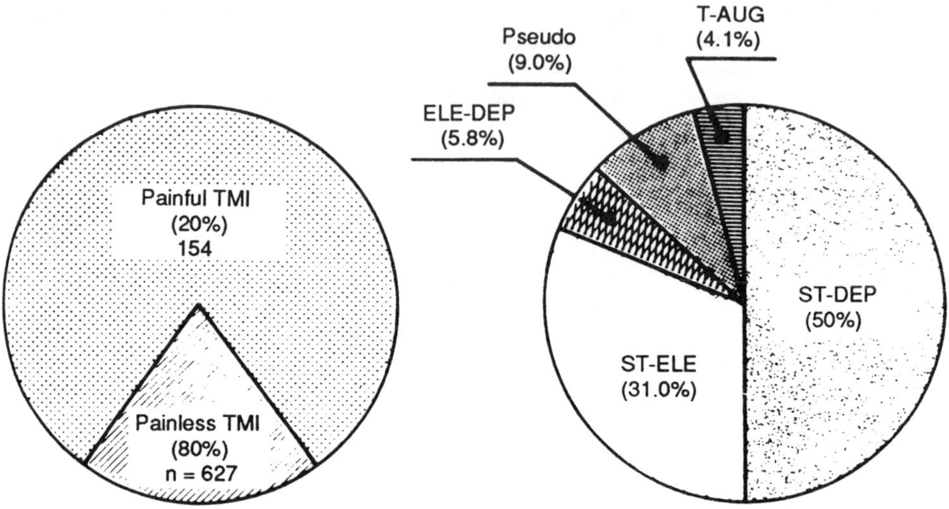

Figure 4 The relative frequency and types of electrocardiographic abnormalities associated with symptomatic and asymptomatic transient myocardial ischemia (TMI) in patients with unstable angina. The most common abnormality is ST-segment depression. T-AUG = T-wave augmentation; pseudo = pseudonormalization of ST-T wave changes; ST-DEP = ST depression; ST-ELE = ST elevation. Therefore, up to 80% of all ischemic episodes in unstable angina may be painless (silent). (Adapted from Ref. 29 with permission.)

up to 90% of all ischemic episodes (15,29). In 1982 Johnson et al. (30) examined the utility of continuous Holter monitoring in 116 patients admitted to the coronary care unit with the diagnosis of unstable angina pectoris. After excluding 24 patients who evolved an acute myocardial infarction during monitoring, 92 patients underwent an average of 21 ± 7 hours of continuous Holter monitoring. Twenty-one patients (23%) were noted to have ST alterations on monitoring, and these patients were compared to the remaining 71 (77%) individuals with no evidence of ST alterations. Patients were followed throughout the course of their hospitalization and for 3 months after hospital discharge (Fig. 5) (30). Patients found to have ST alterations on Holter monitoring were far more likely to have coronary artery disease (94% vs. 58%) or suffer death, myocardial infarction, or severe Class III to IV angina. Unfortunately, these authors did not note the relative proportions of silent versus clinically evident angina, and, therefore, this study is more representative of the degree of active ischemia than of silent ischemia per se. In 1986 Gottlieb et al. addressed this issue more completely in a study of 70 patients with unstable angina (15). These patients were treated in a customary fashion with the exception of continuous electrocardiographic recordings throughout the first 2 days in the coronary care unit. Patients were then divided into either of two groups based on the presence of absence of silent ischemia on continuous monitoring. The first group consisted of 37 patients

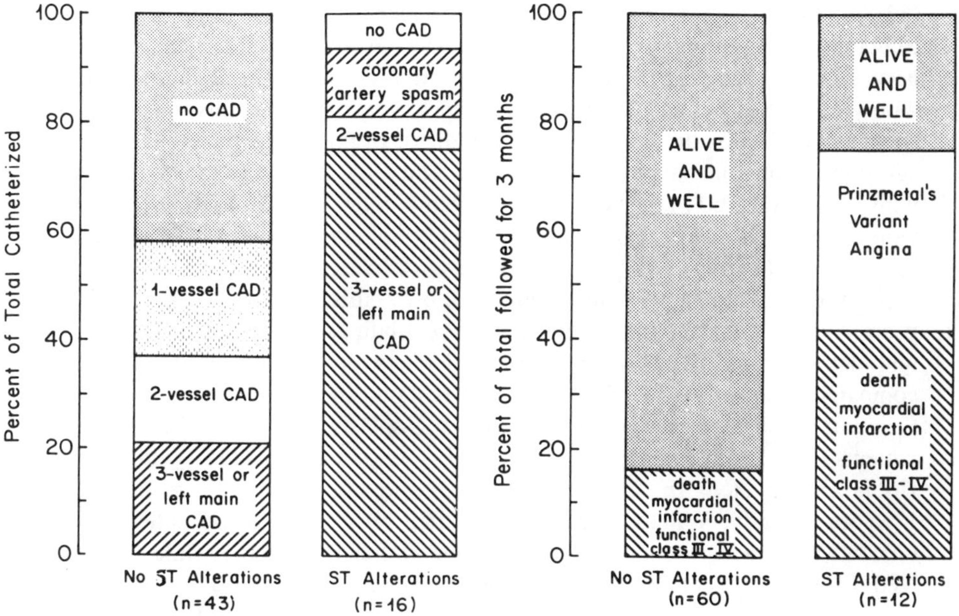

(A) (B)

Figure 5 Findings at cardiac catheterization (A) and the clinical course (B) of patients admitted for unstable angina with and without ST segment alterations on Holter monitoring. Patients with ST alterations were more likely to have severe coronary disease. (B) The clinical course in these patients with (right) and without (left) ST-segment alterations on Holter monitoring after 3 months' follow-up. Death, myocardial infarction, or severe angina was present in 17% of patients without ST changes and 42% of those with ST changes ($p = 0.05$). (Adapted from Ref. 30 with permission.)

(52.8%) with at least one episode of silent ischemia. This group with silent ischemia had significantly higher rates of both myocardial infarction and coronary bypass surgery (16% and 21%, respectively) compared to those patients without silent ischemia (3% and 9%, respectively) (15). In this small study, silent ischemia was the most powerful predictor of poor outcome at 30 days. In addition, among the patients with silent ischemia, the authors found that patients with greater than 60 minutes of silent ischemia in any one 24-hour period had a worse prognosis than patients with less than 20 minutes of silent ischemia in the same period (15).

Gottlieb and colleagues subsequently followed this series of 70 patients for 2 years, further substantiating their short-term findings (31). Of the 37 patients with demonstrable silent ischemia, 10 (27%) developed a myocardial infarction compared with only one of the 33 (3%) without silent ischemia ($p < 0.01$). Coronary bypass surgery or percutaneous angioplasty was required in 11 of 37 patients (28%) with silent ischemia and only 5 of 33 patients (15%) with normal Holter examinations ($p < 0.05$).

More recently, Wilcox et al. (32) reported on a series of 66 patients with unstable angina who underwent continuous Holter monitoring while hospitalized. Episodes of silent ischemia were demonstrated in approximately 11% of the study patients and 70% of all ischemic episodes were noted to be silent. The presence of ischemia on Holter monitor examination possessed a 92% specificity and 25% sensitivity for the combined endpoints of coronary bypass surgery, death, and nonfatal myocardial infarction. Recurrent rest pain alone, however, was 100% sensitive and 49% specific for the same endpoints. It is clear that persistent silent ischemia on ST monitoring of patients with unstable angina does depict an adverse short-term and longer-term clinical outcome. It still remains to be determined whether silent ischemia is contributory to an adverse clinical outcome or is a surrogate marker of patients with more extensive and unstable coronary artery disease.

PROGNOSIS ASSOCIATED WITH THERAPY

The prognostic implications of multiple clinical and diagnostic variables have been discussed and the prognostic implications of the many therapies available for unstable angina will now be reviewed.

For many years, the only available therapy for both chronic and acute coronary artery disease were organic nitrates. Organic nitrates have been shown to be widely effective in the relief of symptoms associated with chronic stable angina so their use in unstable angina seemed obvious. Mulcahy et al. (14) published a series of 101 consecutive cases of unstable angina between the years of 1980 and 1982. This represented 18% of all coronary care unit admissions, and therapy with beta-blockers, calcium channel blockers, and anticoagulants were specifically avoided. Results were reported in terms of early (20-day) and late (1-year) endpoints. In this series, the rates of early and late nonfatal myocardial infarction were 9% and 14%, respectively, while the early and late survival rates were 1% and 9%, respectively. While the results of this observational unrandomized study must be interpreted with some caution, the rates of nonfatal myocardial infarction and death compare favorably with many studies in which the therapy was much more aggressive (9,10,17,21,23,33).

Intravenous nitroglycerin is highly effective in relieving symptoms of chest pain in patients with unstable angina but has yet to demonstrate any effect on survival (34–36). However, meta-analyses of patient population treated with intravenous nitroglycerin for acute myocardial infarction suggest a mortality reduction of 10–30% (37). Therefore, organic nitrates appear to be effective in alleviating the symptoms of unstable angina, but at this time it has not been demonstrated that they affect the prognosis of unstable angina.

Beta-blockers have become the mainstay in the treatment of chronic stable angina. Their use in the treatment of unstable angina pectoris has been less common. The pathophysiology of chronic stable angina is thought to lie in the inability to match coronary oxygen delivery to increases in myocardial oxygen demand. In many patients with unstable angina, however, the primary defect may in fact be related to spontaneous reductions in coronary flow (38). Studies examining the effects of beta-blockers in patients with unstable angina have been inconclusive. Uncontrolled studies have suggested some benefit of beta-blockade when used as monotherapy (38), while randomized trials have failed to report any difference between nitrates and propranolol compared with diltiazem (39) or nifedipine (40) in unstable angina.

In 1986 Gottlieb et al. (41) reported on the effect of propranolol as an addition to therapy with nifedipine with unstable angina pectoris. They studied 81 patients with unstable angina treated with nifedipine in and subsequently randomized to receive propranolol or a placebo. There was no significant effect of propranolol on the incidence of cardiac death, myocardial infarction, or requirement for bypass surgery, although there was a significant effect of propranolol on the number and duration of ischemic episodes and the consumption of nitroglycerin (Fig. 6).

In a similar fashion, any effect of calcium channel blockers on mortality in patients with unstable angina has been difficult to obtain. Just as with beta-blockers, calcium channel blockers reduce the number of ischemic episodes in patients with unstable angina but do not significantly alter the rates of myocardial infarction or death (7,39,40).

Nitrates, calcium channel blockers, and beta-blockers all possess antianginal properties that are due in some measure to a reduction in myocardial oxygen demand. It is this characteristic that renders them effective in the treatment of chronic stable angina. Unstable angina often appears to be a disorder of myocar-

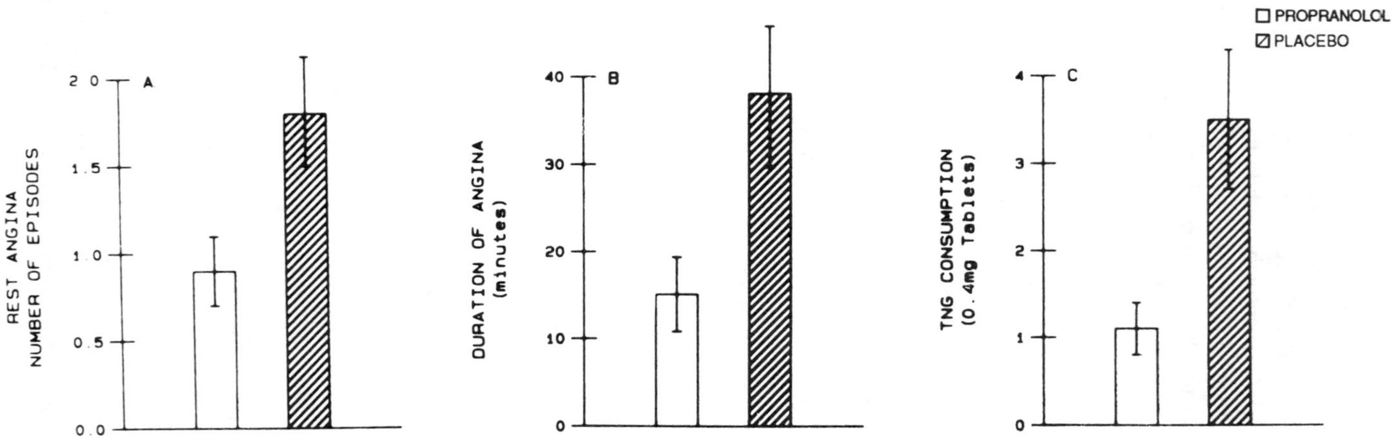

Figure 6 The effect of propranolol on anginal frequency, duration, and nitroglycerin consumption in unstable angina pectoris. (A) Total number of episodes of rest angina during a 48-hour period; propranolol vs. placebo ($p = 0.012$). (B) The duration (minutes) of anginal episodes during a 48-hour period; propranolol vs. placebo ($p = 0.016$). (C) The effect of propranolol therapy on nitroglycerin consumption during a 48-hour period ($p = 0.012$). Therefore, propranolol is effective in reducing the anginal frequency, duration, and nitroglycerin consumption in unstable angina. (Adapted from Ref. 41 with permission.)

dial oxygen supply. Recent pathologic studies have revealed that rupture of an atherosclerotic plaque plays a central role in the development of unstable angina (43). The disrupted atherosclerotic plaque serves as a local stimulus for the recruitment of platelets, activation of thrombin, and subsequent development of thrombus. It is probably this localized environment of platelets, activated thrombin, and clotbound thrombin that serves as a stimulus for further platelet activation and recruitment of thrombus (43). The central role of activated platelets in the pathophysiology of unstable angina is supported by the detection of thromboxane metabolites in the urine of patients during episodes of active ischemia (44).

Fibrinopeptide A is a small peptide produced by the proteolytic cleavage of fibrinogen to fibrin by the enzyme thrombin. Theroux et al. (45) examined 16 consecutive patients with unstable angina and 15 patients with stable angina who were matched for clinical variables. They found that in patients with unstable angina the circulating concentration of fibrinopeptide A was markedly elevated prompting them to conclude that unstable angina is characterized by a relative activation of thrombin and the coagulation system.

Several studies have now addressed the issue of both platelet activation and intravascular thrombus in the setting of unstable angina. The Veterans Administration Cooperative Study of aspirin in unstable angina initiated in 1974 was the first study to directly examine aspirin in unstable angina (8). The principal endpoints were acute myocardial infarction and death at 3 months. The combined endpoints of nonfatal MI and death occurred in 10.1% of the placebo group and 5% of the aspirin group representing a 51% reduction. Nonfatal myocardial infarction was 51% lower in the aspirin group (3.4% vs. 6.9%) (Table 4).

A subsequent study published in 1985 by Cairns et al. examined therapy with aspirin, sulfinpyrazone, both therapies, or neither (9). Patients were enrolled within 8 days of hospitalization and the follow-up period lasted approximately 2 years. Treatment with aspirin afforded a 51% reduction in the incidence of cardiac death and nonfatal MI (8.6% vs. 17.0%). In addition, there was a 71% risk reduction for cardiac death in the groups given aspirin. The authors were unable to find any observed benefit for sulfinpyrazone treatment.

Inhibition of thrombin can be achieved indirectly by administration of heparin, which serves as a cofactor for the enzyme antithrombin III, which subsequently neutralizes thrombin. A number of clinical studies employing heparin for the treatment of unstable angina have been performed. Telford and Wilson conducted a study using heparin and atenolol in patients with unstable angina (6). In all, 214 patients were enrolled and randomized to treatment with heparin, atenolol, both, or neither. The incidence of myocardial infarction in those patients treated with heparin was 3%, compared with an incidence of 15% in patients not treated with heparin. Heparin was given as a 5000-unit intravenous dose every 6 hours. There was no observable benefit with atenolol treatment. This study is difficult to interpret because of the 400 patients entered 186 were

Table 4 Frequency Distribution of Death and Acute Myocardial Infarction During the 12-Week Study Period in 1266 Patients with Unstable Angina

	No. of Patients[a]				
Event	Placebo (n = 641)	Aspirin (n = 625)	Reduction in Aspirin Group (%)	p-Value Unadjusted	p-Value Adjusted[b]
Death or acute myocardial infarction	65 (10.1)	31 (5.0)	51	0.0005	0.0002
Fatal or nonfatal acute myocardial infarction	50 (7.8)	22 (3.5)	55	0.001	0.0003
Nonfatal acute myocardial infarction	44 (6.9)	21 (3.4)	51	0.005	0.002
Death	21 (3.3)	10 (1.6)	51	0.054	0.059

[a]Figures in parentheses represent percentage of group.
[b]Adjusted for baseline characteristics, using logistic regression model.
Source: Ref. 8 with permission.

withdrawn because of incorrect recruitment. A recent study by Theroux et al. examined the effect of both aspirin and heparin in the treatment of unstable angina (11). Four hundred and seventy-nine patients were enrolled in the double-blind, randomized, placebo-controlled trial and treated with aspirin (325 mg/day), heparin (1000 units/hr), or both. Patients were enrolled an average of 8 hours after hospitalization, and the study lasted 6 days (Table 5). The rate of myocardial infarction in patients treated with either aspirin, heparin, or their combination was 4%, 1%, and 2%, respectively. This is to be contrasted with the

Table 5 Endpoints in Unstable Angina Trial

		Myocardial infarction		Refractory angina	
Treatment	n	n	p	n	p
Placebo	118	14		27	
ASA	121	4	0.012	20	0.217
Heparin	118	1	<0.001	10	0.002
ASA + heparin	122	2	0.001	13	0.011

Source: Ref. 11 with permission.

14% rate of myocardial infarction in patients treated with placebo. Recurrent angina, however, was significantly reduced only in those patients treated with heparin. The size of the study precludes any specific direct comparisons between heparin and aspirin, or any comment on the effect of therapy on mortality.

Clinical trials addressing the use of thrombolytic agents in the treatment of unstable angina have been largely disappointing. Some angiographic studies have demonstrated resolution of intracoronary thrombus with thrombolytic therapy, but clinical studies utilizing thrombolytic therapy in the setting of unstable angina have not as yet had sufficient power to demonstrate any significant benefit (46).

CONCLUSIONS

Unstable angina is a common clinical problem with a diverse range of clinical presentations. Patients usually present with some combination of angina at rest or a history of rapidly progressing angina in a setting of shorter periods of activity. Patients presenting with unstable angina generally have electrocardiographic evidence of myocardial ischemia as evidenced by ST-segment depression, T-wave inversion, or, less commonly, ST-segment elevation. Early longitudinal studies demonstrated a very high incidence of both nonfatal myocardial infarction and death.

In patients presenting with unstable angina, the presence of moderate or severe left ventricular dysfunction is associated with an adverse prognosis. In these patients, surgery seems the best alternative given the results of the Veterans Administration Cooperative Study in which patients with unstable angina and left ventricular dysfunction had improved survival after coronary artery bypass grafting compared with medically treated patients. There is also evidence to suggest that the presence of left main coronary artery disease and the percentage of myocardium at risk from diseased vessels is also correlated with an adverse prognosis.

In patients presenting with unstable angina, the presence of T-wave inversions in the anterior precordial leads is highly predictive of a high-grade lesion in the left anterior descending coronary artery. Inferential evidence from a number of studies suggests that these patients require aggressive therapy if myocardial infarction and death are to be avoided. In those patients who stabilize on medical therapy, exercise testing allows for the identification of patients at high risk for subsequent infarction. Furthermore, the presence of multiple ischemic episodes on continuous electrocardiographic monitoring is also a harbinger of a poor prognosis.

In addition to standard therapy with oxygen, sedatives, beta-blockers, nitrates, and calcium channel blockers, it appears that treatment with either aspirin or heparin is particularly effective in preventing mortality, nonfatal MI, and the need for coronary bypass surgery. The role of thrombolytic therapy in the treatment of unstable angina remains to be determined.

In those patients who fail to stabilize with medical therapy, percutaneous transluminal coronary angioplasty and coronary artery bypass surgery remain the most effective therapies for alleviation of symptoms.

REFERENCES

1. Graybiel A. The intermediate coronary syndrome. U.S.N. School of Aviation Medicine Research, Project No. NM 001 0059, 06, 09, September 15, 1954.
2. Vakil RJ. Intermediate coronary syndrome. Circulation 1961; 24:557–71.
3. Levy H. The natural history of changing patterns of angina pectoris. Ann Intern Med 1956; 44:1123–35.
4. Gazes PC, Mobley EM, Faris HM, Duncan RC, Humphries GB. Preinfarction (unstable) angina—a prospective study—ten-year followup. Circulation 1973; 48:331–7.
5. National Cooperative Study Group to Compare Surgery and Medical Therapy. II. In-hospital experience and initial follow-up results in patients with one-, two-, and three-vessel disease. Am J Cardiol 1978; 42:839–48.
6. Telford AM, Wilson C. Trial of heparin versus atenolol in prevention of myocardial infarction in intermediate coronary syndrome. Lancet 1981; 1:1225–8.
7. Gerstenblith G, Ouyang P, Achuff S, et al. Nifedipine in unstable angina. A double-blind, randomized trial. N Engl J Med 1982; 306:885–9.
8. Lewis HD, Davis JW, Archibald DG, et al. Protective effects of aspirin against acute myocardial infarction and death in men with unstable angina: results of a Veterans Administration Cooperative Study. N Engl J Med 1983; 309:396–403.
9. Cairns, JA, Gent M, Singer J, et al. Aspirin, sulfinpyrazone, or both in unstable angina: results of a Canadian multicenter trial. N Engl J Med 1985; 313:1369–75.
10. Scott SM, Luchi RJ, Deupree RH, and the Veterans Administration Unstable Angina Cooperative Study Group. Veterans Administration Cooperative Study for treatment of patients with unstable angina. Circulation 1988; 78(Suppl I):113–121.
11. Théroux P, Ouimet H, McCans J, et al. Aspirin, heparin, or both to treat acute unstable angina. N Engl J Med 1988; 319:1105–11.
12. Harris PJ, Lee KI, Harrell FE Jr, Behar VS, Rosati RA. Outcome in medically treated coronary artery disease: ischemic events: nonfatal infarction and death. Circulation 1980; 62:718–26.
13. Rahimtoola SH, Nunley D, Grunkemeier G, Tepley J, Lambert L, Starr A. Ten-year survival after coronary bypass surgery for unstable angina. N Engl J Med 1983; 308:676–81.
14. Mulcahy R, Awadi AHA, de Buitleor M, Tobin G, Johnson H, Contoy R. Natural history and prognosis of unstable angina. Am Heart J 1985; 109:753–8.
15. Gottlieb SO, Weisfeldt ML, Ouyang P, Mellits ED, Gerstenblith G. Silent ischemia as a marker for early unfavorable outcomes in patients with unstable angina. N Engl J Med 1986; 314:1214–19.

16. Rahimtoola S. Coronary bypass surgery for unstable angina. Circulation 1984; 69:842–8.
17. National Cooperative Study Group to Compare Medical and Surgical Therapy. IV. Results in patients with left anterior descending coronary artery disease. Am J Cardiol 1981; 48:517–24.
18. Selden R, Neill WA, Ritzmann LW, Okies JE, Anderson RP. Medical versus surgical therapy for acute coronary insufficiency: a randomized study. N Engl J Med 1975; 293:1329–33.
19. Bertolasi CA, Tronge JE, Ricitelli MA, Villamayor RM, Zuffardi E. Natural history of unstable angina with medical or surgical therapy. Chest 1976; 70:596–605.
20. DeServi S, Berzuini C, Poma E, et al. Long-term survival and risk stratification in patients with angina at rest undergoing medical treatment. Intl J Cardiol 1989; 22:43–50.
21. Luchi RJ, Scott SM, Deupree RH, et al. Comparison of medical and surgical treatment for unstable angina pectoris: results of a Veterans Administration Cooperative Study. N Engl J Med 1987; 316:977–84.
22. National Cooperative Study Group to Compare Surgical and Medical Therapy. III. Results in patients with ST-T segment elevation during pain. Am J Cardiol 1980; 45:819–24.
23. de Zwaan C, Bär FWHM, Wellens HJJ. Characteristic electrocardiographic pattern indicating a critical stenosis high in left anterior descending coronary artery in patients admitted because of impending myocardial infarction. Am Heart J 1982; 103:730–6.
24. de Zwaan C, Bär FW, Janssen JHA, et al. Angiographic and clinical characteristics of patients with unstable angina showing an ECG pattern indicating critical narrowing of the proximal LAD coronary artery. Am Heart J 1989; 117:657–65.
25. Scarlovsky S, Davidson E, Strasberg B, Lewin RF, Arditti A, Wurtzel M, Agmon J. Unstable angina: the significant of ST-segment elevation or depression in patients without evidence of increased myocardial oxygen demand. Am Heart J 1986; 112:463–7.
26. Butman SM, Olson HG, Butman LK. Early exercise testing after stabilization of unstable angina: correlation with coronary angiographic findings and subsequent cardiac events. Am Heart J 1986; 111:11–18.
27. Swahn E, Areskog M, Wallentin L. Prognostic importance of early exercise testing in men with suspected unstable coronary artery disease. Eur Heart J 1987; 8:861–9.
28. Severi S, Orsini E, Marraccini P, Michelassi C, L'Abbate A. The basal electrocardiogram and the exercise stress test in assessing prognosis in patients with unstable angina. Eur Heart J 1988; 9:441–6.
29. Singh BN, Nademanee K. Prevalence and prognostic significance of silent myocardial ischemia in patients with unstable angina. Circulation 1987; 75(Suppl II):40–42.
30. Johnson SM, Mauritson DR, Winniford MD, Willerson JT, Firth BG, Carey JR, Hillis LD. Continuous electrocardiographic monitoring in patients with unstable angina pectoris: identification of high-risk subgroup with severe coronary disease, variant angina, and/or impaired early prognosis. Am Heart J 1982; 103:4–12.

31. Gottlieb SO, Weisfeldt ML, Ouyang P, Mellits ED, Gerstenblith G. Silent ischemia predicts infarction and death during two-year follow-up of unstable angina. J Am Coll Cardiol 1987; 10:756–60.
32. Wilcox I, Freedman SB, Kelley DT, Harris PJ. Clinical significance of silent ischemia in unstable angina pectoris. Am J Cardiol 1990; 65:1313–6.
33. Scott RS, Baumgartner WA, Soule L, Burkon AM, Gardner TJ, Gott VL, Watkins L Jr, Reitz BA. Predictors of perioperative mortality in patients with unstable postinfarction angina. Circulation 1988; 78(Suppl I):163–165.
34. Hill NS, Antman EM, Green LH. Intravenous nitroglycerin, a review of pharmacology, indications, therapeutic effects, and complications. Chest 1981; 79:69–75.
35. Conti CR. Use of nitrates in unstable angina pectoris. Am J Cardiol 1987; 60:31H–34H.
36. Horowitz JD, Henry CA, Syrjanen ML, Louis WJ, Fish RD, Smith TW, Antman EM. Combined use of nitroglycerin and N-acetylcysteine in the management of unstable angina pectoris. Circulation 1988; 77:787–94.
37. Yusuf S, Wittes J, Friedman L. Overview of results of randomised clinical trials in heart disease. I. Treatments following myocardial infarction. JAMA 1988; 260:2088–93.
38. Guazzi M, Fiorentini C, Polese A, Magrini F, Olivari MI. Treatment of spontaneous angina pectoris with beta-blocking agents. A clinical, electrocardiographic, and hemodynamic appraisal. Br Heart J 1975; 37:1235–9.
39. Théroux P, Taymans Y, Mumsette D, Bosch X, Pelletier GB, Waters DD. A randomized study comparing propranolol and diltiazem in the treatment of unstable angina. J Am Coll Cardiol 1985; 5:717–23.
40. Muller JE, Turi ZG, Pearle DL, Schneider JF, Serfas DH, Morrison J, Stone PH, et al. Nifedipine and conventional therapy for unstable angina pectoris: a randomized, double-blind comparison. Circulation 1989; 69:729–34.
41. Gottlieb SO, Weisfeldt ML, Ouyang P, et al. Effect of the addition of propranolol to therapy with nifedipine for unstable angina pectoris. A randomized, double-blind, placebo-controlled trial. Circulation 1986; 73:331–7.
42. Scheidt S, Frishman WH, Packer M, Mehta J, Parodi O, Subramanian VB. Long-term effectiveness of verapamil in stable and unstable angina pectoris: one-year follow-up of patients treated in placebo-controlled, double-blind, randomized clinical trials. Am J Cardiol 1982; 56:1185–92.
43. Gorlin R, Fuster V, Ambrose JA. Anatomic-physiologic links between acute coronary syndromes. Circulation 1986; 74:6–9.
44. Fitzgerald DJ, Roy L, Catella F, Fitzgerald GA. Platelet activation in unstable coronary disease. N Engl J Med 1986; 315:983–9.
45. Théroux P, Latour JG, Léger-Gauthier C, De Lara J. Fibrinopeptide A and platelet factor levels in unstable angina pectoris. Circulation 1987; 75:156–62.
46. Rutherford JD. Unstable angina and thrombolysis. Chest 1990; 97(Suppl):156–160.
47. Stuart RS, Baumgartner WA, Soule L, Borkon AM, Gardner TJ, Gott VL, Watkins L Jr, Reitz BA. Predictors of perioperative mortality in patients with unstable postinfarction angina. Circulation 1988; (Suppl I):163–165.

Index

About the Editor

JOHN D. RUTHERFORD is Co-director, Clinical Cardiology Service, Department of Medicine, Brigham and Women's Hospital, and Assistant Professor of Medicine, Harvard Medical School, Boston, Massachusetts. The author or coauthor of over 85 journal articles, book chapters, and abstracts, and coauthor of one book, he is an International Fellow of the Council on Clinical Cardiology of the American Heart Association and a Fellow of the American College of Cardiology and Royal Australasian College of Physicians. Dr. Rutherford received the M.B. degree (1969) from the University of Otago Medical School, Dunedin, New Zealand.